Supervision Can
Be Playful

Supervision Can Be Playful

Techniques for Child and Play Therapist Supervisors

Edited by
Athena A. Drewes and Jodi Ann Mullen

JASON ARONSON
Lanham • Boulder • New York • Toronto • Plymouth, UK

Published in the United States of America
by Jason Aronson
An imprint of Rowman & Littlefield Publishers, Inc.

A wholly owned subsidiary of
The Rowman & Littlefield Publishing Group, Inc.
4501 Forbes Boulevard, Suite 200, Lanham, Maryland 20706
www.rowmanlittlefield.com

Estover Road
Plymouth PL6 7PY
United Kingdom

British Library Cataloguing in Publication Information Available

Library of Congress Cataloging-in-Publication Data

Supervision can be playful : techniques for child and play therapist supervisors
/ edited by Athena A. Drewes and Jodi Ann Mullen.
    p. ; cm.
Includes bibliographical references.
ISBN-13: 978-0-7657-0533-4 (cloth : alk. paper)
ISBN-10: 0-7657-0533-8 (cloth : alk. paper)
eISBN-13: 978-0-7657-0606-5
eISBN-10: 0-7657-0606-7
1. Child psychotherapists—Supervision of. 2. Play therapy. 3.
Psychotherapists—Supervision of. 4. Counselors—Supervision of. I. Drewes,
Athena A., 1948– II. Mullen, Jodi Ann.
    [DNLM: 1. Psychotherapy—education. 2. Staff Development—methods. 3.
Counseling—education. 4. Play Therapy—methods. 5. Play and Playthings—
psychology. WM 18 S9596 2008]
    RJ504.S83 2008
    618.92'891653—dc22   2008011253

Printed in the United States of America

∞™ The paper used in this publication meets the minimum requirements of
American National Standard for Information Sciences—Permanence of Paper
for Printed Library Materials, ANSI/NISO Z39.48-1992.

This book is dedicated to our supervisors:

Eva Landauer (October 9, 1917–February 14, 2004), distinguished child psychoanalyst, colleague, and supervisor who worked for 50 years at the Jewish Board of Family and Children's Services in New York City. She trained in London with Anna Freud. Ms. Landauer was my first clinical supervisor (for over five years), and she is credited with having introduced me to and trained me in play therapy, as well as having ignited in me a passion for play therapy. I am forever indebted to her.
~ *Athena A. Drewes*

Rebecca Dayton of Syracuse University and Dave Rodrick of the Victor New York School District—two of my clinical supervisors who taught and facilitated the development of my counseling and play therapy skills and served as role models for the supervisor and person I aspire to be.
~ *Jodi Ann Mullen*

Contents

Part II: Supervising Special Populations

Part III: Facilitating Self-Awareness

Part IV: Potpourri of Playful Techniques

List of Contributors

Sue Bratton, PhD, LPC, RPT-S, associate professor, director, Center for Play Therapy, University of North Texas, Denton

Peggy Ceballos, MEd, coassistant director, Center for Play Therapy, University of North Texas, Denton

David A. Crenshaw, PhD, ABPP, RPT-S, director, Rhinebeck Child and Family Center, LLC, Rhinebeck, New York

Judith M. Dagirmanjian, LCSWR, Family and Child Unit, Ulster County Mental Health, Kingston, New York

Athena A. Drewes, PsyD, RPT-S, director of clinical training and APA internship, The Astor Home for Children, Poughkeepsie, New York

Lennis G. Echterling, PhD, Department of Graduate Psychology, James Madison University, Harrisonburg, Virginia.

Jody J. Fiorini, PhD, associate professor, Counseling and Psychological Services, State University of New York at Oswego

Sandra B. Frick-Helms, PhD, RPT-S, clinical faculty, University of South Carolina School of Medicine, Department of Child and Adolescent Neuropsychiatry and Behavioral Medicine, Columbia; faculty associate, Johns Hopkins University Department of Counseling, Baltimore, Maryland

Ken Gardner, MS, Cpsy, codirector, Rocky Mountain Play Therapy Institute, Calgary, Alberta, Canada

Kristi A. Gibbs, PhD, RPT, assistant professor, Counseling Program, University of Tennessee at Chattanooga

Eliana Gil, PhD, ATR, RPT-S, Childhelp Children's Center of Virginia, Springfield

Eric J. Green, PhD, RPT-S, assistant professor, John Hopkins University, Counseling and Human Services, Baltimore, Maryland

Louise Guerney, PhD, RPT-S, director, National Institute of Relationship Enhancement, Silver Spring, Maryland; professor emerita of human development and counseling psychology, Penn State University

Susan Hansen, LCSWR, RPT-S, Family and Child Unit, Ulster County Mental Health, Kingston, New York

Linda E. Homeyer, PhD, LPC-S, NCC, RPT-S, Texas State University, San Marcos

Melissa Luke, MS, LMHC, Counseling and Human Services, Syracuse University, Syracuse, New York

Mary Morrison, PhD, LPC, NCC, RPT, assistant professor, Texas State University, San Marcos

Jodi Ann Mullen, PhD, LMHC, NCC, RPT-S, Counseling and Psychological Services, State University of New York at Oswego

Evangeline Munns, PhD, RPT-S, King City, Ontario, Canada

Yumiko Ogawa, University of North Texas, Denton

Dee Ray, PhD, LPC, RPT-S, assistant professor, codirector, Child and Family Resource Clinic, University of North Texas, Denton

Arthur Robbins, EdD, professor of art therapy, Pratt Institute, New York, New York

Lawrence Rubin, PhD, LMHC, RPT-S, professor of counselor education, St. Thomas University, Miami, Florida

Angela Sheely, MA, coassistant director, Center for Play Therapy, University of North Texas, Denton

Anne Stewart, PhD, Department of Graduate Psychology, James Madison University, Harrisonburg, Virginia

Lorri Yasenik, MSW, RSW, RPT-S, codirector, Rocky Mountain Play Therapy Institute, Calgary, Alberta, Canada

Acknowledgments

Special thanks to Denise Garafolo, librarian at the Astor Home for Children headquarters in Rhinebeck, New York. No matter how difficult the recovery task, Denise has always come through with the needed articles, books, and material I need for my writing. I truly appreciate your quiet efficiency, along with your warm and cheery demeanor. You never let me down!

Thanks to executive director Dr. Jim McGuirk, medical director Dr. Alice Linder, and the 700-member staff of the Astor Home for Children for the supportive and nurturing environment. Astor is a world-class organization. It is a large, nonprofit, multiservice mental health agency that offers early childhood, outpatient, day treatment, residential care and foster care, and home- and school-based services to children and families throughout Dutchess County in the mid-Hudson area of New York, as well as the Bronx and Orange County. I am proud to be part of this organization. Special thanks for the supervision and collegial support of Dr. David Crenshaw, former clinical director of Astor's Residential Treatment Center, and Andy Fussner, family therapy consultant, formerly of the Philadelphia Child Guidance Clinic. Through your training, support, and role modeling, I have been able to develop and hone my play therapy supervisory skills over the past 16 years. You showed me how it should be done!

Special thanks to Art Pompanio for his encouragement and support at Jason Aronson/Rowman & Littlefield in getting this project off the ground.

Finally, to my family for their always present love, support, and interest: Rev. James R. Bridges, Scott Richard Drewes Bridges, and Seth Andrew Bridges.

~ Athena A. Drewes

I thank Athena Drewes for being my friend and mentor. Athena, I feel blessed that you are part of my life; there is no way this project would have come to fruition without you—thank you!

I have an amazing support system. Thank you to my friends and colleagues who support me unconditionally, my family who are proud of me exponentially, and my husband, Michael, and children, Andrew and Leah, who love me relentlessly.

~ Jodi Ann Mullen

Introduction

This text was born out of our passion and love for play therapy and play, and our belief in its healing power. In conversations together, we both wanted to help pass along to child clinicians, and their supervisors, playful ways to supervise. Play therapy, after all, spans all ages. Play offers curative and therapeutic powers not only *as* therapy or *in* therapy, but *outside* of therapy as well. Adults need to play, too. Perhaps even more so, in order to remain fresh, alive, and involved with our many difficult cases, clients, and supervisees.

It seems contradictory not to have play within the supervision of child and play therapy clinicians who use play-based interventions with their clients. What better way to role model and practice use of play-based interventions with clients than through their actual use during supervision? What better way to help facilitate risk-taking within a supportive, trusting, and inviting supervisory relationship than through the use of play-based techniques that both the supervisor and supervisee can participate in?

Child and play therapists comprise a wide variety of mental health professionals who work in a number of different settings, with diverse populations and diverse levels of supervisees. Some supervisees are beginners to child and play therapy, while other seasoned mental health professionals are new to play therapy. The same scenario is true of supervisors. Some supervisors are new to supervision, while others are new to supervising child and play therapists. In this text we endeavor to offer play-based interventions and strategies to use in the supervision process.

1

Whether read by a person who is a supervisor, a supervisee, or both, this book fills in the gaps in supervision training by university professors of child and play therapists, training directors, and agency and clinic supervisors, as well as private practice supervisors and supervisees wishing to use an experiential approach.

According to the Center for Play Therapy (2005) over one hundred graduate degree programs currently offer at least one graduate course in play therapy. The number of university-based graduate-level courses in play therapy grows substantially each year. This text will be useful to the hundreds of registered play therapist-supervisors (RPT-S), clinicians who require supervision training, as well as graduate school professors and field placement supervisors who need to supervise child therapists-in-training. This text synthesizes what is currently known about what works in clinical supervision with children, provides a method for assessing the supervisory relationship, and, most importantly, provides guidance in selecting creative interventions that are tailored to the needs of the child/play therapy supervisee such that they can provide the highest quality treatment to their clients.

We are proud to have been able to get a diverse cross-section of experts in the field of child and play therapy to share their knowledge and playful interventions with the reader. These contributors have many years of supervisory experience that span a variety of clinical settings that will help the beginner as well as more experienced supervisors in their work. We have organized this text into four parts.

Part I: Supervisory Styles and Critical Considerations contains five chapters devoted to defining terms and discussing the relevant research and models related to clinical supervision. These chapters also address developmental, cross-discipline, population-based, and cultural features related to the supervisory relationship with the supervisee and as well as the client. The focus will also be on the specific challenges faced by child and play therapists. Each chapter includes various play-based techniques that can be immediately applied within supervision to set the stage for a trusting, supportive, and risk-taking environment.

Part II: Supervising Special Populations contains six chapters that examine different types of work settings and client populations encountered by child/play therapist professionals. These chapters reflect issues typically encountered in child and adolescent clinical supervision and treatment and offer unique situations that beginning child clinicians may feel less competent with. Several chapters offer case studies that examine assessment strategies and the application of play-based techniques. Cases and scenarios are examined in terms of relational dynamics, ethical considerations, and intervention choices (supervisee/clinician and supervisor). Play therapy supervisors and supervisors-in-training will be able to learn how to assess and conceptualize the different types of issues in child and play therapy supervision as well as responses to each through the play-based techniques.

Part III: Facilitating Self-Awareness contains four chapters that address the impact of experiencing and providing clinical supervision in child/play therapy as well as how issues of the child/play therapist may emerge as a consequence of participating in clinical supervision. Child/play therapy supervisor and supervisee self-awareness is critical and therefore stressed. When working with child and adult family clients, personal transference and countertransference issues will arise. But similar issues will also come into the supervisor and supervisee relationship. Child and play therapists as well as supervisors must be able to look within as to how these factors may impede a working alliance or the creation of a safe and supportive therapeutic or supervisory setting. The use of expressive arts and sand trays is highlighted in detail that enables both the supervisee and supervisor to use them as joint activities toward self-awareness.

Part IV: Potpourri of Playful Techniques contains two chapters full of unique and playful techniques and activities for use within supervision. Each technique is clearly outlined so that both supervisor and supervisee are able to participate in the activities, with many that can be utilized within a group supervision setting.

We are confident that this book will help to elevate the level of supervision as well as supervisee experience for child and play therapists. In turn, through the use of the play-based techniques offered in this text, the client and his or her family will benefit from a more playful and confident therapist.

Part I

SUPERVISORY STYLES AND CRITICAL CONSIDERATIONS

1

⌘

Supervision

Models, Principles, and Process Issues

Melissa Luke

This chapter defines supervision and introduces three generally accepted categories of supervision models: psychotherapy based, developmental, and social role models. Several supervisory contexts are discussed in more detail, including a rationale for incorporating experiential elements into the supervision of child and play therapy within each. The underlying principles of using experiential and playful interventions within supervision are delineated, with particular emphasis on exploring the supervisory relationship in relation to process issues. Case examples are used to illustrate opportunities for playful supervisory interventions.

Supervision has been recognized as an essential component of the education and training of counselors, psychologists, psychiatrists, psychiatric nurses, social workers, and marriage and family therapists (Bernard & Goodyear, 2004; Watkins, 1995, 1998). Shulman (2005) identified supervision as the "signature pedagogy" across the mental health professions, noting that it has become the primary means of preparation for all clinical practice. Numerous licensing boards and credentialing agencies mandate participation in supervision as a component of their education and training procedures, identifying specific requirements regarding the scope and content of supervision (e.g., American Association for Marriage and Family Therapists, 2002; American Psychological Association, 2000; Association for Play Therapy, 2006; Mascari & Wilson, 2005; National Board for

Certified Counselors, 2000, 2001). As both professional identity development and professional socialization are optimized through supervision provided by a more senior member to a junior member within the same discipline (Bernard & Goodyear, 2004), many organizations maintain requirements for those endorsed to provide approved supervision. For example, the Association for Play Therapy (APT) encourages that supervision be provided by registered play therapist-supervisors (RPT-S) to those applicants seeking credentialing as registered play therapists (RPT) (Association for Play Therapy, 2006).

DEFINITION

Although distinctions between administrative and clinical supervision have been established (Barret & Schmidt, 1986; Dollarhide & Miller, 2006; Henderson & Gysbers, 2006; Sutton & Page, 1994), there remain differing interpretations regarding the standardized characterization, purpose, and processes of clinical supervision (Hart & Nance, 2003; Miller & Dollarhide, 2006; Wilkerson, 2006). The impressive body of literature related to supervision has produced multiple definitions of supervision. However, the most frequently cited definition of supervision is that of Bernard and Goodyear (2004) as follows:

> Supervision is an intervention provided by a more senior member of a profession to a more junior member or members of that same profession. This relationship is evaluative, extends over time, and has the simultaneous purposes of enhancing the professional functioning of the more junior person(s), monitoring the quality of professional services offered to the clients that she, he, or they see, and serving as a gatekeeper for those who are to enter the particular profession (p. 8).

In addition to the functions included in this definition, supervision is also recognized as a social process through which professional mores, attitudes, values, thinking patterns, and problem-solving strategies are acculturated (Auxier, Hughes, & Kline, 2003; Holloway & Wolleat, 1994; O'Byrne & Rosenberg, 1998). For example, supervision provides child and play therapists with experiential opportunities to integrate formal knowledge about child development and theories of change with clinical observation, professional knowledge, and the skills necessary for effective work with children (Drisko, 2000; Zorga, 1997). However, the most fundamental function of all supervision remains facilitating the development of professional counseling skills and ensuring professional gatekeeping and quality control over the counseling services provided to clients (Association for Counselor Education and Supervision, 1990; Bernard & Goodyear, 2004; Bradley & Ladany, 2001).

HISTORICAL CONTEXT

In their comprehensive review of the supervision literature, Leddick and Bernard (1980) noted that it was not until the 1970s that the distinct skills of supervision were organized coherently and in turn propelled the development of various conceptual models of supervision. In the three decades since, there have been many credible models of clinical supervision proposed. Glidden and Tracey (1992) observed that these models provide heuristic value to the practicing supervisor, offering recommendations for how to organize and implement supervision.

A substantive supervision literature has emerged in the past 30 years (Bernard & Goodyear, 2004; Bradley & Ladany, 2001; Falender & Shafranske, 2004), with a wide range of theoretical and empirical content to support and promote clinical supervision (Tyler, Sloan, & King, 2000). Three contemporary journals, *The Clinical Supervisor, Counselor Education and Supervision*, and *Training and Education in Professional Psychology*, are devoted almost exclusively to training and supervision issues. The annual International Interdisciplinary Conference on Clinical Supervision was established in 2005, focusing on core issues in the theory, practice, and research of clinical supervision that cut across professional disciplines (International Interdisciplinary Conference on Clinical Supervision, 2006). These developments support the assertion that supervision is a separate competency distinct from the practice of counseling or therapy (American Counselor Education and Supervision, 1995; American Association for Marriage and Family Therapists, 2002; American Psychological Association, 2002; Dye & Borders, 1990; Holloway, 1995; National Board for Certified Counselors, 2001).

CONCEPTUALIZATIONS OF SUPERVISION

In the first edition of their text *Fundamentals of Clinical Supervision*, Bernard and Goodyear (1992) differentiated among psychotherapy-based, developmental, and conceptual models of supervision. They later deleted their reference to conceptual models and instead referred to social role models (Bernard & Goodyear, 1998, 2004). These three categories are now commonly used to distinguish supervision models (Bernard & Goodyear, 2004; Borders & Brown, 2005; Bradley & Ladany, 2001; Falender & Shafranske, 2004).

Psychotherapy-based Models

Early approaches to supervision emerged out of the various schools of counseling and therapy (Holloway, 1992; Leddick & Bernard, 1980). Prior to formalized theories specific to supervision, supervisors transferred their knowledge about the processes and procedures of a particular theoretical orientation into the domain of supervision. These early conceptualizations of supervision largely depended on models of the counseling relationship, advocating for and influenced by the counseling theories in which they were respectively embedded (Bradley & Gould, 2001).

Eckstein and Wallerstein's (1958) psychoanalytic supervision was among the earliest psychotherapy-based model of supervision, and it noted definitive stages through which the psychodynamic supervisor assisted the supervisee in increasing self-awareness, which, in turn, was theorized to lead to a more effective therapeutic use of self. Other psychotherapy-based models included client-centered supervision, behavioral supervision, and so on. Although child and play therapy is not a specific theoretical orientation, the active learning and symbolic expression inherent in child and play therapy uniquely extend communication beyond verbal means (Rogers, 1957; Sutherland & Bonwell, 1996). It is therefore perplexing that to date there have been no models of supervision to similarly reflect this practice. However, Mullen, Luke, and Drewes (2007) noted that child and play therapy supervisors have a unique opportunity to demonstrate, educate, and promote the potential of experiential and playful interventions, modeling in supervision a professional worldview where play is the language (Ginott, 1959).

Developmental Models

Kell and Mueller (1966) and Boyd (1978) offered the first discussions of supervision that were not attached to a specific theoretical orientation. Underpinning these initial supervisory theories were three intuitive developmental assumptions: clinical skills can be refined through experiential and didactic learning, theory and practice can be integrated through reflective practice, and professional identity is influenced through professional socialization (Bernard & Goodyear, 2004; Dollarhide & Miller, 2006; Holloway & Neufeldt, 1995; Watkins, 1995).

Formalized developmental models of supervision (Littrell, Lee-Borden, & Lorenz, 1979; Loganbill, Hardy, & Delworth, 1982) propose a sequence of hierarchical stages of increasing skill and awareness. These models suggest that the varied but predictable developmental needs of the supervisee determine the supervisory activity (Neufeldt, 1994). Though Holloway (1987) described developmental models of supervision as having become "the zeitgeist of supervision thinking and research" (p. 209), several reviews of the related literature concluded that there remains empirical uncertainty regarding their validity (Goodyear & Robyak, 1982; Holloway, 1992; Steven, Goodyear, & Robertson, 1998; Worthington, 1987).

Social Role Models

While developmental models of supervision hinge upon the evolving needs of the supervisee, social role models of supervision summarize supervisory behaviors, particularly the component tasks and processes related to the role of the supervisor (Bernard & Goodyear, 2004). As early as 1958, Apfelbaum introduced the roles of the critic, model, and nurturer to distinguish varied therapeutic approaches. Much the same way, social role models (Bernard, 1979, 1997; Hawkins & Shohet, 1992; Holloway, 1995), sometimes characterized as eclectic, integrated, and process-based models (Borders & Leddick, 1987; Bradley & Ladany, 2001; Falender & Shafranske, 2004), describe the supervisory foci, goals, functions, roles, and styles used within supervision. Though the referent terminology varies, there is general agreement that the included models serve as "conceptual tools for understanding the interrelated forces that contribute to the process of supervision" (Falender & Shafranske, 2004, p. 19).

While supervisors may have a predilection for a particular role or style of supervision (Bernard, 1981; Holloway, 1995; Putney, Worthington, & McCullough, 1992), research has not supported a clear supervisee preference for any one supervisory role or style (Fernando & Hulse-Killacky, 2005; Shechtman & Wirtzberger, 1999), nor have there been consistently reported advantages attributed to a particular role in terms of productivity, efficiency, or learning (Holloway & Wampold, 1983). As social role models tend to be atheoretical, they can be used in conjunction with developmental approaches and within various other theoretically aligned models, possibly contributing to the considerable contemporary discussion and application of social role models of supervision (Pearson, 2001, 2004, 2006).

INCORPORATION OF EXPERIENTIAL ELEMENTS

Contemporary supervisory theory recognizes clinical supervision as a unique intervention that differs from teaching, counseling, or consultation (Bernard & Goodyear, 2004). Though interpersonal communication often takes place through means other than just words (Pedersen, 1994; Sue & Sue, 1999), supervisory intervention has historically been constrained to verbal methods across all existing models of supervision (Mullen, Luke, & Drewes, 2007). However, when supervisory intervention is expanded to include experiential and play therapy interventions, there may be an increased emergence of a childlike playfulness, more risk-taking, and a deeper reflective process. Furthermore, Fall and Sutton (2003) contend that communication is expanded when supervision intentionally includes mechanisms for symbolic expression. The following illustrates three familiar supervisory contexts in which the supervision of child and play therapists can incorporate playful and experiential techniques.

Practicum and Internship

The Discrimination Model (Bernard, 1979, 1997) is one of the most widely used models of supervision in training settings (Borders & Benshoff, 1999; Borders & Brown, 2005). Developed as "the simplest of maps" (Bernard, 1997, p. 310) for supervisors-in-training to conceptualize their supervisory interventions, the Discrimination Model (Bernard, 1979) proposed three focuses of supervision (intervention skills, originally labeled as process skills; conceptualization skills; and personalization skills) and three role postures for the supervisor (teacher, counselor, and consultant). Because each role can be used to effectively address each focus, the Discrimination Model offers abundant possibilities to include experiential techniques within the supervision of child and play therapy practitioners-in-training.

Using the role of teacher, a supervisor may simply demonstrate experiential techniques to expand the child or play therapist-in-training's intervention skill repertoire. From the same role, the supervisor could also evaluate the ways in which the supervisee is conceptualizing the case. Similarly, to elicit more information about how the child or play therapist-in-training is conceptualizing a client, the supervisor may use the role of counselor and ask the supervisee to symbolically represent their understanding and awareness of the client's experience. Further, because it is not uncommon for practitioners-in-training to have more than one supervisor (e.g., instructor, site-supervisor, clinical supervisor), the supervisor can use the counselor or consultant role to attend to the supervisee's phenomenological experience (i.e., personalization) of potentially receiving multiple supervisory directives.

School

Although counselors, psychologists, social workers, and sometimes teachers provide mental health services to children within a school setting, the professional literature has consistently indicated that supervision has yet to establish itself as common practice within the school context (Luke & Bernard, 2006). Without supervision, these practitioners may be missing opportunities for the established benefits of supervision, which include: increased effectiveness and accountability; improved counseling skills and understanding of role expectations; enhanced professional development; and improved job performance, confidence, and awareness of the multifaceted role of the school counselor (Agnew, Vaught, Getz, & Fortune, 2000; Brott & Meyers, 1999; Crutchfield & Borders, 1997; Dahir, 2000; Herlihy, Gray, & McCollom, 2002). Contrary to these benefits, many practitioners receiving supervision have reported that the supervision they did receive was unsatisfactory (Coll, 1995), raising questions as to whether the current practice of traditionally verbal methods for supervision adequately meet the needs of supervisees practicing within a school context.

In discussing the school counseling supervision, Struder (2005) contended that the preferred supervisor fluctuated between the various supervisory foci and roles, depending upon the developmental, contextual, and situational needs of the supervisee. Given that many practitioners working in a school provide conventional child and play therapy services, incorporating the same experiential and playful interventions into their supervision may increase the supervisor's flexibility to meet the needs of these supervisees. Though expressive techniques have been utilized for centuries to promote symbolic communication (Heiney & Darr-Hope, 1999), their use within supervision has only recently begun to appear in the literature (Drisko, 2000; Mullen, Luke, & Drewes, 2007). This could be accomplished by providing the school-based practitioner with expressive means that take into consideration the school context (e.g., toy school house and figures). Moreover, providing parallel opportunities for supervisees to engage with and communicate their experiences in supervision via means other than verbal expression may increase their empathy for their child clients. For example, it could be helpful for the supervisee to play out their excitement, frustration, isolation, sense of responsibility, and so on related to being one of the only practitioners in the school to be providing child and play therapy.

Group

Hayes, Blackman, & Brennan (2001) noted that in defining group supervision it is important to differentiate between the context in which the supervisees compose the group and the context "in which the object of supervision is the leadership of a group" (p. 185). However, in either instance the use of experiential and playful interventions that are grounded in developmental learning and inter-personal, relational theory can increase the effectiveness of supervision (Mullen, Luke, & Drewes, 2007).

Supervisors promote the growth of their supervisees through communicating, modeling, and directly teaching the skills necessary within a particular therapeutic discipline and theoretical orientation (Dye & Borders, 1990; White & Russell, 1995). Although play therapy is not a specific theoretical orientation, it has been argued that the shared worldview that embraces symbolic expression and playful interventions can be promoted when the supervisee can genuinely engage these within supervision (Mullen, Luke, & Drewes, 2007). In a group supervision context, supervisees can authentically experience these interventions for the purposes of exploring the important group systemic levels, including the intra-personal, inter-personal, and whole group. For example, a supervisee may be asked to select a ball and move it between objects that represent the internal voice, communication between self and other select group members, as well as the overall group considered together. Within a group, supervisees can spontaneously "unmask" themselves through playful interventions and therapeutically share a play space with one another, as well as the supervisor, in turn liberating "the spirit of growth and development" (Drisko, 2000, p. 157).

UNDERPINNINGS AND FOUNDATIONAL PRINCIPLES

The empirical literature has produced differing constructs on which selection of supervisory interventions are based, and include the working alliance (Martin, Garske, & Davis, 2000), social influence attributes such as expertness, trustworthiness, and attractiveness (Neufeldt, Beutler, & Ranchero, 1997), supervisee development (Ellis & Dell, 1986; Ellis, Dell, & Good, 1988; Gysbers & Johnston, 1965; Heppner & Roehlke, 1984), and theoretical orientation (Goodyear, Abadie, & Efros, 1984; Goodyear & Bradley, 1983; Goodyear & Robyak, 1982; Putney, Worthington, & McCollough, 1992; Whitman, Ryan, & Rubenstein, 2001). Regardless of how selected, each supervisory intervention implies a distinctive distribution of power between the supervisor and supervisee (Holloway, 1995). This includes experiential and playful interventions as well.

As early as 1957 Rogers posited that experiential learning was the only learning directly related to effective counseling (p. 78). In discussing experiential learning, Kolb (1984) noted that the effective supervisor needed to use a range of methods to assist the supervisee in reflection, conceptualization, and the implementation of professional skills. More recently, it was suggested that "students are simply more likely to internalize, understand, and remember material learned through active engagement in the learning process" (Sutherland & Bonwell, 1996, p. 3). Though future investigation of the efficacy is warranted, it seems that incorporating active symbolic communication into one's supervisory repertoire holds promise for enhancing supervisory, as well as child and play therapy, outcomes.

PROCESS ISSUES

Although no research could be identified that examined the effects of implementing experiential and expressive activities in supervision, several studies suggest that the choice of supervisory intervention may affect the process of supervision (Milne & James, 2002; Worthington & Roehkle, 1979). Because nonverbal behavior is thought to be the language of emotions and relationship (Kiesler, 1988), it follows that purposeful use of experiential and playful nonverbal interventions within supervision may assist in illuminating the dynamics of the supervisory relationship and processes.

It has been further speculated that the supervisory relationship itself, as well as the experience of this relationship, contributes to the content of and processes within supervision (Bordin, 1983; Eckstein & Wallerstein, 1958; Holloway, 1992, 1995). As such, a supervisor using symbolic communication, nonverbal expressive modalities, and playful interventions may be developing a more positive working alliance with supervisees, and therefore be providing more comprehensive and effective supervision. However, future studies are needed to explore these relationships.

CASE EXAMPLES

What follows is an overview of three clinical supervision cases wherein the author created and utilized playful interventions to address specific supervisory content. The active symbolic expression that occurred through the use of such experiential techniques appeared to benefit the child or play therapist supervisee and is offered as a representation of how similar playful interventions may enhance the supervision provided to child and play therapists in general.

Supervisee in the Hat

While attending the First Timers luncheon at the 2006 American Counseling Association convention, this author had the good fortune to meet then-ACA President-Elect Marie Wakefield, who was donning a Dr.

Seuss–like *Cat in the Hat*–type hat. Soon after this encounter, during which Wakefield discussed having hundreds of hats, each representative of different occupations, moods, and occasions, the usefulness of hats as a means of symbolic expression was evident. This author began working with a new supervisee named Cheyenne, and the use of hats would become relevant.

Cheyenne was a 24-year-old Latina woman enrolled in a school counseling program, completing her first practicum placement at an urban elementary school. During our fourth weekly supervision session, she expressed reluctance to identify measurable goals for the children with whom she had just begun working. Furthermore, when asked, Cheyenne did not know how I as a supervisor might help her to reach university-specified objectives by the end of the semester. After some querying, I sensed that in order to assist Cheyenne in developing and articulating either therapeutic or supervisory goals, we were going to need to first discuss our relationship and interpersonal expectations.

Instead of addressing this material verbally with Cheyenne, I took inspiration from Wakefield and her hats. Pointing to boxes of human figures and clothing apparel that indeed included many hats, I asked Cheyenne to represent herself as she had thus far appeared in supervision, her hopes for me as a supervisor, her fears for me as a supervisor, her hidden self in supervision, herself at the end of the semester, herself as a school counselor, myself as a supervisor while she was at practicum, not present with me, and so on. After each selection was made, we took turns describing what we saw and felt and our associations with both. I purposefully avoided making any interpretations. I then switched "roles" with Cheyenne, asking her to decide upon the stems for my selection of figures and apparel. Her requests included my representation of a good supervisee, a bad supervisee, myself as supervisor when I was pleased, and myself as supervisor when I was negatively evaluating a supervisee. Again we processed our thoughts and affect in response to each.

Following this experiential, playful intervention, I suggested to Cheyenne that something between us had shifted and asked her if she was able to put words to what this was. Without a pause, she responded, "Oh yes, Melissa, we became known today and now I can see how you can help me with my counseling skills." And with that, she selected a form from one of the boxes. It was one figure, but of two people in a canoe. Cheyenne put a party hat on one of the people and a mortar board on the head of the other saying, "I'm not sure who's who, but I think this is us, doing what we did today, paddling together toward graduation."

Without further prompting by me, Cheyenne was able to collaborate with her elementary school clients to identify specific areas in which their work would focus. She could articulate in her case notes how she was using the therapeutic relationship, modeling, and expressive play techniques to facilitate clients' engagement in the therapeutic process.

Obstacle Course

Stephan was a 42-year-old white male, working full time as a night supervisor at an auto manufacturing plant, while also attending part-time graduate school in rehabilitation counseling. Though Stephan was extremely conscientious in his studies, he was struggling to balance his roles as father, husband, employee, coach, student, and rehabilitation counseling intern. In our twelfth weekly supervision session, Stephan presented an audio tape of a two-part intake session that he conducted with a mildly cognitively delayed twelve-year-old biracial boy named Julius, mandated to alcohol treatment. It was immediately clear that though Stephan was hearing his client's words, he was unable to access Julius's emotional experience. Given the way Stephan had previously established connections with similar clients, I was struck by his lack of emotional availability with respect to this client. After some discussion about this, it was apparent that Stephan's assessment of his connection to and understanding of Julius significantly differed from mine. I asked him if he would be willing to do a little experiment, and he quickly agreed.

I suggested to Stephan that the next time he met with Julius, instead of asking him about his day or previous week, that he might try to have him act it out, as if it were charades. Stephan and I then talked about some of the advantages to this approach and how it fit into the theoretical framework from which he was working. Stephan's dialogue then digressed, with him commenting about how his own eight- and eleven-year-old children enjoyed games called *Caboodle* and *Cranium*. The following supervision session, Stephan was quite excited to show me a diagram that he had drawn of an obstacle course made by Julius. Instead of charades, Julius asked to construct a three-dimensional maze, representing his recent experiences. Stephan played an audio tape of this session, reflecting Julius's experiences while making the obstacle course, and eliciting exponentially more therapeutic material than he had in the two previous talk-based sessions.

Consistent with principles of symbolic expression and experiential technique, Stephan asked Julius to lead him through the obstacle course as he told him about what each object represented. When asked in supervision about his kinesthetic experience while traversing Julius's obstacle course, Stephan reported that he was reminded of being back in college on a football scholarship and being required to do drills in double practice sessions to the point of literal exhaustion in the August heat and humidity. I shared aloud my amazement at Stephan's powerful association.

Further, I deduced how he might have been hesitant to vicariously experience such a laborious and possibly overwhelming undertaking, joining Julius in his phenomenological experience. Stephan's eyes glossed over and he said, "You know, he's a year older than my son. I think what is hard for me to stay with is that Julius is just a kid." However, following this session, Stephan did relate to Julius, emotionally connecting to him as the child that he was.

Sand Storm

Raina and I had been working together as part of a live supervisory reflecting team at a community marriage and family therapy training clinic for almost a year. In this capacity, four experienced clinicians were each paired with a student co-therapist to provide services to uninsured clients. While each co-therapist worked with their respective couples and families, the remaining six therapists composed the reflecting team, observing behind the one-way mirror and intermittently delivering interventions.

Raina and her co-therapist Linda had been working with a mother, Beth, and her four-and-a-half-year-old son, Josh, for about six months, regarding adjustment and separation issues resulting from husband/father Romando's deployment to Afghanistan. Having just returned from his tour, Romando was present in this session, seated on the couch next to Beth. Josh was playing silently in the sand tray at his parents' feet. Throughout the first half of the session, Raina and Linda independently worked with Beth and Romando, helping them express their mixed feelings regarding their separation, reunion, and expectations for the future. However, it seemed that the co-therapists were out of synch, for when one moved in one direction, the other often went in the opposite direction. Although out of the awareness of either of his parents or the co-therapists, Josh acted out scenes in the sand tray corresponding to the affective content of the adults' verbalizations. At several points in the session, Raina and Romando both tried to verbally engage Josh, who mutely remained engrossed in his work on floor.

When the reflecting team and family switched rooms, it was suggested that one of us take the perspective of each family member, exaggerating the myriad inter-personal reactions occurring in the session thus far. I chose Josh, and amplified his physical and verbal detachedness from everyone in the room, as well as his emotional reactivity within the sand tray. Others on the reflecting team sculpted the couples' approach-avoidance dance and the co-therapist dyad's parallel of the same. The only verbalized intervention to the family and co-therapists was as we passed in the hall, asking, "How would you like all that to change?"

Once back to our original rooms, the physical changes were notable. Romando sat on the floor next to Josh and together they co-constructed a battle scene, while Beth sat on the couch above them both, taking turns rubbing her husband's shoulder and her son's head as she tracked their activities. During this time, Raina and Linda were able to work in tandem, focusing equally on each family member. In the last few minutes of the session, Raina got down next to the sand tray and asked Josh to share what he and his dad had been playing. In a voice of only a four and a half year old, Josh proudly exclaimed that they were the good guys, but they were at war. He went on to address through his "play" many of the same issues that had been discussed earlier in the family session. These included how the family was renegotiating boundaries and rules, intimacy and separation, as well as communication styles. When asked to name his sand tray, Josh called it "Sand Storm" and then qualified this designation by saying, "But the storm is over. My dad and I are on the same side now."

CONCLUSION

Supervision has its own history, theoretical knowledge base, models, and related contemporary issues (Bernard & Goodyear, 2004). Yet, it could be said that the science of supervision has not yet caught up to the practice, meaning that many of the models, methods, and processes of supervision have not been adequately investigated. Worse, the extant research in supervision has been soundly criticized. Primarily there are isolated and unrelated studies that narrowly focus on the supervision of students' practicum experiences conducted within a university community context (Ellis & Ladany, 1997; Lambert & Ogles, 1997; Leddick & Bernard, 1980; Watkins, 1995). It has also been noted that the majority of supervision studies are descriptive, rely upon survey research, and are plagued by numerous methodological flaws (Gruman & Nelson, 2008). These identified omissions in the present supervision knowledge base raise questions about the appropriateness of generalizing findings to the supervision of child and play therapists-in-training.

As a result, Ellis, Ladany, Krengel, and Schult (1996) recommend that future supervision research carefully attend to the use of appropriate theoretical grounding, unambiguous hypotheses, and minimization of threats to validity. Additionally, it has been suggested that in efforts toward a comprehensive research program in supervision, investigations use a range of methodologies, including self-report, experimental, single-subject, repeated measures, and qualitative designs, to assess the multiple dimensions of the supervision process (Falender & Shafranske, 2004). Finally, as a large amount of the supervision includes the work of child and play therapists, research specifically examining such supervision is warranted. Such future investigations should also consider the relationships between the inclusion of experiential and playful interventions within supervision. Supervisory outcomes could be assessed by instruments such as the Supervisee Perception of Supervision (Olk & Freidlander, 1992), Working Alliance Inventory (Hovrath, 1982), Supervisor Rating Form (Barak & LaCrosse, 1975), and the Play Therapy Skills Checklist (PTSC) (Ray, 2004).

REFERENCES

Agnew, T., Vaught, C. C., Getz, H. G., & Fortune, J. (2000). Peer group clinical supervision program fosters confidence and professionalism. *Professional School Counseling, 4*(1), 6–12.

American Association for Marriage Family Therapists. (2002). *Approved supervisor designation: Standards and responsibilities handbook.* Alexandria, VA: American Association for Marriage Family Therapists.

American Psychological Association. (2000). *Office of Program Consultation and Accreditation guidelines and principles for accreditation of programs in professional psychology* (Rev. ed.). Washington, DC: American Psychological Association.

American Psychological Association. (2002). Ethical principles of psychologists and code of conduct. *American Psychologist, 57,* 1060–73.

Apfelbaum, B. (1958). *Dimensions of transference in psychotherapy.* Berkley: University of California Press.

Association for Counselor Education and Supervision, Supervision Interest Network. (1990). Standards for counseling supervisors. *Journal of Counseling & Development, 69,* 30–32.

Association for Counselor Education and Supervision. (1995). Ethical guidelines for counseling supervisors. *Counselor Education and Supervision, 34,* 270–76.

Association for Play Therapy. (2006). www.a4pt.org/.

Auxier, C. R., Hughes, F. R., & Kline, W. B. (2003). Identity development in counselors-in-training. *Counselor Education and Supervision, 43,* 25–38.

Barak, A., & LaCrosse, M. B. (1975). Multidimensional perception of counselor behavior. *Journal of Counseling Psychology, 22,* 471–76.

Barret, B. G., & J. J. Schmidt (1986). School counselor certification and supervision: Overlooked professional issues. *Counselor Education and Supervision, 26,* 50–55.

Bernard, J. M. (1979). Supervisor training: A discrimination model. *Counselor Education and Supervision, 19,* 60–68.

Bernard, J. M. (1981). In-service training for clinical supervisors. *Professional Psychology, 12*(6), 740–48.

Bernard, J. M. (1992). Training master's level counseling students in the fundamentals of clinical supervision. *The Clinical Supervisor, 10*(1), 133–43.

Bernard, J. M. (1997). The discrimination model. In C. E. Watkins, Jr. (Ed.), *Handbook of psychotherapy supervision* (310–27). New York: Wiley.

Bernard, J. M., & Goodyear, R. K. (1992). *Fundamentals of clinical supervision.* Boston: Allyn & Bacon.

Bernard, J. M., & Goodyear, R. K. (1998). *Fundamentals of clinical supervision* (2nd ed.). Boston: Allyn & Bacon.

Bernard, J. M., & Goodyear, R. K. (2004). *Fundamentals of clinical supervision* (3rd ed.). Boston: Allyn & Bacon.

Borders, L. D., & Benshoff, J. (1999). *Clinical supervision: Learning to think like a supervisor.* Video production sponsored by the Association for Counselor Education and Supervision.

Borders, L. D., & Brown, L. L. (2005). *The new handbook of counseling supervision.* Malwah, NJ: Lawrence Erlbaum Associates.

Borders, L. D., & Leddick, G. R. (1987). *Handbook of counseling supervision.* Alexandria, VA: Association for Counselor Education and Supervision.

Bordin, E. S. (1983). A working alliance-based model of supervision. *The Counseling Psychologist, 11,* 35–42.

Boyd, J. D. (1978). *Counselor supervision: Approaching preparation practices.* Muncie, IN: Accelerated Development.

Bradley, L. J., & Gould, L. J. (2001). Psychotherapy-based models of counselor supervision. In L. J. Bradley, & N. Ladany (Eds.), *Counselor supervision* (3rd ed., 147–82). Philadelphia: Brunner-Routledge.

Bradley, L. J., & Ladany, N. (Eds.). (2001). *Counselor supervision* (3rd ed.). Philadelphia: Brunner-Routledge.

Brott, P. E., & Meyers, J. E. (1999). Development of professional school counselor identity: A grounded theory. *Professional School Counseling, 2*(5), 339–48.

Coll, K. M. (1995). Clinical supervision of community college counselors: Current and preferred practices. *Counselor Education and Supervision, 35,* 11–117.

Crutchfield, L. B., & Borders, L. D. (1997). Impact of two clinical peer supervision models on practicing school counselors. *Journal of Counseling and Development, 75,* 219–30.

Dahir, C. A. (2000). The national standards for school counseling programs: A partnership in preparing students for the new millennium. *NASSP Bulletin, 84*(616), 68–75.

Dollarhide, C. T., & Miller, G. M. (2006). Supervision for preparation and practice of school counselors: Pathways to excellence. *Counselor Education and Supervision, 4,* 242–52.

Drisko, J. W. (2000). Super-vision insights: Brief commentaries on supervision. *The Clinical Supervisor, 19,* 153–65.

Dye, H. A., & Borders, L. D. (1990). Counseling supervisors: Standards for preparation and practice. *Journal of Counseling and Development, 69,* 27–32.

Eckstein, R., & Wallerstein, R. S. (1958). *The teaching and learning of psychotherapy.* New York: International Universities Press.

Ellis, M. V., & Dell, D. M. (1986). Dimensionality of supervisor roles: Supervisors' perceptions of supervision. *Journal of Counseling Psychology, 33,* 282–91.

Ellis, M. V., Dell, D. M., & Good, G. E. (1988). Counselor trainees' perceptions of supervisor roles: Two studies testing the dimensionality of supervision. *Journal of Counseling Psychology, 35,* 315–24.

Ellis, M. V., & Ladany, N. (1997). Inferences concerning supervisees and clients in clinical supervision: An integrative review. In C. E. Watkins, Jr. (Ed.), *Handbook of psychotherapy supervision* (447–507). New York: Wiley.

Ellis, M. V., Ladany, N., Krengel, M., & Schult, D. (1996). Clinical supervision research from 1981 to 1993: A methodological critique. *Journal of Counseling Psychology, 43*, 35–50.

Falender, C. A., & Shafranske, E. P. (2004). Clinical supervision: A competency-based approach. Washington, DC: American Psychological Association.

Fall, M., & Sutton, J. M. (2003). Supervision of entry level licensed counselors: A descriptive study. *The Clinical Supervisor, 22*(2), 139–51.

Fernando, D. M., & Hulse-Killacky, D. (2005). The relationship of supervisory styles to satisfaction with supervision and the perceived self-efficacy of master's-level counseling students. *Counselor Education and Supervision, 44*, 293–304.

Ginott, H. G. (1959). The theory and practice of "therapeutic intervention" in child treatment. *Journal of Consulting Psychology, 23*, 160–66.

Glidden, C. E., & Tracey, T. J. (1992). A multidimensional scaling analysis of supervisory dimensions and their perceived relevance across trainee experience levels. *Professional Psychology: Research and Practice, 23*, 151–57.

Goodyear, R. K., Abadie, P. D., & Efros, F. (1984). Supervisory theory into practice: Differential perception of supervision by Ekstein, Ellis, Polster, and Rogers. *Journal of Counseling Psychology, 31*, 228–37.

Goodyear, R. K., & Bradley, F. O. (1983). Theories of counselor supervision: Points of convergence and divergence. *The Counseling Psychologist, 11*, 59–67.

Goodyear, R. K., & Robyak, J. E. (1982). Supervisors' theory and experience in supervisory focus. *Psychological Reports, 51*, 978.

Gruman, D., & Nelson, M. L. (2008). Supervision of professional school counselors. In H. K. Coleman & C. Yeh (Eds.), *Handbook of school counseling*. New York: Erlbaum.

Gysbers, N. C., & Johnston, J. A. (1965). Expectations of a practicum supervisor's role. *Counselor Education and Supervision, 4*, 68–74.

Hart, G. M., & Nance, D. (2003). Style of supervision as perceived by supervisors and supervisees. *Counselor Education and Supervision, 43*, 146–58.

Hawkins, P., & Shohet, R. (1989) *Supervision in the helping professions. An individual, group and organizational approach*. Milton Keynes, UK: Open University Press.

Hayes, R. L., Blackman, L. S., & Brennan, C. (2001). Group supervision. In L. J. Bradley & N. Ladany (Eds.), *Counselor supervision* (3rd ed., 183–206). Philadelphia: Brunner-Routledge.

Heiney, S. P., & Darr-Hope, H. (1999). Healing icons: Art support programs for patients with cancer. *Cancer Practice, 7*(4), 183–89.

Henderson, P., & Gysbers, N. C. (2006). Providing administrative and counseling supervision for school counselors. In G. A. Waltz, J. C. Bleuer, & R. K. Yep (Eds.), *Vistas: Compelling perspectives on counseling* (161–64). Alexandria, VA: American Counseling Association.

Heppner, P. P., & Roehlke, H. J. (1984). Differences among supervisees at different levels of training: Implications for a developmental model of supervision. *Journal of Counseling Psychology, 31*, 76–90.

Herlihy, B., Gray, N., & McCollom, V. (2002). Legal and ethical issues in school counselor supervision. *Professional School Counseling, 6,* 55–60.

Holloway, E. L. (1987). Developmental models of supervision: Is it development? *Professional Psychology: Research and Practice, 18,* 209–16.

Holloway, E. L. (1992). Supervision: A way of teaching and learning. In S. D. Brown & R. W. Lent (Eds.), *Handbook of counseling psychology* (2nd ed., 177–214). New York: John Wiley.

Holloway, E. L. (1995). *Clinical supervision: A systems approach.* Thousand Oaks, CA: Sage.

Holloway, E. L., & Neufeldt, S. A. (1995). Supervision: Its contributions to treatment efficacy. *Journal of Consulting and Clinical Psychology, 63*(2), 207–13.

Holloway, E. L., & Wampold, B. E. (1983). Patterns of verbal behavior and judgments of satisfaction in the supervision interview. *Journal of Counseling Psychology, 30,* 227–34.

Holloway, E. L., & Wolleat, P. L. (1994). Supervision: The pragmatics of empowerment. *Journal of Educational and Psychological Consultation, 5*(1), 23–43.

Hovrath, A. O. (1982). *Working alliance inventory* (Rev. ed.). Vancouver, BC: Simon Fraiser University.

International Interdisciplinary Conference on Clinical Supervision. (2006). Retrieved October 28, 2006, from www.socialwork.buffalo.edu/csconference.

Kell, B. L., & Mueller, W. J. (1966). *Impact and chance: A study of counseling relationships.* Englewood Cliffs, NJ: Prentice-Hall.

Kiesler, D. J. (1988). *Therapeutic metacommunication: Therapist impact disclosure as feedback in psychotherapy.* Palo Alto, CA: Consulting Psychologists Press.

Kolb, D. A. (1984). Experiential learning: Experience as the source of learning and development. Englewood Cliffs, NJ: Prentice-Hall.

Lambert, M. J., & Ogles, B. M. (1997). Researching psychotherapy supervision. In C. W. Watkins, Jr. (Ed.), *Handbook of psychotherapy* (421–46). New York: Wiley.

Leddick, G. R., & Bernard, J. M. (1980). The history of supervision: A critical review. *Counselor Education and Supervision, 20,* 186–96.

Littrell, J. M., Lee-Borden, N., & Lorenz, J. A. (1979). A developmental framework for counseling supervision. *Counselor Education and Supervision, 19,* 119–36.

Loganbill, C., Hardy, E., & Delworth, U. (1982). Supervision: A conceptual model. *Counseling Psychologist, 10,* 3–42.

Luke, M., & Bernard, J. M. (2006). The school counselor supervision model: An extension of the discrimination model. *Counselor Education and Supervision, 45,* 282–95.

Martin, D. J., Garske, J. P., & Davis, M. K. (2000). Relation of the therapeutic alliance with outcome and other variables: A meta-analytic review. *Journal of Consulting and Clinical Psychology, 68,* 438–50.

Mascari, J. B., & Wilson, J. (2005). Current state licensing trends: Credits, supervision and threats to counselor identity. Presented at American Association for State Counseling Boards Annual Conference. Savannah, GA (available online at www.aascb.org/extras/aascb/pdfs/05conf/proceedings.pdf and www.aascb.org/extras/aascb/pdfs/updatestateinformation.pdf).

Miller, G. M., & Dollarhide, C. T. (2006). Supervision in schools: Building pathways to excellence. *Counselor Education and Supervision, 45,* 296–303.

Milne, D. L., & James, I. A. (2002). The observed impact of training on competence in clinical supervision. *British Journal of Clinical Psychology, 41,* 55–72.

Mullen, J. A., Luke, M., & Drewes, A. (2007). Supervision can be playful too: Play therapy techniques that enhance supervision. *International Journal for Play Therapy, 16*(1), 69–85.

National Board for Certified Counselors. (2000). *NBCC eligibility requirements.* Retrieved October 27, 2006, from www.nbcc.org.

National Board for Certified Counselors. (2001). *Approved clinical supervisor requirements.* Retrieved March 2, 2007, from www.cce-global.org/credentials -offered/acs/art_acsrequirements.

Neufeldt, S. A. (1994). Use of a manual to train supervisors. *Counselor Education and Supervision, 33,* 327–36.

Neufeldt, S. A., Beutler, L. E., & Ranchero, R. (1997). Research on supervisor variables in psychotherapy supervision. In C. E. Watkins, Jr. (Ed.), *Handbook of psychotherapy supervision.* New York: Wiley.

O'Byrne, K., & Rosenberg, J. I. (1998). The practice of supervision: A socio-cultural perspective. *Counselor Education and Supervision, 38,* 34–42.

Olk, M., & Freidlander, M. L. (1992). Trainees' experiences of role conflict and role ambiguity in supervisory relationships. *Journal of Counseling Psychology, 39,* 389–97.

Pearson, Q. M. (2001). A case in clinical supervision: A framework for putting theory into practice. *Journal of Mental Health Counseling, 23,* 174–83.

Pearson, Q. M. (2004). Getting the most out of clinical supervision: Strategies for mental health counseling students. *Journal of Mental Health Counseling, 26,* 361–73.

Pearson, Q. M. (2006). Psychotherapy-driven supervision: Integrating counseling theories into role-based supervision. *Journal of Mental Health Counseling, 28,* 241–53.

Pedersen, P. (1994). *A handbook for developing multicultural awareness* (2nd ed.). Alexandria, VA: American Counseling Association.

Putney, M. W., Worthington, E. L., & McCullough, M. E. (1992). Effects of supervisor and supervisee theoretical orientation and supervisor-supervisee matching on interns' perceptions of supervision. *Journal of Counseling Psychology, 39*(2), 258–65.

Ray, D. (2004). Supervision of basic and advanced skills in play therapy. *Journal of Professional Counseling: Practice, Theory & Research, 32*(2), 28–41.

Rogers, C. R. (1957). Training individuals to engage in the therapeutic process. In C. R. Strother (Ed.), *Psychology and Mental Health* (76–92). Washington, DC: American Psychological Association.

Shechtman, Z., & Wirzberger, A. (1999). Needs and preferred style of supervision among Israeli school counselors at different stages of professional development. *Journal of Counseling and Development, 77*(4), 556–64.

Shulman, L. (February 6–8, 2005). The signature pedagogies of the professions of law, medicine, engineering and the clergy: Potential lessons for the education of teachers. Paper presented at the Math Science Partnerships (MSP) Workshop:

"Teacher Education for Effective Teaching and Learning," Hosted by the National Research Council's Center for Education. Irvine, CA (available online at hub.mspnet.org/media/data/Shulman_Signature_Pedagogies.pdf?media_000000001297.pdf).

Steven, D. T., Goodyear, R. K., Robertson, P. (1998). Supervisor development: An exploratory study of change in stance and emphasis. *Clinical Supervisor, 16,* 73–88.

Struder, J. R. (2005). Supervising counselors-in-training: A guide for field supervisors. *Professional School Counseling, 8,* 353–59.

Sue, D., & Sue, D. (1999). *Counseling the culturally different: Theory and practice* (3rd ed.). New York: Wiley.

Sutherland, T. E., & Bonwell, C. C. (1996). *Using active learning in college classes: A range of options for faculty.* San Francisco, CA: Josey Bass.

Sutton, J. M., & Page, B. J. (1994). Post-degree clinical supervision of school counselors. *The School Counselor, 42,* 32–39.

Tyler, J. D., Sloan, L. L., & King, A. R. (2000). Psychotherapy supervision practices of academic faculty: A national survey. *Psychotherapy, 37,* 98–101.

Watkins, C. E. (1995). Psychotherapy supervision in the 1990's: Some observations and reflections. *American Journal of Psychotherapy, 49,* 568–81.

Watkins, C. E. (1998). Psychotherapy supervision in the 21st century: Some pressing needs and impressing possibilities. *Journal of Psychotherapy Practice and Research, 7,* 93–101.

White, M. B., & Russell, C. S. (1995). The essential elements of supervisory systems: A modified Delphi study. *Journal of Marital and Family Therapy, 21,* 33–54.

Whitman, S. M., Ryan, B., & Rubenstein, D. F. (2001). Psychotherapy supervisor training: Differences between psychiatry and other mental health disciplines. *Academic Psychiatry, 25*(3), 156–61.

Wilkerson, K. (2006). Peer supervision for the professional development of school counselors: Toward an understanding of terms and findings. *Counselor Education and Supervision, 46,* 59–67.

Worthington, E. L., Jr. (1987). Changes in supervision as counselors and supervisors gain experience: A review. *Professional Psychology: Research and Practice, 18,* 189–208.

Worthington, E. L., & Roehlke, H. J. (1979). Effective supervision as perceived by beginning counselors-in-training. *Journal of Counseling Psychology, 26,* 64–73.

Zorga, S. (1997). Supervision process seen as a process of experiential learning. *The Clinical Supervisor, 16*(1), 145–61.

2

⌒∞⌒

Sanding in Supervision

A Sand Tray Technique for Clinical Supervisors

Kristi A. Gibbs and Eric J. Green

Clinical supervision is a task that a majority of mental health professionals are required to do at various intervals in their careers (Bernard & Goodyear, 2004; Scott, et al., 2000). Regardless of whether the mental health practitioner is maintaining a private practice or teaching in a graduate program, therapists typically provide supervision to junior members of the profession. However, most graduate degree programs that prepare mental health professionals preclude a course in supervision (Navin, Beamish, & Johanson, 1995). As a result, training in supervision is not standardized, and clinicians often assume the role of supervisor without sufficient preparation (Scott, et al., 2000).

Mental health professionals typically receive instruction on various theories of counseling and are encouraged to develop a personal theory in an effort to conceptualize clients' issues. Frequently this is referred to as a "roadmap," which clinicians utilize to effectively counsel clients. Clinical supervision, similarly, requires that clinicians formulate a detailed roadmap to conceptualize supervisees' concerns. However, many clinicians who engage in supervision have not been adequately trained in specific models of clinical supervision. Unfortunately, when a supervisor has not received sufficient preparation they are inadequately prepared to advise members of the next generation of therapists (Magnuson, Norem, & Bradley, 2001).

In this chapter an overview of two widely used models of supervision will be presented: the Integrated Developmental Model (Stoltenberg,

McNeill, & Delworth, 1998) and the Discrimination Model (Bernard, 1979). Additionally, a sand tray technique created by the authors, *sanding in supervision*, will be discussed to provide the reader with an experiential activity, along with a case study illustrating its utility.

CLINICAL SUPERVISION IN THE MENTAL HEALTH FIELD

Bernard and Goodyear (2004) defined supervision as an intervention that is provided by a senior member of a profession to a more junior member of that same profession. The purpose of this relationship is to guide the supervisee in his acquisition and practice of new skills. To be effective, a supervision relationship is "evaluative, extends over time, and has the simultaneous purposes of enhancing the professional functioning of the more junior person(s), monitoring the quality of professional services offered to the clients that she, he, or they see, and serving as a gatekeeper for those who are to enter the particular profession" (p. 8).

There are many paradigms of clinical supervision, two of which will be discussed fully in this chapter: *developmental* and *social role*. Developmental models focus primarily on the supervisee's stage of development (i.e., the differences between a student in the first practicum versus a post-master's supervisee who is halfway through the hours needed for licensure); social role models focus on the role that the supervisor engages in during supervision (i.e., teacher, counselor, consultant).

Integrated Developmental Model

Stoltenberg (1981) developed the Integrated Developmental Model (IDM) of supervision. Because this is a developmental model of supervision, the IDM places the focus of the supervisory relationship on how supervisees increase their clinical efficacy by augmenting their training skills through engagement in supervised counseling experiences. Using this model Chagnon and Russell (1995) conceptualized the supervisee through a lens in which they assert two basic assumptions about the development of supervisees. The first assumption is that supervisees move through qualitatively different stages as they gain skill and knowledge in the practice of counseling. The second suggests that supervisees require diverse supervision environments as they move through levels of development in their own skill and training.

The Integrated Developmental Model (Stoltenberg, McNeill, & Delworth, 1998) describes counselor development as occurring through four different stages. In the first stage, level 1, the supervisee has limited training or limited experience and is dependent on the supervisor. The supervisee in this first stage may be a student or possibly a more seasoned clinician who has a distinctive proclivity to obtain new skills. For example, it is typical for a clinician who has primarily counseled adult clients to become overly reliant upon his supervisor when deciding to change client populations and switch to counseling children.

At the next stage, level 2, the supervisee is fluctuating between dependency and autonomy. The supervisee in stage 2 might also be a student, but this supervisee has typically received advanced training in the field or has more work experience in mental health counseling. During the third level the focus switches to developing personal judgment, and the supervisory relationship becomes more collegial. A stage 3 supervisee typically possesses a graduate degree and may be working toward mental health licensure. Last, upon reaching level 4, the supervisee has become a master counselor, aware of personal strengths and limitations. The relationship at this level is more consultant rather than supervisory. The supervisee has probably obtained licensure as a mental health professional and is practicing independently.

Knowing where a supervisee is in terms of development is integral to facilitating a productive supervision experience. It is important to provide a different, developmentally appropriate environment as a supervisee progresses through the different stages of development. One way to assess developmental level is to ask the supervisee, "How are you feeling with these skills?" or "What do you need from me in supervision?" Often seasoned clinicians forget how intimidating it can be in the early stages of clinical development. This model helps the supervisor evaluate the supervisee's developmental level, which can enhance learning and provide a framework conducive to effective supervision.

The Discrimination Model

The Discrimination Model (Bernard, 1979) is a social role model that attends to the role the supervisor takes as well as to three different focus areas for supervision. The roles include teacher, counselor, or consultant; and the focus areas include *intervention skills, conceptualization skills,* and *personalization skills.* According to the Discrimination Model it is cogent for the supervisor to determine which focus area(s) should be addressed at any given time during a session, keeping in mind that the focus area may shift multiple times during one supervision session.

The first focus area identified by Bernard (1979) is intervention skills, originally labeled process skills. Intervention skills are observable behaviors and include the basic counseling skills that most therapists learn early in their training. Examples include opening a session, probes, reflections, restatements, or summaries. Bernard indicated that "these behaviors, most noticed by the client, become indicators that counseling has begun and social chit-chat has ended" (p. 62).

Bernard (1979) named the second focus area conceptualization skills. These are less observable, more covert behaviors. "Conceptualization skills are those that reflect deliberate thinking and case analysis by the counselor" (p. 62). These skills involve the therapist's ability to understand what the client is saying in session and identify themes across sessions.

The third and final focus area is personalization skills. Personalization skills include both overt behaviors as well as behaviors that are more subtle in nature. Examples include ability and comfort assuming the role of counselor, ability to be challenged without becoming overly defensive, and engagement in the counseling relationship without bringing personal issues into the session (Bernard, 1979).

Once the focus area has been identified, the supervisor will respond from one of three roles. Bernard (1979) stated that it is important to choose the role in a deliberate manner, tailored to an individual supervisee's needs, rather than simply as a result of personal preference. The three basic roles are teacher, counselor, and consultant.

> The supervisor as teacher focuses on some knowledge or expertise that he or she wishes to transmit to the counselor. The supervisor as counselor places priority on the counselor's personal needs, with the belief that this focus will allow the counselor to overcome the nervousness or self-doubt that impedes natural development. The supervisor as consultant focuses on a relationship with the counselor that is explorative in nature and assumes that the counselor has the ability to express his or her supervision needs (p. 64).

The Discrimination Model offers the supervisor a myriad of choices for intervening and establishing goals in the supervision session.

Goals of Supervision

Bernard and Goodyear (2004) identified three primary goals of supervision: enhancing the professional functioning of the supervisee, monitoring client care, and serving as a gatekeeper to the profession. Enhancing the professional functioning of the supervisee is a broad goal that should be discussed between each individual supervisor and supervisee. According to Bernard and Goodyear, this objective is typically influenced by the supervisor's own theory or model and the supervisee's developmental needs and expressed wishes. For example, a supervisee may express a desire to learn skills unique to counseling children without any specific knowledge about what those skills are. The training and education provided by the supervisor will be largely influenced by the supervisor's own beliefs about how best to counsel children. On the other hand, someone seeking to be trained specifically in play therapy will probably seek out a supervisor who has training in that area. So, both the supervisee's wishes and the supervisor's theoretical orientation should influence the first goal of supervision.

Monitoring client care and serving as gatekeeper to the profession may be the most important responsibilities of any supervisor. Bernard and Goodyear (2004) stated that these objectives can be difficult, especially when the supervisor suspects harm to a client. While supervisors often see themselves as allies with their supervisee, "they must be prepared, should they see harm being done to clients, to risk bruising the egos of their supervisees" (p. 14). As gatekeeper, occasionally a supervisor may find it necessary to steer a supervisee out of the profession.

Serving as gatekeeper to the profession may be particularly challenging when supervising mental health professionals who counsel children. Counselor competence is one of four ethical concerns identified most often when children are involved in counseling (Croxton, Churchill, & Fellin, 1988; Hendrix, 1991; Henkelman & Everall, 2001; Huey, 1996; Koocher & Keith-Speigal, 1990; Lawrence & Robinson Kurpius, 2000; Remley & Herlihy, 2007; Sweeney, 2001). Lawrence and Robinson Kurpius (2000) stated that children are a special population, requiring unique knowledge and skills and that, therefore, ethical practice mandates distinct education, training, and supervised practice before beginning independent counseling with children. Several authors have asserted a belief that most mental health professionals will, at some time in their careers, counsel children without having received appropriate training (Lawrence & Robinson Kurpius, 2000; Stern & Newland, 1994). When this is the case, it is the duty of the supervisor to fill the gatekeeping role and either steer the supervisee toward appropriate training or counsel them out of the field.

In order to execute the aforementioned goals of supervision, it is imperative that the supervisee receive feedback. Bernard and Goodyear (2004) assert that experience in the practice of counseling is rarely sufficient for learning unless it is accompanied by clear, systematic feedback. A supervisor's knowledge of at least one model of supervision can increase the likelihood that the supervision relationship will be successful as the supervisor becomes more knowledgeable with skills such as giving feedback. Also, a clinician trained in supervisory skills may be more likely to establish a clear roadmap including setting goals for the supervisory relationship. Supervision of clinicians who counsel children will likely include goals specific to that population as well.

Supervision Issues Specific to Counseling Children

As indicated previously, the professional literature points to a belief that most therapists will, at some time in their careers, counsel with children (Lawrence & Robinson Kurpius, 2000; Stern & Newland, 1994). Lawrence and Robinson Kurpius (2000) have also noted that "a counselor's effectiveness in working with adults does not mean that effectiveness will transfer to minors. There are special areas of knowledge and skills that are unique to working with children" (p. 132).

When supervising someone who is learning to counsel children, it is particularly important to remember two things: the supervisee may not have received prior training in skills unique to counseling children and the supervisee may not be aware of the specialized training that is necessary to counsel children. It is common for a student to graduate from a training program in mental health with limited skills training in the area of counseling children (Gibbs, 2004). Unfortunately, some clinicians may believe erroneously that child clients are miniature adults and can be effectively counseled with the same verbal techniques used with adolescent or adult clients (Lawrence & Robinson Kurpius, 2000). Children, consistent with their development, communicate through play: toys are their words and play is their language (Axline, 1947). Therefore, it is important to assess the skills someone has with counseling children at the onset of the supervision relationship and to explain the unique set of skills necessary for counseling children. For example, it is important for a child therapist to be willing and able to use play as a vehicle for communication with children (Kottman, 2001).

Another consideration is the clinician who has mastered skills with one population, and perhaps has practiced for many years with this population, but is making a change to acquire new skill sets with a diverse clientele. For example, someone who has become a master counselor in their practice with adults may temporarily revert to an earlier developmental level during a transition to learn new skills for counseling children.

So far, this chapter has defined clinical supervision within the mental health field, provided two discrete models of supervision, and covered special issues in supervision, including the supervision of mental health practitioners working with minors. The next section will examine a specific supervision technique that clinical supervisors may utilize to bolster the supervisory relationship with supervisees working with a specialized population: children.

UTILIZING SAND TRAY IN CLINICAL SUPERVISION

Developmental and psychosocial deficits may limit an adult's ability to express emotions accurately and completely. Sand tray provides a medium for supervisees to discover and articulate intensely felt emotions that may otherwise be difficult to express verbally (Mitchell & Friedman,

2003). Also, sand tray allows the supervisee to experience play in a way that may provide more insight into child clients.

The use of a sand tray in therapy with children was first developed by Margaret Lowenfeld (1979). She provided child clients with a shallow box filled with sand and various small toys, which could be placed in the sand to "build a world." Later Dora Kalff, having trained with Carl Jung, integrated Jung's approach with Lowenfeld's work in the sand and named it *sandplay* (Mitchell & Friedman, 2003). Sandplay refers to the Jungian approach developed by Dora Kalff (1980) that recognizes individuation as the goal, in an analytic process, grounded in the life-world of the client. The therapist using sandplay has ideally studied Jung's psychology and has completed personal work in sand therapy. *Sand tray* is a common use of sand and toys that permits a clinician to engage with the client in play. The client's play may be conceptualized through numerous theories such as humanistic-existential, cognitive behavioral, and psychodynamic.

Sandplay is a nonverbal form of therapy that reaches a profound preverbal level of the psyche (Green & Ironside, 2004). Deep in the unconscious humans strive for wholeness and inner psychic reparation. Sandplay encourages a creative regression and enables the self-healing archetype within the individual's psyche to appear (Green & Ironside, 2005; Weinrib, 1983). Sandplay is an activity that integrates play with sand, and choice and inclusion of water or miniature objects. It is a means of activating fantasy and embodying it through expressive means, depicting the unconscious of the individual symbolically through sand manifestations (Green, 2006; Steinhardt, 2000).

Sanding in Supervision: A Technique for Clinical Supervisors

Sanding in supervision (Green & Gibbs, 2006) is a technique that the authors based on Margaret Lowenfeld's World Technique, in which she asked child clients to create world pictures. To use this intervention in a supervision session, the supervisor must first have a sand tray filled with sand and a selection of miniatures from which the supervisee may choose. The supervisee will then insert miniature objects into the sand and create a scene of his choosing, telling a story with the objects similar to an artist's painting. The session can take place in the office where supervision typically occurs or in another location where the supervisor has already assembled the sand tray and miniatures. Having access to a play room that has a sand tray is another alternative that may imbue its own curative qualities.

Once the supervisee is seated in the room where the sanding will occur, the authors recommend saying, "Today I am going to ask that you build something in the sand tray for me. You may use any of the miniatures that you see in these bins. I am going to give you up to 30 minutes to complete this project, and then I'll ask you to tell me about it." Two suggestions are listed below, but it is ultimately up to the supervisor to find a comfortable medium and discern what fits the dynamics specific to the supervisor-supervisee relationship (Green & Gibbs, 2006).

Example 1: "Think about your most challenging client. Based on information you know, as well as your larger conceptualization of the client, build your client's world." Rationale: This version allows the supervisee to explore the world of a client that may be posing some particular challenges, and the hoped-for result is an increased understanding of the client.

Example 2: "Think back to the time before you started your training in mental health. Reflect on your experiences along the way as you have completed your degree. Build your journey along the path of becoming the person you are today." Rationale: This version can be particularly helpful with students who are nearing the end of their training program. In the authors' experience, the result of students completing this exercise was increased insight regarding how much learning occurred in the training program and thereby improved confidence regarding clinical skills. In the case study that follows, this technique will be further clarified.

CASE STUDY: CAROLINE

Caroline is a 41-year-old student in the final semester of her master's degree program in community counseling. Currently she is completing an internship in a community mental health agency where she counsels children, adolescents, and adults. Caroline comes into supervision on this day looking particularly distressed. She enters the playroom with her supervisor and receives the following directions: "I want you to spend some time thinking about and conceptualizing your most perplexing or challenging client. Build your client's world for me in the sand." Caroline is told that she can use any of the miniatures in the sand, and she asks, "What about other things?" to which her supervisor responds, "Anything you see in here is for placing in the sand with the exception of the puppets."

The supervisor does not comment or ask Caroline questions as she is building but rather waits for Caroline to state that the world is complete. This allows the supervisee to create freely her world without interruption. Half an hour later Caroline declares, "It's done!" The supervisor responds, "Please tell me about the world you have created."

The supervisor notices that Caroline has not confined her world to the sandbox. She has placed items under the sandbox, on the table beyond the sandbox, and in every available area of the sandbox. Under the sandbox sits a yellow tub, which previously held Play-Doh, turned upside down with a skeleton on top. On the table sit various people all facing the world that has been built in the sandbox. On the ledge of the sandbox appear to be angels and elderly people. Finally the sandbox is filled with people, army men, red discs (originally pieces to a game in the playroom), trees, pipe cleaners, and a black piece of construction paper that appears to be covering something.

Caroline identifies her sand scene as the world of her 10-year-old female client who was physically abused and neglected from the ages of two to five. She says that the client felt as if she were drowning and could not remember much of her earlier years. Caroline adds that the client was locked in the closet (there was a puppet trapped under the yellow tub that was under the sandbox) a lot as a child. The red discs represent the client's anger, directed particularly at her mother. The black construction paper represents a memory lapse. When the paper is removed there is a shark underneath that Caroline identifies as the client's father.

Caroline seems to be growing increasingly sympathetic toward her client at this point and states, "I guess I can see why her life is so chaotic." Caroline takes a deep breath and continues with her explanation of the world she has created, "The people on the table represent five years of therapist hopping, and the things around the edge of the sandbox represent good things which she [the client] won't allow in." Caroline is in the sandbox with the client, but there is a fence placed between the two of them.

When Caroline is finished with her explanation of the sand scene, the supervisor asks, "What might it be like to live in this world?" Caroline replies, "Wow! It must be tough to be her. I never really thought about all of this stuff that she is carrying around. No wonder she is all over the place when we are in session." Caroline sits for a moment, absorbing the images contained within the world she created. She seems to need a moment to process what has happened, as she seems content with observing the scene and makes no eye contact toward the supervisor. After a minute or so, the supervisor asks Caroline what she has learned in the process of this exercise. Caroline responds, "You know, this is that client that I always dread. She exhausts me, and I wonder if she is really doing any work. Every week we talk about the same thing, and she never seems to take any responsibility for what she can change. Ugh! But now, I believe that I have more insight into her inner world. I think I can be more patient with her. And now, maybe I can help her." Caroline has a smile on her face and seems relieved to have gained this new awareness about her client.

Caroline's supervisor asks one last question, "How has this experience been for you?" She responds, "Great! When you first asked me to do this

I thought it was pointless. But after I became involved, the time passed quickly. When I examine what I have created in the sand, I know that I could not have gained that sort of insight about my client just by talking to her. This was incredible!"

Caroline's supervisor believed the depiction in the sandbox to be just as representative of Caroline as it was of her client. Although she did not share this with Caroline, in many ways, the supervisor experienced frustration with Caroline just as she did with her client. This dynamic, called parallel process, occurs in the supervision relationship when the supervisee presents similar feelings and behaviors as the client presents to the supervisee during the counseling session (Friedlander, Siegel, & Brenock, 1989). Caroline had disclosed information on previous occasions regarding her own personal experiences with "therapist hopping," and the supervisor knew that she had some history of trauma. Caroline learned something about her client that day, and she also learned something about herself. Caroline said that she believed she could be more empathic with her client having become more aware of the chaos that surrounds her client's life. She also said that she believed that at 41 she may have more in common with a 10-year-old than she previously believed. "We are a lot alike, my client and me. Building that world helped me realize just how much I can relate to her."

CONCLUSION

This chapter has provided a basic overview of supervision, providing a definition of clinical supervision in the mental health field and describing the Integrated Developmental Model (Stoltenberg, McNeill, & Delworth, 1998) and the Discrimination Model (Bernard, 1979). The chapter also illustrated a case example of a technique for using sandplay in supervision. There are many benefits to using the technique of sanding in supervision in the context of clinical supervision (Carey, 2006; Markos & Hyatt, 1999; Green & Gibbs, 2006). A supervisee's clinical skills may be advanced if they are provided a safe and supportive supervisory relationship in which sand techniques are utilized to encourage creativity and autonomy (Carey, 2006; Green & Gibbs, 2006). Sanding in supervision also facilitates the supervisee's understanding of her client's inner world and provides for the healthy expression of difficult emotions (Allan, 2004). Finally, parallel learning occurs in the supervisee's therapeutic relationship with the client when the supervisor utilizes sanding in supervision, as illustrated in the case study (Markos & Hyatt, 1999). Utilizing sand tray activities in clinical supervision is one method clinical supervisors may utilize to foster development in the supervisory dyad, in which safety, warmth, and creative expression engender clinical efficacy to both the supervisee and the client, who is affected indirectly.

REFERENCES

Allan, J. (2004). *Inscapes of the child's world: Jungian counseling in schools and clinics.* Dallas, TX: Spring Publications, Inc.

Axline, V. (1947). *Play therapy.* New York: Ballantine.

Bernard, J. M. (1979). Supervisor training: A discrimination model. *Counselor Education and Supervision, 19*, 60–68.

Bernard, J. M., & Goodyear, R. K. (2004). *Fundamentals of clinical supervision.* Boston: Allyn & Bacon.

Carey, L. (Ed.). (2006). *Expressive and creative arts methods for trauma survivors.* Philadelphia: Jessica Kingsley Publishers.

Chagnon, J., & Russell, R. K. (1995). Assessment of supervisee developmental level and supervision environment across supervisor experience. *Journal of Counseling and Development, 73*, 553–58.

Croxton, T. A., Churchill, S. R., & Fellin, P. (1988). Counseling minors without parental consent. *Child Welfare, 67*, 3–14.

Friedlander, M. L., Siegel, S. M., & Brenock, K. (1989). Parallel process in counseling and supervision: A case study. *Journal of Counseling Psychology, 36*, 149–57.

Gibbs, K. (2004). Counselor educators' perceptions of training students to counsel children in non-school settings (Doctoral dissertation, University of New Orleans, 2004).

Green, E. J. (2006). Jungian play therapy: Activating the self-healing archetype in children affected by sexual abuse. *Louisiana Journal of Counseling, 8*, 1–11.

Green, E., & Gibbs, K. (October 14, 2006). *Utilizing play in supervision.* Association for Play Therapy Annual Conference, Toronto, Ontario, Canada.

Green, E. J., & Ironside, D. (2004). Archetypes, symbols, and Jungian sandplay: An innovative approach to school counseling. *Counselor's Classroom.* Retrieved September 22, 2006, from www.guidancechannel.com.

Green, E. J., & Ironside, D. (January 29, 2005). *Jungian sandplay in family therapy: Implications for marriage and family counselors.* International Association of Marriage and Family Counselors World Conference, New Orleans, LA.

Hendrix, D. H. (1991). Ethics and intrafamily confidentiality in counseling with children. *Journal of Mental Health Counseling, 13*, 323–33.

Henkelman, J. J., & Everall, R. D. (2001). Informed consent with children: Ethical and practical implications. *Canadian Journal of Counseling, 35*, 109–21.

Huey, W. C. (1996). Counseling minor clients. In B. Herlihy & G. Corey (Eds.), *ACA ethical standards casebook* (5th ed., 241–45). Alexandria, VA: American Counseling Association.

Kalff, D. (1980). *Sandplay: A psychotherapeutic approach to the psyche.* Boston: Sigo Press.

Koocher, G. P., & Keith-Spiegal, P. C. (1990). *Children, ethics, and law.* Lincoln: University of Nebraska Press.

Kottman, T. (2001). *Play therapy: Basics and beyond*. Alexandria, VA: American Counseling Association.

Lawrence, G., & Robinson Kurpius, S. E. (2000). Legal and ethical issues involved when counseling minors in nonschool settings. *Journal of Counseling and Development, 78*, 130–36.

Lowenfeld, M. (1979). *The World Technique*. London: George Allen & Unwin.

Magnuson, S., Norem, K. & Bradley, L. J. (2001). Supervising school counselors. In L. J. Bradley and N. Ladany (Eds.), *Counselor supervision: Principles, process, & practice* (3rd ed., 207–21). Philadelphia: Brunner-Routledge.

Markos, P. A., & Hyatt, C. J. (1999). Play or supervision: Using sandplay with beginning practicum students. *Guidance and Counseling, 14*(4), 3–6.

Mitchell, R. R., & Friedman, H. S. (2003). Using sandplay in therapy with adults. In C. E. Schaefer (Ed.), *Play therapy with adults*. Hoboken, NJ: Wiley.

Navin, S., Beamish, P., & Johanson, G. (1995). Ethical practices of field-based mental health counselor supervisors. *Journal of Mental Health Counseling, 17*, 243–53.

Remley, T. P., Jr., & Herlihy, B. (2007). *Ethical, legal, and professional issues in counseling* (2nd ed.). Upper Saddle River, NJ: Merrill Prentice Hall.

Scott, K. J., Ingram, K. M., Vitanza, S. A., & Smith, N. G. (2000). Training in supervision: A survey of current practices. *The Counseling Psychologist, 28*, 403–22.

Steinhardt, L. (2000). Foundation and form in Jungian sandplay. London: Jessica Kingsley Publishers.

Stern, M., & Newland, L. M. (1994). Working with children: Providing a framework for the roles of counseling psychologists. *The Counseling Psychologist, 22*, 402–25.

Stoltenberg, C. D. (1981). Approaching supervision from a developmental perspective: The counselor-complexity model. *Journal of Counseling Psychologists, 28*, 59–65.

Stoltenberg, C. D., McNeill, B. W., & Delworth, U. (1998). *IDM: An integrated developmental model for supervising counselors and therapists*. San Francisco: Jossey-Bass.

Sweeney, D. S. (2001). Legal and ethical issues in play therapy. In G. Landreth (Ed.), *Innovations in play therapy: Issues, process and special populations* (65–81). Philadelphia: Brunner-Routledge.

Weinrib, E. L. (1983). *Images of the self*. Boston: Sigo Press.

3

⸎

When Approaches Collide

A Decision-Making Model for Play Therapists

Ken Gardner and Lorri Yasenik

RATIONALE FOR A DEFINED PLAY THERAPY SUPERVISION MODEL

The field of play therapy has expanded significantly in the past eight years. National and international play therapy organizations have grown in membership to include thousands of trained professionals in the field of play therapy. In addition to increased membership in play therapy organizations world wide, institutions of higher education are now offering specialized courses and programs in play therapy (University of York England, University of South Africa, University of North Texas, Texas State University–San Marcos, International Christian University Tokyo, Alliant International University, Loma Linda University [Canadian Campus], State University of New York–Oswego, and Fairleigh Dickinson University).

Play therapy organizations (Association for Play Therapy, Canadian Association for Child and Play Therapy, British Association of Play Therapists, Play Therapy United Kingdom, Play Therapy International) have identified the fact that most members come from various professions such as clinical social work, youth and child care, psychology, nursing, marriage and family therapy, psychiatry, and expressive therapies such as art therapy and music therapy. Those entering into the field of play therapy with degrees from other primary professions tend to belong to a professional association that regulates their *general* practice. Various regulatory bodies have identified the skills and competencies necessary to provide general mental health services. Although training in general counseling is an essential requirement prior to gaining specialized play therapy training, general counseling training does not provide adequate practical and ethical guidance to competently practice as a play therapist.

Professional competencies for play therapists must be acknowledged and underscored. Various professional organizations and authors have identified specific lists of competencies that a play therapist needs to work toward to be able to practice safely and ethically as a play therapist. For instance, the Delphi Technique (Dalkey & Helmer, 1962) was used by Landreth and Joiner (2005) to establish core skills/methods and practical experiences that are considered essential in the education of play therapists. This information was obtained through questionnaires provided to experts in the field of play therapy and from play therapy professors. As an outcome of this study, approximately ten goal areas were identified to help guide the training and practice of play therapy in the United States. Play Therapy United Kingdom (*Professional structures model*, 2002), Play Therapy International, and the British Association for Play Therapy have also developed areas of core competencies. Generally, the global areas of concern for those granting certification and/or registration in play therapy include: play therapy knowledge, play therapy skills, and professional and personal attributes and attitudes related to being a play therapist. All organizations emphasize the requirement of receiving skilled supervision related to the discrete domains that are essential to play therapy practice. This having been said, it is critical that those in the field of play therapy supervision adopt a systematic use of a supervision model to guide the supervision process. Not unlike the necessity of having a systematic use of a theoretical model to establish an interpersonal process (part of the definition of play therapy itself), those delivering and receiving supervision should also be able to describe their model so that they are operating in a predictable way that provides a reliable framework for supervisees.

Specialized supervision is necessary to avoid the dangers of random eclecticism. Students may be trained in one approach to play therapy or they may be trained across a number of approaches. Both APT and PTUK recommend core training courses for play therapists that require students to compare and contrast from five to eight modern play therapy theories such as child-centered play therapy, Adlerian play therapy, cognitive-behavioral play therapy, theraplay, gestalt play therapy, relationship play therapy and filial play therapy, and nondirective play therapy. Students of play therapy are therefore leaving training with knowledge about a number of different ways to approach children in the play therapy setting. Depending on the play therapy settings for the practical experience component of training, the student may emerge with strengths in one or more ways of approaching the play therapy process. Supervisees generally bring diversified training experiences to supervision, therefore supervisors need a way to meet the supervisee in an inclusive manner. Supervisors then need a specialized play therapy supervision model that accepts and supports all approaches to play therapy.

The goals for play therapy supervisors are to provide: (1) objective feedback and guidance, (2) input for clinical situations (including techniques, special topics, and process), (3) consultation and direction regarding ethical issues and dilemmas, and (4) consultation and direction regarding legal issues (British Association of Play Therapists, 2006, Association for Play Therapy, 2006).

The dilemma in providing specialized play therapy supervision appears to be how the supervisor will meet the above goals and address core play therapy competencies if she does not have a highly inclusive model that will honor all ways of working with children. Furthermore, Schaefer (2003) notes that practitioners are selecting from various theories those strategies and techniques that appear best fitted for the child client's presenting problem. Phillips and Landreth (1995) found that an eclectic, multitheoretical orientation was, by far, the most common approach reported by respondents. How does the supervisor provide an organizing structure to address this growing trend?

THE PLAY THERAPY DIMENSIONS MODEL

The Play Therapy Dimensions Model (PTDM) (Yasenik & Gardner, 2004) evolved from this dilemma. The PTDM recognizes that there are fundamental philosophical differences as well as shared viewpoints between schools of play therapy. The model is a decision-making and treatment-planning tool. It is useful to most play therapists in that it allows for the reflection on and use of numerous theoretical models, making it eclectic in nature. There are three overriding assumptions. First, each child is unique regarding his or her skills and abilities; second, all children follow a common developmental pathway; third, the play therapist has a central role in facilitating change and optimizing growth (Yasenik & Gardner, 2004). As each child seen in therapy is unique, this requires the play therapist to tailor interventions to the *child* and the *child's* needs. The model is not prescriptive, but it is intended to provide a way for the therapist to conceptualize the play therapy process and to answer the *who, what, when, why,* and *how* of the play therapy process. The direction gained by the therapist to answer the above questions is, again, driven by the *child.*

The PTDM identifies two primary dimensions—*consciousness* and *directiveness*—and highlights the ways in which existing theories and techniques in play therapy interact within these two dimensions.

The consciousness dimension (figure 3.1) reflects the child's representation of consciousness in play. Consciousness can be represented in the child's play activities and verbalizations. Children often have a need for emotional distance from the issues, worries, and concerns they are attempting to reorganize. A weaving process can be observed in children's play, which is represented by the movement up and down the consciousness dimension, moving from greater levels of consciousness to lesser levels or vice versa (Yasenik & Gardner, 2004). When children experience disruption through an outside experience, their mental schemas may be distorted and conflicted in relation to the way they see themselves or others. Dissociated thoughts and feelings can be made conscious through symbolic play. Wilson, Kendrick, and Ryan (1992) refer to symbolic play and its role in play therapy and note Piaget's (1977) developmental theories of adaptation, assimilation, and accommodation. Symbolic play is often at the semi-conscious or experiential level, and children make use of symbols to organize cognitive schemas and assimilate new possibilities into a past representation, which then leads them to potential growth and change. Children need to be viewed from a developmental perspective when discussing *consciousness*. Each child will present with a different capacity for conscious awareness because, for instance, the very young child's language and cognitive schemas are still developing. To consider the degree of consciousness represented in a given play therapy session is critical as the play therapist tracks the child's process.

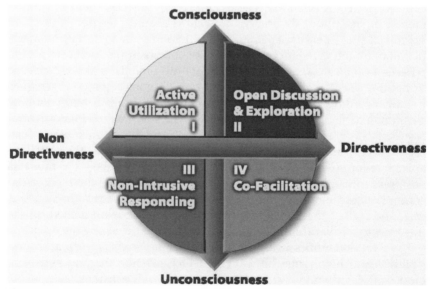

Figure 3.1.   Play Therapy Dimensions Diagram.

Psychodynamic theorists and Jungian analytical play therapy (Peery, 2003) support the notion that children project internal energy onto play objects whether they are consciously aware of it or not. If the play objects or materials are viewed by the therapist as symbolizing internal energy, the therapist may choose to make use of an interpretation. Jungian play therapists will identify conscious and unconscious influences and may at times make interpretive comments and identify observed themes in the play. The concept of deintegration would be considered and the therapist may explore possible regression to access deeper unconscious material. Although some play therapy theories fully explore the levels of consciousness in therapy, others may not. The degree to which consciousness is acknowledged and explored is still a decision-making factor for all play therapists.

Critical to the consciousness dimension is the therapist's knowledge of coping strategies used by children who have experienced traumatic events or life-threatening experiences. Regardless of the referral request, play therapists must exercise sound clinical judgment when making decisions about facilitating greater degrees of conscious representation of dissociated thoughts and feelings. Pynoos and Eth (1986) in their study of children who had witnessed homicide observed the following coping strategies: repression, fixation on the trauma, displacement, denial-in-fantasy (child imagines a positive rather than the traumatic one), and identification (child identifies him/herself with a parent or helper figure). Terr (1993) related compulsive repetition of the abduction scene in her description of sessions with the children of Chowchilla who had been abducted and buried alive in their school bus. Play therapists must make observations that are developmentally anchored when considering the level of consciousness in the play and the ability and capacity of the child to move in the direction of increased conscious awareness.

The consciousness dimension is therefore one area of concern for the play therapist. Directive play therapists may choose to name possible feelings, behaviors, and future actions during a play session, or they may structure play activities for the child as related to the interrupting events. Those working on the lower end of the consciousness continuum would not interrupt the child's process; rather they would follow the child's lead and trust the inner drive of the child to reorganize his or her experiences without using interpretive comments to bring the issues to conscious awareness. Neither approach is wrong. The PTDM encourages play therapists to answer the when, why, and how (directed by knowing and observing the child) when exploring greater degrees of consciousness in a given play therapy session.

The next primary dimension as outlined by the PTDM is *directiveness* (figure 3.1). This dimension represents the therapist's activity with respect to the degree of immersion (the degree to which the therapist enters and directs the play) and level of interpretation made by the therapist. Therapists working on the far left side of the directiveness continuum would be viewed as least immersed in the play and the child would be fully directing the play. Many play therapists have been trained in nondirective play therapy approaches and have been influenced by pioneers in the field such as Axline (1969) and Rogers (1951). Axline (1969) described the principles of the relationship between the child and therapist, which emphasized the *child's* role in making decisions and eliciting change. Landreth and Sweeney (1999) further emphasize Axline's nondirective work when describing the child-centered approach to play therapy. They focus on the person of the child and the nondiagnostic, nonprescriptive involvement of the therapist, and highlight the innate capacity of children to direct their own growth and healing. In child-centered play therapy, the therapist works to understand the *child's* perception of his or her reality rather than to inject the therapist's view of the child's reality. Axline (1969) and Landreth (2002) follow the Rogerian personality constructs of (1) the person, (2) the phenomenal field, and (3) the self. These theorists, among others, describe the hallmarks of the nondirective end of the directiveness dimension.

On the far right side of figure 3.1, the therapist would be viewed as fully immersed, as evidenced by the child *and* the therapist's involvement in a play activity structured by the therapist. Adlerian play therapy (Kottman, 2003) may demonstrate the directiveness dimension in that the therapist may initially work with a child nondirectively and over time more directively by modeling and teaching prosocial skills to aid the child in connecting with others. Examples of therapeutic activities include practicing family drawing techniques, asking the child questions about early recollections, helping the child gain personal insight, and using metacommunication (in which the therapist makes a direct interpretation about an observed interactional pattern). The structured phases of treatment highlight this play therapy approach. Other structured theoretical approaches to play therapy include gestalt play therapy (Oaklander, 2003), theraplay (Munns, 2000), ecosystemic play therapy (O'Connor, 1997), cognitive behavioral play therapy (Knell, 1999 & 2003), and prescriptive play therapy (Schaefer, 2003). They may all be represented by the far right end of the directiveness dimension. It must also be recognized that therapists practicing these approaches to play therapy may also make decisions about the *degree* of directiveness at any given time during the therapy process. They may be seen as more or less directive and more or less immersed in the play process with the child. When examining degree of directiveness, it is apparent that relationships are two way, and although there are times when the child needs to choose and direct the play activity, there may also be times when the child becomes immobilized and looks to the therapist to provide structure or direction.

The PTDM offers a way for therapists trained both directively and nondirectively to anchor and discuss their approaches in supervision. Supervisors (regardless of training background) can approach the supervisee from the points of view of consciousness and directiveness. This allows the supervisee and supervisor the freedom to view both on a continuum and supports the weaving process of the play in the directions of consciousness and directiveness as signaled by the child.

The PTDM therefore comprises the two primary dimensions, consciousness and directiveness, that intersect to create four quadrants. Each quadrant can be viewed in figure 3.1. The quadrants provide an organizing structure for play therapists regardless of theoretical orientation. The quadrants assist all play therapists in identifying their level of directiveness, immersion, and degree to which they facilitate the child's conscious awareness of emerging play themes and activities. The quadrants are not meant to simply identify different approaches or ways of practicing play therapy; rather they are a way to view any given play therapy session or sessions. The quadrants provide a window for looking at the possibility of using many play therapy models and interventions during one session or across sessions. The quadrants also provide a way to conceptualize movement during a play therapy session. The same therapist may work in all four quadrants during one session or over time depending on the style of the child, the presenting need, the capacity for play, and the child's developmental stage. Based on the fact that child clients inform play therapists of their needs, there is no prescribed order to work in of any of the quadrants. Supervisors have a way to discuss and explore with the supervisee what quadrant they began in and why.

Quadrant 1 is called *Active Utilization* and can be found in the upper left corner of figure 3.1. This quadrant is situated in the nondirective, yet conscious, space on the diagram. In this quadrant, the child initiates the play using his or her own metaphors, symbols, and/or concrete verbalizations. Working in this quadrant is different than working in Quadrant III (which is also placed on the nondirective side of the diagram) in that intermittent interpretive comments initiated by the therapist trigger conscious responses from the child. The therapist (in brief ways and at various timely points in the therapy process) enters the play with the child and expands the play into the realm of conscious awareness. Therapists who make various levels of interpretation typically do this in a quick manner and do not continue with an open discussion of the issue unless the child is inclined to want to continue this way. Rather, the therapist may make an interpretation about a character or motivation of a character, or the therapist may make a more direct interpretation that links the play scene with something known to be similar to what happened to the child. Therapists do not stay in Quadrant 1, *Active Utilization*, for very long. The therapist will soon be seen working back in Quadrant III, *Nonintrusive Responding*, in which the child continues to direct and lead the play or, if the interpretation has brought a matter forward in a highly conscious way for the child, the child may want to talk more about his or her experiences, causing the therapist to move to Quadrant II, *Open Discussion and Exploration*. Supervisors can help supervisees track their movement between quadrants (as brief and quick as the movement may be) when discussing a play session or when reviewing videotaped sessions.

Mills and Crowley (1986) draw on Ericksonian theory and emphasize that the term *utilization* connotes a profound respect for the validity and integrity of the child's presenting behavior. Central to the technique of utilization is the discrete set of skills and abilities to observe, participate in, and reframe what the child presents. In play therapy, the process of active utilization denotes that the therapist brings key elements of the child's play into the realm of conscious awareness by offering verbal, interpretive context to explore and potentially resolve specific issues.

Quadrant I, *Active Utilization*, signifies the belief that play therapists are working with the whole child, meaning that therapeutic activities impact the child at various levels: cognitively, affectively, and linguistically. Harter (1999) supports the fact that emergence of language in children brings forward the ability to construct a narrative of their life story and influences the development of an enduring portrait of the self. O'Connor (2002) points out the strong correlation between children's mental health and their use of language. In part, the child's ability to use language as a bridge from action to symbol to thought, as well as language's central function in emotional self-regulation, suggests that language should play a central role in the treatment process.

Quadrant II, *Open Discussion and Exploration*, can be found on the upper right side of the figure 3.1. It is placed on the conscious and directive part of the diagram, indicating that the therapist working in this quadrant would be observed as initiating and structuring the play activity relative to the child's presenting problem. Therapists working in this quadrant will likely be using a developmentally sensitive, cognitive play therapy approach and will engage in conscious processing of the child's presenting issue. Structured play-based activities may include therapeutic board games, drawing exercises, externalizing activities, role-playing, sandplay reenactment, feeling card games, and so forth. Therapists may choose to work in this quadrant when a child is in need of more structure, feeling language, or if the child has been unable to reorganize a traumatic event through the normal course of play. Play therapists may not always practice in Quadrant III; rather, they may have found that during the course of nondirective play therapy, the child has signaled that they need more discussion and direction and in fact may have led the therapist in that direction.

Sometimes work in Quadrant II, *Open Discussion and Exploration*, has been driven by brief therapy approaches or settings that demand limited time spent with children, such as school-based play therapy. Although directive and conscious approaches to play therapy may not meet the needs of all children, some settings are focused on symptom relief, and Quadrant II lends itself to emphasizing an open dialogue of thoughts and feelings that often leads to exploration of new choices though active problem-solving or the rehearsal of new coping skills. There are many good reasons to work with children in Quadrant II. Greenspan (1997) stresses that problem solving follows an emotional pathway and that it is not until a child arrives at an intuitive emotionally mediated response or idea that *feels* right that he will actually be able to make use of the resolution. Play therapists (even though directive and using conscious material) understand that the playing through until it *feels* right is part of the healing process. This knowledge and skill distinguishes the cognitive and directive play therapist from other therapists not trained in the curative powers of play.

Quadrant III, *Nonintrusive Responding*, is perhaps the best understood quadrant by play therapists. It is found on the bottom left side of figure 3.1. Those therapists trained in nondirective work will recognize that this quadrant is both in the unconscious and nondirective place on the diagram. The child leads the play, and the therapist and child remain in the metaphor of the play. In Quadrant III, the child is encouraged to accept responsibility for herself, and essentially chooses the themes and play content, and drives the play therapy process. Landreth (2001) notes the therapist does not attempt to interpret what is happening in the play or bring up issues in a conscious way with the child, as it is through the use of symbolic materials that a child can distance herself from traumatic experiences, while retaining a sense of control.

The terms *nonintrusive responding* and *nondirective play therapy* are not one in the same. *Nonintrusive responding* describes therapeutic activities and roles while working in Quadrant III, whereas *nondirective play therapy* is viewed as a play therapy model based on the philosophical beliefs of client-centered or Rogerian psychotherapy. To complicate matters, nondirective play therapy has been implemented in various ways, and as a result, has been subject to misinterpretation (Wilson, Kendrick & Ryan, 1992). Nondirective approaches have been mistaken to imply therapist *inactivity*; however, Rogers's descriptions of therapy sessions clearly indicate that person-centered therapists provide direction and set limits. Direction might come in the form of providing a safe and protected space to "be" and behaviorally responding to the child in a consistent and supportive manner. Broadly speaking, the term *nondirective* is used to describe an essential part of the process that recognizes that children have within themselves a basic drive toward health and are able to solve their problems if offered the opportunity. It is the goal of nondirective play therapy approaches to allow the child to become more self-actualized. Quadrant III, *Nonintrusive Responding*, makes room for many different interpretations of nondirective play therapy approaches and, through supervision, the supervisee may explore the differences between child-centered play therapy and other forms of nondirective play therapy approaches, for instance.

Most therapists who begin their sessions with the child directing and leading the play claim to work primarily in Quadrant III. For some play therapists, this is true and very little to no movement to other quadrants may be observed due to their nondirective approach, while for others, movement occurs, but the therapist did not have a way to conceptualize the movement.

Quadrant IV, *Co-Facilitation* is found on the bottom right side of figure 3.1. Work in this quadrant is viewed as more directive, but continuing to honor the child's need for distance and the unconscious drive and nature of the play. Initially, the child is observed as directing the play, but the child may direct or invite the therapist into the play. The therapist will enter the play and may make use of previous tracking of themes and patterns to make a decision to test a hypothesis or elaborate the play by inserting comments, actions, and soft interpretations while staying in the metaphor. This activity is what makes Quadrant IV more directive, but the therapist is still in the realm of working with the themes and characters represented by the child. The directiveness is noted due to the fact that the therapist will make comments and give a voice or degree of affect to a character or situation that the child has not directly instructed the therapist to do. The therapist will stay in the play and assist in elaborating the play. Elaboration may be very effective for those children who have been demonstrating a looping process (circular, incomplete segments of play) or compulsive repetition. In Quadrant IV, *Co-Facilitation*, the therapist is *co-facilitative* in that they use the material, play themes, and scenarios of the child, but they add to the play in some way so that new avenues are opened for the child to express, process, and internally differentiate emotions and experiences.

Children's play can be observed as naturally co-facilitative. During cooperative play, for instance, each child adds to and elaborates their playmate's ideas, affect, themes, and characterization of objects and dramatic representations. A storyline evolves, and children project into it new ideas, themes, conflicts, and resolutions. Normal child's play is interactive and relational, which makes it fun. When working in Quadrant IV, the therapist stays in the fantasy and symbolism of the child's play and may be seen engaging in activities like introducing new characters (not directed for use by the child) such as helper figures or helpless figures, or use more than one character to demonstrate a child's inner conflict. Supervisors may assist supervisees to enter the play when it appears to be appropriate and to help supervisees read the child client responses to any elaborations. Children's responses (verbal and nonverbal) will assist the supervisee in knowing whether continuing to work in Quadrant IV is indicated or contraindicated.

The four quadrants help play therapists organize and identify how they are intervening with child clients. Furthermore, from a supervision point of view, supervisors can help supervisees answer the *who, what, when, and why* based primarily on child responses.

DEVELOPMENTAL FRAMEWORK FOR SUPERVISION

Utilizing a developmental framework in combination with the PTDM provides play therapy supervisors with a way to (1) identify the stage of development of the supervisee, (2) design supervision activities that match the needs of the supervisee, (3) assist the supervisee in talking about the play therapy process, and (4) support the supervisee to avoid the practice of random eclecticism.

How each supervisee makes use of the PTDM will be linked to their stage of development as a play therapist. As the play therapist developmentally progresses, she will make use of the PTDM in more complex ways. It appears that everyone is on a growth continuum, with no stage being better or worse than another; rather it is *just where one is.* Many developmental models (in addition to facilitative, behavioral, skills training, and reflective approaches) of supervision are cited in the literature and have generated a considerable amount of research interest (Milton, 2001). Stoltenberg, McNeill, and Delworth (1998) and other developmentally focused supervisors have conceptualized therapist development as occurring in stages, levels, or phases. After some review of various conceptualizations, a three-phase approach was adapted for play therapists (Yasenik & Gardner, 2004).

Phase I

Beginning play therapist is the first phase of play therapist development. Play therapy is a specialized form of therapeutic intervention with children; therefore although therapists may have been trained in adult models of treatment, they soon realize that adult training is not easily generalized

to work with children. Most institutions still do not provide full programs in child and play therapy; rather, both students and seasoned
therapists interested in working with children have typically been exposed to a single, non-practice-based play therapy course. Learning
about the power of play and the symbolic nature of the child's way of
communicating cannot be rushed. The unique skill set and personal
awareness necessary to work with children cannot be achieved by fast-
tracking the learning process.

One of the hallmarks of Phase I is that supervisees are inclined to want
to move quickly from novice to expert in the field of play therapy. This is
generally driven by a high level of anxiety and uncertainty about the
process. Beginning play therapy supervisees are interested in the "best"
and "correct" approach. Therapist self-awareness is typically limited
while self-focus in sessions is high as therapists are preoccupied about
how they are doing. When learning new skills, it is difficult to hold parts
of the greater whole in mind.

Phase I play therapists are usually task and technique oriented. There
is high concern about evaluation and the therapist in this phase is relatively unaware of his strengths and weaknesses. Confidence levels sometimes exceed skill, or emerging skill is identified with little accompanying confidence. General competencies include play therapy assessment
techniques, interpersonal assessment, play therapy case conceptualization, identifying individual child differences and child moderating factors, contrasting at least five play therapy theoretical approaches, identifying treatment goals/plans, and professional ethics related to child
therapy.

When working with Phase I play therapists, supervisors will need to focus on a number of bridging activities. These are purposeful supervision
activities designed to increase the skills, knowledge, and experience of the
supervisees. Bridging activities during supervision include such things as
spending extra time increasing intensity and frequency of theoretical discussions, exploring personal practice models, reviewing recorded play
therapy sessions, introducing play therapy techniques, observing practical skill demonstration by the supervisor in the play therapy room, introducing self-development exercises using expressive play-based modalities, and providing positive feedback.

Movement from Phase I to Phase II is indicated by a decrease in need
for techniques, while self-focus decreases and client focus increases. Supervisors will identify an increase in supervisee autonomy with greater
levels of confidence when working with more complex cases. The supervisee will demonstrate an increased comfort in utilizing tools and techniques, and there will be greater independence in problem solving.

Phase II

Phase II is imitation of experts, and it is here that the supervisee enters the middle stage or adolescentlike stage of development. This phase of development is marked by a separation/autonomy conflict. At times the conflict can lead to a false sense of autonomy and confidence. When things go well, they go very well and when they do not, the Phase II therapist's confidence is shaken. The ambivalence is further emphasized by the play therapist's fluctuation between thoughts of extreme incompetence and thoughts of not needing any help at all. During this phase, supervisees typically ask for help with difficult clients. Regardless of the supervisee's abilities, he is challenged within some of the domains of his functioning. Supervisors can identify Phase II supervisees by their general evasiveness and intermittent nonacceptance of supervisors' suggestions for some of their clients while at the same time demonstrating a need to rely on the supervisor fully for others.

The Phase II supervisee is better aware of the client's needs and more able to identify the child client's worldview. Increased overall awareness means that supervisees will also be more vulnerable to their own fragility as well as the vulnerability of the child clients. Therapists at this phase of development are better able to be challenged to be in touch with their own childhoods. It is in this phase that the supervisor learns about the supervisee's tolerance, patience, and capacity for empathy. One of the most confusing aspects of Phase II is that the expectations for integration of broad-based knowledge are much higher, and the relief of feeling competent is churned up with additional pressure to keep adding to the learning experience. The ambivalent nature of this phase of development can lead to feelings of frustration and subsequent projection of those feelings onto the supervisor.

Supervision bridging activities to enhance growth include encouraging risk taking and creativity, shifting from a "tell me" to "show me" approach (it is time to stop providing all the suggestions), decreasing the high level of supervision structure by encouraging more independence, expecting mixed success (experiences gained in one case may not always generalize to other cases), emphasizing the therapy *process* versus therapy techniques, increasing co-consultation approaches, assigning more complex cases, and providing more supportive confrontation (even though ambivalence is evidenced, supervisors should not avoid challenging the supervisee). This can be a difficult phase for both supervisors and supervisees, but perhaps more so for the supervisor. The supervisor must continue to support the supervisee in her growth and development in spite of being intermittently rejected by the supervisee. Supervisees will both seek proximity to the supervisor and avoid it at the same time.

Supervisors will not likely experience supervising someone in their movement from Phase I to Phase II unless the supervisor has a primary supervisory relationship with a supervisee for more than a two-year period. The other complicating factor for supervisors is they must developmentally be at least a Phase II supervisor to adequately assist the supervisee's growth and development. Phase II supervisors will have received supervision from a professional who is more clinically advanced than they are. Additionally, Phase II supervisors will ensure they receive supervision on their supervision.

Evidence of movement from Phase II to Phase III is observed when Phase I and II learning objectives have been integrated. Phase II therapists have developed a conceptual framework from which to work with children and families. A drop in ambivalence will be noted, and the supervisee may offer more in the way of collegial interaction. Those exiting Phase II are more interested in self-evaluation and self-exploration. An openness to different conceptual frameworks emerges, and supervisees begin to own their own decision making. A heightened independence is observed, and advanced Phase II supervisees do not take it personally when a difficult situation with a client does not work out.

Phase III

Phase III is considered an advanced play therapist. It is during this phase that a supervisee often begins to identify an area of specialization. At this level a play therapist has accumulated a broad knowledge base and is focused on diverse ways of conceptualizing cases. Advanced play therapists know how they are making use of the self in play therapy sessions and how to quickly identify the needs of the child and appropriately respond. They are aware of the dimensions of directiveness and consciousness represented during any given play therapy session. The Phase III therapist is capable of identifying multiple factors for consideration when evaluating a play therapy session or play process. This level of development is also evidenced by the ability to use structured and unstructured play therapy tools and approaches for formal assessment and observation. Additionally, the supervisee at this developmental phase can simultaneously keep in mind the unique qualities of the child, the presenting problem, and the numerous ways to address specific referral issues. Phase III supervisees have studied special childhood problems and childhood diagnoses.

In supervising an advanced play therapist, Phase III requires the supervisor to also be advanced in his or her own practice knowledge, skills, and experience. Although supervisees are more autonomous, supervisors must not remove themselves from the supervision process; rather it is important to continue to provide all the support offered at the Phase II developmental stage in addition to setting the stage to provide additional growth opportunities.

Phase III objectives for supervision include giving the supervisee more independence while finding ways to be there for critical moments; focusing on global client and personal development issues including systemic, political, legal, and specialized case consultations; and spending more time referring to spirituality. It is a time for building co-collaborative relationships, including shared evaluations, and helping to identify all the domains of functioning as a play therapist and highlighting the areas that require more development than others. In this phase, the supervisor continues to make use of experiential activities by encouraging original technique design and development based on accumulated experience (supervisees are never too experienced to learn experientially and when experiential learning stops, so then does therapist development), challenges and provides supportive confrontation (you cannot grow without being challenged), and continues to address all previous clinical objectives such as intervention skills, play therapy assessment techniques, and so forth.

Post Phase III

Movement from Phase III to an experienced play therapist is observed when the Phase III therapist consistently functions across all therapeutic domains. At this time, supervisees solidify their professional identities. They have a heightened sense of personal awareness and understanding, and they are more capable of monitoring the impact of their professional lives on their personal lives. Although many experienced play therapists have developed an area of specialization, they have also reached a point that they realize that the more they learn, the more they don't know. Learning is the constant building of new cognitive schemas. Experienced play therapists are typically trained in a number of play therapy models and approaches and are skilled in identifying efficacy in practice as well as intuition and the magic of play therapy. The experienced play therapist has had considerable practical experience and can draw on literally hundreds of examples of children who present with similar problems but have needed different things during the therapy process. The experienced play therapist respects the need for ongoing supervision and learning in spite of his or her confidence and cumulative play therapy experience. No amount of book learning and training programs can replace the experience gained in repetition. Books and training programs enhance experience, but they do not replace it. The Post-Phase III therapist has come to understand that in addition to all the layers of learning and development of core play therapy competencies, something unexplainable happens in the play therapy process that cannot be fully known. The aerodynamic laws state that the bumblebee cannot fly, but the bee ignores these laws and flies anyway.

AVOIDING COLLISION POINTS IN PLAY THERAPY: SUPERVISION MECHANISMS AND TOOLS

During clinical supervision many aspects of the therapy process must be attended to and coordinated to avoid unfortunate collision points. The PTDM encourages supervisors and supervisees to examine both client and therapist moderating factors. Increased understanding of these critical factors optimizes treatment planning and outcomes, and supports therapist growth and development.

Most play therapists would agree that children should be viewed from a developmental perspective. At the same time, play therapists typically emphasize that each child is unique. Therefore, supervision activities must move beyond an examination of critical aspects of development and capture certain unique qualities of the child. For example, if a supervisee fails to understand the play capacity of the child, he or she could misinterpret the child's play behavior as one of disengagement, versus a fundamental constriction in their overall play capacity. Failure to fully consider the child's attachment organization could lead to limited or improper interpretations of critical themes evidenced in the child's play.

Within the PTDM, several supervision tools are available to assist the supervisor in quickly identifying a supervisee's level of client understanding. A composite of one tool is the Child Client Moderating Factors Scale (Yasenik & Gardner, 2004). While dozens of factors could be considered, this would become unwieldy for the supervisee to keep in mind. Accordingly, eleven factors were selected based on the authors' clinical experience and review of play therapy models. While supervisors might weigh the importance of these factors differently according to their primary theoretical model, knowing about these moderating factors is essential to supervision and clinical decision-making as these factors impact the pacing, timing, and nature of interventions.

When a supervisee meets with a caregiver prior to seeing the child for the first time in the play therapy room, the supervisee should be able to provide a preliminary score for some of the factors on the Child Client Moderating Factors Scale. Once the child is seen in session, the supervisee can revisit their ratings and look for discrepancies between the caregivers' view of the child and what was noted during the session. An experienced Phase II therapist, compared to a Phase I therapist, will likely be able to rate most areas after seeing the child one or two times. As the Phase I therapist gains experience using this tool, she will likely remember the factors more easily and be able to rapidly update or complete the scale after a few clinical sessions.

As noted earlier, the child client informs the play therapist about the need for movement between the four quadrants on an ongoing basis. Therefore, using the Child Client Moderating Factors Scale over time will assist the supervisee to look for and respond to critical indicators of the child's need to stay in one quadrant or move to another. For instance, if the supervisee notices that the child's verbal communication, emotional capacity, self-regulation, and relational capacity are all high, she will recognize that the child has the need or capacity to work in a more conscious manner and in a more directive way, potentially moving from Quadrant III, Nonintrusive Responding, to Quadrant II, Open Discussion and Exploration (see table 3.1).

Knowing one's self is an essential underpinning of clinical work with children, as one's inner child is instantly awakened and present during play therapy. Not only must a supervisee constantly work on knowing the self, but she must also work to use self-understanding in the most appropriate and meaningful way, therapeutically. Accordingly, supervisors should be prepared to facilitate supervisee self-understanding and actively assist the supervisee's conscious use of self in the play therapy process.

The Therapist Degree of Immersion Scale was developed to strengthen therapists' awareness of the impact they have on child clients and to support appropriate decision-making. Typically, this scale is completed by the supervisee in advance of a supervision session. As this is a challenging topic to address in supervision, as well as difficult to approach in a general way, specific therapist behavior and interaction is described as *immersion*. To explore the degree to which they are immersed in the play, and what impact this has on the child, supervisees are asked to look at six categories of immersion, and rate the level to which they were immersed in each category, as well as the child's response to their immersion. This follows from the basic assumption that it is the child's needs that drive the therapy process. Higher levels of immersion are not necessarily better. Instead, the degree and type of immersion must be carefully examined for each child, and in relation to the overall therapy process.

After each rating, the supervisee is asked to provide three clinical indications of the effectiveness of their use of self. When used regularly in supervision, the immersion scale keeps supervisees on track by continually reflecting on the interaction between them and the client. Understanding what happens in the space between themselves and the child client at various moments in the play therapy process builds the supervisee's attunement to the child, and strengthens their decision-making. In many cases, it also supports the supervisee's awareness of certain markers of transference and countertransference, and the impact of these issues on the play process (see table 3.2).

Table 3.1. Child Client Moderating Factors Scale

Please consider the child you are working with and mark on the line to establish a scale score.

Play Capacity

1	2	3	4	5
Very low play capacity; child is significantly delayed or demonstrates severe trauma response.		Moderate play capacity; some imaginative play.	High play capacity; creative, imaginative complex themes.	

Ability to Communicate (rate verbal and nonverbal communication separately)

1	2	3	4	5
Limited ability to communicate—cognitive, emotional delays lead to markedly low levels of self-expression.		Moderate communication ability—some verbal or nonverbal ability to self-express.	High ability to communicate—demonstrates self-understanding/expression—some conscious awareness.	

Developmental Stage (rate each area separately)

1	2	3	4	5
Severe delay in cognitive, emotional, and/or physical development.		Moderate delay in cognitive, emotional and/or physical development.	Developmentally on track or advanced in one or more areas.	

Emotional Capacity (verbal and nonverbal expression)

1	2	3	4	5
Low capacity to express emotional states.		Moderate capacity for emotional expression.	High capacity for emotional expression.	

Self-Regulation Ability

1	2	3	4	5
Low ability to self-regulate lability, impulsivity, emotionality or abreactive etc.		Moderate ability, can manage to self-regulate.	High ability to self-regulate most of time.	

Attachment Organization

1	2	3	4	5
Significant attachment difficulties noted—may be diagnosed as disordered or caregivers may report significant relationship difficulties related to attachment.		Some attachment difficulties reported/observed. Has at least one primary or secondary attachment figure. Some level of security with that person observed.	Secure attachment relationships reported/observed. No attachment difficulties reported.	

Relational Capacity

1	2	3	4	5
Reported difficulties in numerous relationships —peers, family members; low reported/observed relational capacity; low reported positive engagement skills.		Moderate difficulties reported with at least one significant relationship or relationship group.		High capacity for positive engagement with others; good relationship skills reported overall.

World-View: Cognitive Schema

1	2	3	4	5
Child has negative world view, negative sense of self and others; does not view world as a safe place; may not trust others; views self as having little control or as needing to take control.		Moderate negative world view may be context-specific or person-specific.		Positive world view—even in the face of adversity; reframes experiences into positive.

Defense Mechanisms

1	2	3	4	5
Significant defense mechanisms observed or reported. May be signs of reactive defenses such as denial, sublimation, dissociation, aggression.		Some evidence of defense mechanisms in place— may be context-specific or person-specific.		Positive use of defense mechanisms; not interfering with daily functioning.

Resilience

1	2	3	4	5
Low resilience, fragile overall self-definition and response pattern to adversity. Slow to recover from difficult, hurtful experiences and defines self negatively in the face of these experiences.		Some evidence of moderate recovery from adverse circumstances. Selective ability to regroup.		High resilience—quick recovery with positive, nondebilitating outcome.

Support Network

1	2	3	4	5
Very few long-term supports available. Uncertain plan re: caregiving. Isolated, lack of acceptance of support, few resources.		A few reliable support services or supportive people exist. The child accepts help and care from these supports, including friends.		Significant supports exist in the child's immediate environment; supports are viewed as acceptable and important.

Table 3.2. Therapist Degree of Immersion Scale

Please consider the different ways in which you are immersed in the play and make use of your self. Mark on each line to establish a scale score.

(1) Verbal Discussion: During the session, what was the degree to which you were involved in verbal discussion about the child's life or with the child (outside of the play activity)?

1 Low	2	3 Moderate	4	5 High
No open discussion		Some open discussion occurred	Spent significant part of session outside play in direct discussion Primarily therapist initiated.	

Child's Response: Please rate the effectiveness of use of **verbal discussion**.

☐ Low ☐ Medium ☐ High

(2) Reflective Statements: During the session, how were you involved in making reflective statements in relation to tracking the child's emotions, nonverbal behavior, play activities, verbal content, sequences or metaphors?

1 Low	2	3 Moderate	4	5 High
Infrequent use of statements		Moderate use of reflective statements but primarily used one or two types of reflections during the play.	Made frequent use of reflective statements.	

Child's Response: Please rate the effectiveness of use of *reflective statements*.

☐ Low ☐ Medium ☐ High

(3) Emotionality: What is the degree to which you provided emotionally based responses (either directly to the child or through the play metaphor) during the session?

1 Low	2	3 Moderate	4	5 High
Primarily observed child. Rarely reflected emotions of child. Did not interject emotional responses.		Intermittently mirrored emotions of child or the play character.	Interjected comments/ emotional responses to elaborate emotional expression of child.	

Child's Response: Please rate the effectiveness of use of **emotionality**.

☐ Low ☐ Medium ☐ High

(4) Emotional Self: What is the degree to which you were emotionally involved during the session?

1	2	3	4	5
Low		Moderate		High
I did not feel particularly emotionally involved. I felt some empathy, but my feelings remained neutral.		I felt moderately emotionally involved. I noticed I had some of my own feelings related to the client material.		I felt highly emotionally involved and affected by the client's presentation and/or client disclosure.

Child's Response: Please rate the impact of **your emotionality**.

☐ Low   ☐ Medium   ☐ High

(5) Physical Self: What is the degree to which you were physically involved during the session? Physical self includes: physical movement in play activities, physical proximity or touch, level of physical energy.

1	2	3	4	5
Low		Moderate		High
Almost not at all. Primarily observed child. Did not engage in activities even when approached by the child.		Engaged in physical play only when directly invited to do so. Some physical play with moderate contact.		Frequently engaged in physical play with close proximity and physical contact.

Child's Response: Please rate the effectiveness of use of **physical self**.

☐ Low   ☐ Medium   ☐ High

(6) Interpretations: What is the degree to which you used **interpretations** during the session? Interpretations are purposeful comments initiated by the therapist that elicit, or have the potential to elicit, higher degrees of consciousness in the child.

1	2	3	4	5
Low		Moderate		High
Not at all		Have formulated a number of soft hypotheses and am now using characters to test hypotheses and make interpretations—this is done within the play metaphor.		Directly stated an observation or hypothesis to bring a matter to conscious awareness.

Child's Response: Please rate the effectiveness of use of **interpretations**.

☐ Low   ☐ Medium   ☐ High

(*continued*)

Table 3.2.   (continued)

(7) Interpretation Frequency: During the session how frequently did you make interpretive responses?

1	2	3	4	5
Low		Moderate		High
Never—just held interpretations and continued to be nonintrusive throughout.		Intermittently made interpretive comments within the play and/or intermittently made direct interpretations.	Much of session was interpretive. nonintrusive.	

Child's Response: Please rate the effectiveness of use of **interpretations**.

☐ Low   ☐ Medium   ☐ High

Case Study: Sarah and Carlos

The application of the Child Client Moderating Factors Scale and the Therapist Degree of Immersion Scale in supervision is illustrated though the case example of Carlos, an eight-year-old boy who is working with Sarah, his play therapist.

Sarah is a skilled counselor working in a rural setting. Although Sarah has been involved in adolescent addictions counseling for several years, she is relatively new to the field of play therapy. Sarah recently transitioned from an addictions treatment center to a community mental health center. At this point, Sarah's caseload shifted from working exclusively with adolescents to working with young children and their parents. Although Sarah is excited by this change, she is concerned that her current supervisor, who is highly skilled in the area of family therapy, is not a qualified play therapist or play therapy supervisor. Accordingly, Sarah has made specific arrangements to receive distance supervision from a qualified play therapy supervisor.

Carlos currently resides in a foster home and has limited contact with his biological mother, Lyn. According to reports on file, Lyn has chronic issues with drug and alcohol abuse. Carlos was apprehended from his mother's care one year before due to emotional neglect and repeated exposure to domestic violence. Carlos has not seen his biological father for approximately four years.

Sarah's play therapy supervisor, Katherine, asked Sarah to forward videotapes of the first four sessions with Carlos, as well as ratings on the Child Client Moderating Factors and the Therapist Degree of Immersion scales. After interviewing Sarah, Katherine viewed Sarah as a Phase I play therapist, based on Sarah's recent entry to the field of play therapy, her level of concern or anxiety about the process of play therapy, and the concerns she presented regarding the possibility of being evaluated through videotaped sessions. At the same time, Katherine recognized that Sarah had numerous strengths as a counselor and was eager to learn new skills.

During the telephone supervision conference, Sarah reported that she initially allowed Carlos to take the lead in the playroom and chose to make use of reflective statements. When asked which quadrant she was working in, Sarah responded that she thought she was working in Quadrant III, Nonintrusive Responding, as Carlos maintained the lead throughout the session. Interestingly, Sarah indicated that during the first session Carlos barely explored the playroom, although at one point Carlos went to the sand tray and repetitively buried and uncovered objects that he grabbed off the shelf. In the second session, Carlos chose to use swords, and dressed up as a warrior. At this point, Carlos directed Sarah to get a sword and fight. Recognizing that Carlos's drive or direction was to move toward this type of play, Sarah maintained a nonintrusive style of responding. Sarah reported that as Carlos began to strike harder and harder, she responded with a therapeutic limit about maintaining safety in the play session. Following this, Carlos suddenly abandoned his play activity and went back to burying objects in the sand. Sarah reported that this same pattern occurred in their third session.

When asked how she felt about working with Carlos, Sarah commented that she was bored at certain points and wondered if Carlos was ready for play therapy because his play style and play activities seemed limited. When Katherine asked if sword fighting would be appropriate for his age, Sarah said it was probably typical of boys Carlos's age, but commented that Carlos's aggressiveness might indicate that he would do better in an anger management group for children, particularly because anger outbursts were identified as a primary concern by the referral source. Katherine used this comment as an opportunity to explore potential indicators of Carlos's need or readiness to enter Quadrant II, Open Discussion and Exploration. Katherine asked Sarah to review certain factors on the Child Client Moderating Factors Scale, such as the ability to communicate and emotional capacity. In discussing these factors, Sarah commented that Carlos did not seem very verbally communicative and in fact tended to "shut down" any conversations about his family or home setting. Although Sarah immediately rated Carlos as low for emotional capacity, as she discussed examples of what occurred in their sessions, she changed this rating to moderate, as there were certain instances in which Carlos, through the drama of the play, became more animated and emotionally expressive. Based on this discussion, Katherine suggested that there were several markers indicating that Carlos's drive and direction were in the area of less conscious expression of feelings or experiences, versus demonstrating a need to openly discuss experiences. Katherine also raised the point that Carlos's ego strength may not be at a level at which he could tolerate open discussions or directed activities on issues such as loss. Given these observations, Sarah noted that perhaps it was better to remain in the field of play with Carlos, working at lower levels of consciousness.

Katherine asked Sarah to prioritize her ratings on the Child Client Moderating Factors Scale, according to the degree of importance certain factors held in understanding Carlos's needs and potential directions in play therapy. Sarah chose Carlos's self-regulation ability, play capacity, and ability to communicate as three factors that required focus. Sarah rated Carlos's self-regulation ability as low, stating that it was somewhere between a one and two on this scale. When her ratings were explored, it was apparent that Sarah based her ratings on external reports of Carlos's anger outbursts. In fact, during session, Carlos consistently responded to therapeutic limits to slow down his sword fighting, demonstrating an ability to regulate quite quickly. Sarah also gave an example in which Carlos accepted limits for dumping and throwing sand. Through this discussion, Sarah began to realize that Carlos's ability to self-regulate was perhaps in the moderate range. Once this was understood, Sarah commented that she felt more hopeful, as she was worried that Carlos would become more aggressive and ultimately would revert to aggressive behaviors as a means of testing, or ending, the therapeutic relationship. Katherine took note of this discussion and decided to return to it later during a discussion of transference and countertransference issues.

While discussing Sarah's low ratings of Carlos's play capacity, Sarah commented that Carlos showed little interest in exploring the play environment and kept returning to two activities, sword fighting and sandplay. Furthermore, his engagement in these activities appeared limited. Katherine asked that Sarah follow up with Carlos's foster parents to obtain more information concerning Carlos's play preferences and style at their home. Katherine also asked Sarah to comment on what transpired each time Carlos shifted from playing with swords to sandplay. Sarah stated that each shift appeared sudden and unplanned. When Katherine probed further, it became clear that Carlos was moving from high-intensity play to an activity that was calming and soothing. Once again this highlighted Carlos's potential for self-regulation. While discussing this pattern Katherine asked Sarah to examine the ratings she provided concerning Carlos's worldview. Although Sarah had rated this factor when she first completed the Child Client Moderating Factors Scale, she had not weighted it as a high-priority area. Katherine's invitation to explore this rating was purposeful as she hoped to increase Sarah's understanding of Carlos from a phenomenological perspective. Sarah had some awareness of the impact of addictions on children, given her previous work experience, and carried this as a global presupposition in her sessions with Carlos. However, discussions in supervision revealed that Sarah never used this understanding as a jumping-off point to understand Carlos's unique experiences and what might transpire in his play, thematically. As indicated by Gil (1991), only the child can communicate or show the meaning of their experiences. Katherine invited Sarah to first explore whether she viewed Carlos as a survivor or a victim. Through this discussion, Sarah commented that she automatically thought that he was a victim, but had not really thought of the possibility that Carlos might show or tell her otherwise. Was it possible that Carlos was resilient in ways that others had yet to understand? If this were the case, it would be important to work with, or strengthen, certain factors that contribute to Carlos's resiliency. By history, Carlos had experienced nurturing experiences with a maternal aunt and had spent a considerable amount of time in her care. This may have given Carlos a positive internal working model for relationships, one that could be accessed or mobilized in play therapy.

Although neither Sarah nor Katherine fully understood the significance of Carlos's repetitive burying of objects in the sand, Katherine invited Sarah to view this play as an opportunity to explore Carlos's worldview. On the videotape that Sarah provided, Katherine noticed that Sarah stopped tracking Carlos for segments of this play. Sarah commented that at first she tried to stay "with it" but became discouraged and bored by the repetitive nature of Carlos's actions. Katherine highlighted Carlos's burying of objects as representing a need to have some form of emotional experience. Katherine also pointed out the importance of Sarah reflecting Carlos's emotional drive by either noticing or reflecting his actions and intent, or by responding with an increased emotional valence when certain characters were experiencing something, such as no longer being able to see or hear what was around them. Katherine reminded Sarah that these represent forms of immersion in the play. Katherine further advised that Sarah could also simply "wonder" what these burying experiences might feel like. These interventions were framed as soft hypotheses that would inform Sarah whether Carlos could tolerate heightened levels of emotionality in the play. If Sarah shifted the form and emotional intensity of reflective statements or responses, would these play segments extend or deepen, allowing Carlos an opportunity to express or re-organize certain feelings and experiences? Katherine also worked with Sarah to consider these as indicators of Carlos's readiness and need to move toward Quadrant IV, Co-Facilitation. Therapist-led shifts, while subtle in nature, could still occur in the unconscious dimension, but would also allow Carlos to process certain experiences. In fact, there would likely be a weaving, back-and-forth process in this quadrant, with Carlos taking the lead and Sarah briefly inserting or elaborating certain elements of the play.

Regarding the other factors on the Therapist Degree of Immersion Scale, Katherine asked Sarah to comment on which components of immersion she would increase or decrease, and state why this would be helpful. Sarah immediately commented that she was uncertain whether any of these factors should change as she worried this would shift the process away from Quadrant III, Nonintrusive Responding. Katherine reassured Sarah that a small shift in one's use of self would not necessarily entail a shift to another quadrant. To illustrate this, Katherine asked Sarah to examine a segment of swordplay during the fourth session when Carlos suddenly appeared more animated and playful. Specifically, Katherine asked Sarah to rate the degree of emotionality and her emotional use of self. Sarah commented that she purposefully kept these levels low as she was worried Carlos would become more aggressive in his play if she increased her actions, physically, or became more animated and emotionally involved. In fact, Carlos's movement from swordplay to sandplay occurred at a time when he appeared uninterested and verbalized that it wasn't very fun. Katherine asked Sarah to reconsider what might happen if she were to increase her physical and emotional use of self, by becoming more animated and playful, essentially matching Carlos's initial energy levels and direction in play. Would this mean taking the lead away from Carlos? Sarah soon realized that what was missing was her own emotional involvement in the play. Rather than supporting Carlos's ownership of play activities, Sarah's concern for being too emotionally present in the play might have inhibited his drive and direction for the play to become more adventurous and emotional. The result of this discussion was that Sarah planned to monitor these aspects of immersion. In the next session Sarah looked for possibilities to increase these components of immersion, while carefully tracking Carlos's responses.

Near the end of the supervision session Katherine asked Sarah about potential transference and countertransference issues. Sarah responded that she hadn't really thought much about these issues but acknowledged that when Carlos was first referred she wondered whether a male therapist would be more helpful as Carlos lacked male role models in his life. When asked whether the loss of his mother was a significant event for Carlos, Sarah readily agreed it was a central issue for Carlos and might even be triggering his acting-out behaviors. Katherine wondered what it would be like for Sarah if Carlos moved to a stage in the therapy process at which he showed high levels of dependency on her, or projected conflicting emotions such as anger, sadness, and mistrust, transferring his unmet needs toward Sarah in her role as therapist. Sarah immediately replied that this would be fine, as it would signal that Carlos was really processing issues. However, when Katherine provided examples of the ways in which children represent unmet dependency needs, Sarah felt discomfort but was uncertain why she was feeling this way. Katherine briefly commented that this likely represented an emotional blind spot, indicating that therapists often experience these at various points in the play therapy process. Together with Sarah, Katherine began to explore what dependency needs might feel like and mean to Sarah. Sarah's first response was it would mean a high level of responsibility. Sarah went on to comment that she really liked the idea of supporting others' growth in counseling and had never felt uneasy with the notion of carrying a burden of responsibility for their well-being. As it turned out, Sarah had been in a position as a younger child of caring for a parent with complicated health issues. Recognition of the emotional pull of this issue for Sarah, in the form of countertransference, would become an important milestone in Sarah's development as a therapist. Certainly one discussion in supervision would not be enough, but with Katherine's support Sarah might avoid some of the potential pitfalls of automatically responding to Carlos's needs without an awareness of what was triggering her responses. Future supervision sessions focused on certain aspects of transference and countertransference; it turned out that Carlos was an excellent teacher for Sarah with respect to these issues.

CONCLUSION

The Play Therapy Dimensions Model evolved from the recognition that an increasing number of play therapists work from a multitheoretical orientation, and because of this, they require an organizing structure to guide effective clinical decision-making. Even if supervisees and supervisors share similar theoretical orientations, unless there is process for reflection and decision-making, there is the potential for a number of collision points in supervision. By focusing on the unique needs of the child, as well as the therapist's use of self or immersion in the play therapy process, supervisors and supervisees from diverse schools of play therapy can share certain landmarks for understanding movement in play therapy. When coupled with a developmental framework for supervision, supervisors are better equipped to advance the skill base of the supervisee, moving him or her toward higher levels of autonomous decision-making and self-awareness as a play therapist. Over time, the supervisee will move from a practitioner who is highly focused on the next best technique or approach, to a self-reflecting practitioner who is able to critically examine a number of approaches, in relation to their use of self and the unique needs of the child. As our profession is progressing in the delineation of core competencies for play therapists, a similar progression must now occur in articulating the essential elements of clinical decision-making for play therapists. It is hoped that the Play Therapy Dimensions Model offers supervisors additional tools for identifying and actively supervising to these essential ingredients.

REFERENCES

Association for Play Therapy. (2006). *Registered play therapist: Criteria for registration*. Fresno, CA: Association for Play Therapy.

Axline, V. (1969/1987). *Play therapy*. New York: Ballantine Books.

British Association of Play Therapists. (2006). *Clinical supervision requirements*. UK: British Association of Play Therapists.

Canadian Association for Child and Play Therapy. (2006). *Certification as a child psychotherapist and play therapist*. Toronto, ON: Canadian Association for Child and Play Therapy.

Dalkey, N., & Helmer, O. (1962). An experimental application of the Delphi method to the use of experts. *Management Science, 9*, 458–67.

Gil, E. (1991). *The healing power of play: Working with abused children*. New York: Guilford Press.

Greenspan, S. I. (1997). *The growth of the mind and the endangered origins of intelligence*. Cambridge, MA: Perseus Books.

Harter, S. (1999). *The construction of the self: A developmental perspective*. New York: Guilford Press.

Knell, S. M. (1999). Cognitive-behavioral play therapy. In K. O'Connor & C. Schaefer (Eds.), *Play therapy theory and practice: A comparative presentation* (79–99). New York: Wiley.

Knell, S. M. (2003). Cognitive-behavioral play therapy. In C. E. Schaefer (Ed.), *Foundations of play therapy* (175–91). New Jersey: John Wiley & Sons, Inc.

Kottman, T. (2003). Adlerian play therapy. In C. Schaefer (Ed.), *Foundations of play therapy* (55–75). New York: John Wiley & Sons, Inc.

Landreth, G. (2001). Facilitative dimensions of play in the play therapy process. In G. Landreth (Ed.), *Innovations in play therapy: Issues, process, and special populations* (3–22). Philadelphia: Brunner Routledge.

Landreth, G. (2002). *The art of the relationship* (2nd ed.). Philadelphia: Brunner/Routledge.

Landreth, G., & Joiner, K. (2005). A model based on objectives developed by the Delphi Technique. *International Journal of Play Therapy, 14*(2), 49–68.

Landreth, G., & Sweeney, D. (1999). The freedom to be: Child-centered group play therapy. In D. Sweeney & L. Homeyer (Eds.), *Handbook of group play therapy* (39–64). San Francisco: Jossey-Bass.

Mills, J., & Crowley, R. (1986). *Therapeutic metaphors for children and the child within*. Philadelphia, PA: Brunner/Mazel.

Milton, M. (2001). Supervision: Researching therapeutic practice. In M. Carroll & M. Tholstrup (Eds.), *Integrative approaches to supervision* (183–91). London: Jessica Kingsley Publishers Ltd.

Munns, E. (2000). Traditional family and group theraplay. In E. Munns (Ed.), *Theraplay: Innovations in attachment-enhancing play therapy* (9–26). Northvale, NJ: Aronson.

Oaklander, V. (2003). Gestalt play therapy. In C. E. Schaefer (Ed.), *Foundations of play therapy* (143–55). New York: John Wiley & Sons, Inc.

O'Connor, K. J. (1997). Ecosystemic play therapy. In K. O'Connor & L. Braverman (Eds.), *Play therapy theory and practice: A comparative presentation* (234–84). New York: Wiley.

O'Connor, K. J. (2002). The value and use of interpretation in play therapy. *Professional Psychology: Research and Practice, 33*(6), 523–28.

Peery, C. (2003). Jungian analytical play therapy. In C. E. Schaefer (Ed.), *Foundations of play therapy* (14–54). New York: John Wiley & Sons, Inc.

Phillips, R., & Landreth, G. (1995). Play therapists on play therapy I: A report of methods, demographics and professional/practice issues. *International Journal of Play Therapy, 4*(1), 1–26.

Piaget, J. (1977). *The language and thought of the child*. London: Routledge & Kegan Paul.

Play Therapy International. (2006). *International standards for certification in child psychotherapy and play therapy*. UK: Play Therapy International.

Play Therapy United Kingdom. (2002). *Professional structures model*. UK: Play Therapy United Kingdom.

Pynoos, R., & Eth, S. (1986). Witness to violence: The child interview. *Journal of the American Academy of Child Psychiatry, 25*(3): 306–19.

Rogers, C. (1951). *Client-centered therapy*. Boston: Houghton Mifflin.

Schaefer, C. E. (2003). Prescriptive play therapy. In C. E. Schaefer (Ed.), *Foundations of play therapy* (306–20). New York: John Wiley & Sons, Inc.

Stoltenberg, C., McNeill, B., & Delworth, U. (1998). *IDM supervision: An integrated developmental model for supervising counselors and therapists*. San Francisco: Jossey-Bass Inc.

Terr, L. (1983). Time sense following psychic trauma: A clinical study of ten adults and twenty children. *American Journal of Orthopsychiatry, 53*, 244–61.

Wilson, K., Kendrick, P., & Ryan, V. (1992). *Play therapy: A nondirective approach for children and adolescents*. London: Ballerie Tindall.

Yasenik, L., & Gardner, K. (2004). *Play therapy dimensions model: A decision-making guide for therapists*. Calgary: Rocky Mountain Play Therapy Institute.

4

⟨∞⟩

Through a
Cross-Cultural Lens

*How Viewing Childhood as a Distinct
Culture Impacts Supervision*

Jodi Ann Mullen

*Debbie came to supervision flustered. Before she even sat down she began telling me
what a disaster her first session was with Roberto. Roberto, she explained, was a
four-year-old boy of Latino descent. His parents were first-generation Americans.
His four grandparents all had emigrated from Mexico. Roberto was referred for counseling by his pre-school teacher. His parents were relieved by the worries of the school
representative; they too had concerns. Roberto was impaired by his need for order. He
became irate when things were not just so. Debbie shared, "His mother said if she
doesn't lay out his pajamas prior to his bath, he will hold his breath until he passes
out—can you believe that?" I smiled and said, "That Roberto is some communica-
tor, impressive." Debbie looked irritated with my remark and added, "I bet you will
be impressed that he held his breath and passed out in session too!"*

Mental health practitioners who work with adults are, or at least feel
that they are, ill-prepared to work with children (Corey, Corey, &
Callahan, 1993; Erikson, 1985; Mullen, 2003). Graduate programs prepare
counselors through practice, at least initially, with peers. The pre-service
experience therefore leaves professional mental health neophytes scrap-
ing to adapt adult-centric counseling skills for use with children because
the clinical skills they learned and practiced were not designed for children. The skills counselors are trained in typically do not consider the
chronological age of the client as a salient (or perhaps the most salient)
component of the client's culture. Therefore students in mental health
professions are led to believe that a mere adaptation of adult-centric counseling skills is enough for counselors to feel (or be) clinically capable
when working with children.

There certainly are skills and interventions that are well-suited to working with adults as well as children; however, I am arguing in this chapter that it requires not an adaptation of skills and techniques, but an adjustment of philosophical paradigms to successfully work with children in a clinical context. If childhood, and therefore children, can be viewed from a multicultural perspective, our ability to serve the mental health needs of children is greatly enhanced.

I choose to make this argument here, in a text focusing on supervision, because I find that many of my supervisees and students struggle in their clinical work with children because they view children and childhood from an adult-centric perspective—a perspective that marginalizes children and devalues the unique aspects of the culture of childhood. I believe that it is my role as the clinical supervisor to aid my supervisees and students to reframe their perspective of child counseling and play therapy as cross-cultural counseling. Conceptualizing their clinical relationships in this way will help provide mental health services that are respectful of the clients' most salient cultural features.

DEFINING THE CULTURE OF CHILDHOOD

The culture of childhood can be conceptualized as the shared experiences children have in particular societies and subcultures and to the social construction of childhood itself (Mullen, 2003). Childhood as a culture has distinct values, rules, customs, status, and even language.

Values define the boundaries between cultures by aiding in communication because they are shared among group members. Values are often sources of disagreement between cultural groups, as each group experiences the situation from their own perspective (Pedersen & Ivey, 1993). Think, for example, about the different ways children and adults perceive time. For instance, I say to my four-year-old son, "I will get you more apple juice in a second." He replies "One." Children value a concrete definition of time, whereas the culture I am a part of, adulthood, values a looser, less literal definition of time. This may lead to disputes in some instances, and at the very least it can lead to confusion or misunderstanding between cultures.

Rules are another cultural component that need to be illuminated to appreciate the rich diversity that is evident when viewing culture through a lens of development. Rules in cultures guide conduct and action. One example in the culture of childhood is the rule with regard to possession: Possession is the law. If you have it in your hand it is yours; "finders keepers, losers weepers." How would that work in the culture of adulthood? Let's say you are borrowing this book from a colleague and he asks for it back; how would the "finders keepers" rule work? Not well I suppose, but it is a legitimate rule among second graders (Mullen, 2007).

Customs are also essential elements of a particular culture. Customs are long-standing practices or conventions that regulate social life. In the culture of childhood some games can be considered customs. For example, teams are frequently selected through the customary practice of "One potato, two potato . . ." or "Rocks, paper, scissors" (Mullen, 2007).

Language is also a defining cultural component. In the culture of childhood, communication through language is more comprehensive than the primarily verbal language that is relied on in the culture of adulthood. Children communicate through play, nonverbal behavior, and nonsense (like sound effects). Older children often serve as child language interpreters of younger children to parents and other adults.

Individual cultures define the status of members within the culture differently. In the culture of childhood, size matters; children who are taller and/or look older (more like members of the dominant culture of adulthood) seem to achieve greater status within the culture of childhood. Status also comes with knowledge of the dominant culture. Children who know about, or have experiences with, elements of adolescent or adulthood cultures achieve higher status in their own culture (Mullen, 2007).

In this section I briefly described how childhood could be viewed as a distinct culture. The examples offered were intended to clarify some of the distinctions between the culture of our supervisees' clients, namely childhood—a culture we and our supervisees have left behind—and the culture of adulthood. It would be remiss and even unethical for counselors to not consider and honor the culture of their clients. Counselors who work with children are at risk for adult-centrism.

Assessing Supervisees' Cross-Cultural Skills

If mental health practitioners are going to be effective in their work with children, some essential skills are necessary for this particular cross-cultural counseling endeavor. Many of these skills will need to be developed in supervision because the mental health practitioner (1) has not been prepared to work cross-culturally with children, (2) has been prepared but has had only minimal experience with the members of this culture (children), or (3) has been prepared, has some practical experience, and continues to demonstrate adult centricism. Consequently, supervisors of child counselors and play therapists need to assess each supervisee's cross-cultural skills. In this section I will describe some counseling skills that are well developed in culturally competent child counselors and play therapists. Additionally, I will offer some ways of assessing the skills and cultural competencies of supervisees, as well as provide a number of exercises or activities designed to improve the skills and competencies that enhance professional child counseling and play therapy practice.

Many counseling skills that are considered both basic and essential in counseling adults are also cornerstones to effective counseling with children. Child counselors need to be able to listen and to demonstrate and communicate to child clients that they are listening and understanding the client. In verbal-based counseling this is done through active listening skills.

The skills of encouraging, reflective listening, paraphrasing, clarifying, and summarizing are part of the foundation of counseling children. However, these skills look different in practice with child clients than in clinical practice with adults or adolescents. Counselors who use active listening skills in their sessions with children will have to respond to children's verbal *and* nonverbal communication. Additionally clinical responses will have to be succinct and language suited to the developmental, cognitive, cultural, and sub-cultural positions of the client. Some supervisees and students struggle with this.

Active listening skills are particularly important with clients who are members of the culture of childhood. Members of this culture have a great deal of experience with being devalued. Members of the dominant culture (adults) routinely minimize and deny the experiences of children (Fiorini & Mullen, 2006). A child who states that she hates her sister is responded to, but not listened to: "You don't hate your sister." Feelings and experiences of children are also minimized by adults, as if a little person means little problem. Therefore when a child shares with us through his play or verbalizations that he is enraged, we are likely to respond in a way that does not capture the magnitude of the feeling or experience, like: "You are a little upset." Active listening skills are thus the foundation for creating solid clinical relationships with children. Mental health professionals who do not listen to children are not able to create a cross-cultural relationship.

Assessment of active listening skills with regard to working clinically with children can be done a number of ways. Review of recorded sessions, transcripts of sessions, and observations of sessions will provide supervisors with knowledge about their supervisees' abilities. Additionally, listening for particular supervisee questions and self-report will help assess supervisees' abilities. For example, when supervisees raise concerns that the child is not talking, or not talking enough, in a given session, I am alerted. This says to me that the supervisee is not paying close enough attention to nonverbal communications. To help supervisees develop this critical counseling skill of listening and responding to nonverbal communications, supervisors can employ various strategies. Here is an example of a supervision intervention intended to illustrate the necessity of this skill while simultaneously offering direct instruction. The supervisee is shown a series of photographs of children. The photographs only show the face of a child. The supervisee is asked to make a listening response based only on the facial expression of the child (Mullen, 2007). This is a difficult exercise for many supervisees and typically requires the supervisor to provide an example and guidance. The benefit of this authentic learning activity is that supervisees learn the importance of focusing on children's facial expressions and have an experience with making responses in the simultaneously safe and pressured atmosphere of supervision.

Similarly, supervisees often need assistance in keeping responses succinct and culturally relevant to child clients. The following intervention is intended to demonstrate why these skills look different in clinical practice with children and adults. Supervisees are presented with a list of feeling words. The task for the supervisee is to translate the feeling words into child language (Mullen, 2007). By this I mean, the supervisee is encouraged to use interjections, facial responses, and simple feeling word responses in order to translate the feeling word into a response a child will be able to understand and integrate. An example illustrates the task at hand. The instructions go something like this, "Supervisee, here is a list of feeling words. What I would like you to do for each word on the list is to come up with a child-centric response. When actively listening to children we cannot use the same responses we can with adults. I'll do the first one for you. The word is frustrated. Many children know what frustrated means, but some very young ones might not, or you may just be over-using it. So we need to think of other ways to communicate to the child that as their counselor or play therapist we understand that they are frustrated. I might say instead, "You are fed-up," or "That bugs you," or "I might just sort of growl." "Now you try with the remainder of the list. Remember, don't limit yourself to words and keep each alternative response less than five words; you lose children after that."

Supervisees' stereotypes regarding the culture of childhood and the sub-cultures of their child clients need to be assessed and addressed. A clinician who believes that "Children are to be seen not heard" clearly is not culturally sensitive with regard to the culture of childhood. (It is possible that any particular cultural belief about children is salient to the counselor's culture. So, it is likely that some significant energy will need to focus on the impact cultural beliefs have on the child client–counselor relationship.) It's not just skills that enhance child counselor competency but perspective and frankly, personality. This may seem like an over-simplification, but child counselors should like children. Supervisors can assess this by asking supervisees, "What do you like about this child?" Not all clinicians are meant to work with children, and many whose intentions are good are not well-suited because of their own pains, emotional un-availability, and adult centricism. This should be talked about openly in supervision.

Landreth (2002) provides a thorough discussion of personality charac-teristics of play therapists that create opportunities for children to grow and develop. To attain, have, and maintain these personality characteris-tics is an ambitious and arduous task. Landreth eloquently suggests that having these characteristics is not as important as the continuous, thoughtful, and sometimes painstaking motivation needed to incorporate these dimensions into our relationships with children. Intentionality is therefore an essential part of the foundation of the personality of a play therapist. The personality characteristics that Landreth discusses are not limited to play therapists, but also to child counselors who do not profes-sionally identify as play therapists and to other professionals who work with children as well. The effective child counselor is objective, flexible, and has an ability to see the child's perspective. The ability to see a child's perspective is evidenced by the counselor's ability to cross the cultural barriers between the cultures of adulthood and childhood.

HOW TO HONOR THE CULTURE OF CHILDHOOD IN MENTAL HEALTH

Skilled play therapists and child counselors are able to effectively navi-gate the cultural barriers between adulthood and childhood. Because of this unique skill, play therapists should anticipate a more complex role in their relationships with children. Play therapists will have the added re-sponsibility of serving as translators between these two cultures (Mullen, 2003). This is a precarious position.

Being in counseling relationships with children is both an honor and re-sponsibility. It is a distinct honor to be invited into the world of any child. Supervisees and students can think of each child as a teacher with a par-ticular lesson to teach. Although the supervisee is not privy to the course outline, which certainly will include tests, the lesson will emerge out of obfuscation when the counselor or play therapist is open to learning from the child-teacher. To illuminate the lessons being learned, it is useful to ask supervisees, "What lesson is your teacher focusing on with you now?" Supervisees will typically stare at me for a minute or two as they wonder what teacher, what lesson, and various other questions about my competency or sense of reality. Once the supervisee realizes the child is the teacher and we dialogue about the lesson being taught and learned, I can then expand on the metaphor. Supervisees can be asked if there is a theme song that represents their lesson or a title that would be appropriate. I also have asked supervisees to show me the lesson using art mediums or a sand tray. I want to know what it will look like when the lesson is over, and I might have the supervisee use a narrative approach to write a letter to the lesson or the theme of the lesson. Framing the relationship in this way enhances the supervisees' level of respect of the child as a person, client, and member of another culture.

As those lessons are being taught and integrated, another process is simultaneously taking place. Supervisees are recognizing the responsibility of working with children. It matters what you communicate to their parents and other invested adults, but the *how and why* of the communication needs to be thoughtful. Communicating with other adults, including parents, about children in counseling and play therapy is a complex task. Historically, this is viewed as the biggest challenge for my students and supervisees.

Supervisees will need direction and support in handling many of the situations that require them to represent and share about their primary client. Furthermore supervision tends to be a breeding ground for intense transference and countertransference dynamics. Supervisees and students (as well as some of us more seasoned practitioners) tend to blame parents for the troubles of their child clients. It's hard not to. Parents of children who need mental health services have often made poor choices with regard to their children. It is necessary, though, to move past blame to collaboration. Our time and relationships with our child clients are limited in ways that parental relationships are not. It behooves child counselors and play therapists to deal with transference and countertransference issues head on in supervision.

One activity that can be used in supervision to help child counselors and these professional helpers connect with parents is a role play. The supervisee is asked to take on the role of the parent and to talk about how difficult it is to be a parent. While the supervisee is in role I will ask a few questions that I hope facilitate a deeper understanding of the parent's perspective. "Can you tell me about how much you love your child?" "What is special about your relationship with your child?" "Can you name three things that are awesome about your child?" As I listen to the responses of supervisees in the role of parent, I am sure to communicate accurate empathic understanding. It is through this exchange that supervisees come to know and accept the parents of their child clients.

As supervisors of child counselors and play therapists, we are well aware of the complex and complicated facets of our helping profession. We know that working with children requires a view of children that is respectful and thoughtful. We know that developmental differences between childhood and adulthood have to be considered as these differences impact all aspects of our work with children. Seldom do beginning child counselors and play therapists appreciate the diversity between the cultures of childhood and adulthood. We can anticipate this as most of the professional literature that focuses on cultural perspectives has excluded children and childhood (Vargas & Koss-Choino, 1992). We are in a position to honor the culture of childhood as we provide supervision that embraces childhood culture and provides multiple ways for our supervisees to learn in authentic ways how to avoid adult-centricism.

REFERENCES

Corey, G., Corey, M. S., & Callahan, P. (1993). *Issues and ethics in the helping professions*. (4th ed.). Pacific Grove, CA: Brooks/Cole.

Erikson, J. M. (1985). Sources of lifelong learning. *Journal of Education, 167*(3), 85–96.

Fiorini, J., & Mullen, J. A. (2006). *Counseling children and adolescents through grief and loss*. Champaign, IL: Research Press.

Landreth, G. (2002). *Play therapy: The art of the relationship*. New York: Brunner Mazel.

Mullen, J. A. (2003). Speaking of children: A study of how play therapists make meaning of children. (Doctoral dissertation, Syracuse University, 2003). *Dissertation Abstracts International, 64*, 11A.

Mullen, J. A. (2007). *Play therapy basic training: A guide to learning and living the child-centered play therapy philosophy*. Oswego, NY: Integrative Counseling Services.

Pedersen, P. B., & Ivey, A. (1993). *Culture-centered counseling and interviewing skills*. Connecticut: Praeger.

Vargas, L. A., & Koss-Choino, J. D. (1992). *Working with culture: Psychotherapeutic interventions with ethnic minority children and adolescents*. San Francisco: Jossey-Bass.

5

⚜

Culturally Competent Supervision of Child and Play Therapists

Athena A. Drewes

It is important for clinicians to have a multicultural perspective in all aspects of counseling and treatment (Fong, 1994). It is more essential than ever, for, by 2010, 12 of the most populated states, which make up half of the nation's population, will have significant minority populations (Hodgkinson, 1992). We can expect that the supervision constellation of client, therapist, and supervisor will, in all likelihood, contain persons of differing racial-ethnic backgrounds and will be dealing with problems and concerns in a diverse social environment (Fong, 1994). Becoming cross-culturally and multiculturally competent as a supervisor and supervisee requires commitment and follow-through (Gil, 2005) along with self-examination and self-disclosure.

In supervision there are at least three relationships: client-supervisee, supervisee-supervisor, and client-supervisor. Any one of these constellations may be culturally different, and all three may even be culturally different from each other (Ryde, 2000). Working in a culturally sensitive way is never easy. The therapist cannot be and is not culturally neutral as we each view the world inevitably from our own cultural perspective (Ryde, 2000). Personal assumptions, which shape our world view, are the result of many characteristics such as "race, ethnicity, gender, class, sexual orientation, age, religion, nationality, physical ability" (Robinson & Howard-Hamilton, 2000, cited in Garrett et al., 2001, p. 151), as well as acculturation, geographic location, and socioeconomic status.

Consequently, the role of the supervisor is even more critical in being responsible for assuring that multicultural issues receive focus in supervision (Bernard and Goodyear, 1992). It is the supervisor who needs to assist the supervisee in identifying cultural awareness; in identifying cultural influences as they impact on the client's behavior; in counselor-client interactions and in the supervisory relationship; and in providing a culturally sensitive, supportive, and challenging environment for the supervisee (Fong, 1994). Further, in order for multicultural competence to be demonstrated by therapists, they need to be able to display cultural awareness, knowledge, and skills in working with culturally diverse clients (Sue, Arredondo, & McDavis, 1992). Working with cultural difference is challenging and demanding. While formal casework is the useful way such competence can be obtained, the supervision of clinical cases is even more critical for therapists so they can take their knowledge and put it into culturally sensitive practice (Bernard & Goodyear, 1998; Inman, 2005). Thus, supervisors play a significant role in helping trainees and even practicing therapists to develop their multicultural concepts, diagnoses, and treatment skills (Lawless, Gale, & Bacigalupe, 2001; Inman, 2005).

Child and play therapists, whether in training or already actively practicing, are influenced by cultural and racial-ethnic aspects that shape their core assumptions, attitudes, and values of their work, as well as interactions with clients and the supervisor (Fong, 1994). Clinical work is challenging, especially when cultural issues are present (Gallon, Hausotter, & Bryan, 2005). The role of the supervisor is to promote the supervisee's growth by challenging these cultural assumptions, encouraging the supervisee in emotional expression, and being able to validate the conflict of attitudes and values (Fong, 1994).

UNIQUE ASPECTS OF SUPERVISION

Being an effective, culturally competent therapist does not automatically make you a culturally competent supervisor. There are unique skill sets that are relevant to culturally competent therapy and separately for culturally competent supervision (Constantine, 2005). The development of multicultural supervision competence is an ongoing, multifaceted, and multilayered process (Constantine, 2005). Supervision sessions will need to have planned discussion of culture and its importance in counseling, along with the space to explore supervisee and supervisor cultural backgrounds. Modeling by the supervisor and experiential play-based exercises are methods that can be used in individual and group supervision to assist in raising cultural sensitivity and awareness. Only within a safe environment that allows the supervisee to establish a comfort level can learning be encouraged through risk-taking, exploration, and experimentation. In such an environment the supervisee can disclose feelings, conflicts, and actions (Gallon, Hausotter, & Bryan, 2005; Inman, 2006). When polled, supervisees value being directly taught in a supportive and facilitative relationship (Gallon, Hausotter, & Bryan, 2005).

High-quality supervision allows for conflict resolution, open disclosure, mentoring, and overt discussions of culture and gender that are willingly addressed by the supervisor and faced by the supervisee (Gallon, Hausotter, & Bryan, 2005). Rather than waiting for the supervisee to bring up issues, the supervisor needs to identify problems and initiate discussion of them. Through trust and communication, which are essential to the supervisory alliance, both the supervisor and supervisee need to be willing to disclose. This is most important around culture and diversity issues.

Research

Research supports the positive relationship between supervisor multicultural competence and the supervisory relationship (Inman, 2006). Factors such as the openness of the supervisor and attention to cultural factors, along with guidance on culture-specific issues, have specifically been determined to be important to a culturally responsive supervisory relationship (Fukuyama, 1994; Hird et al., 2001). In addition, the supervisee's perception of a strong working alliance is related to the processing of cultural issues within the supervision dyad (Inman, 2006). Having common belief systems (high racial identity levels) about cultural issues, along with the supervisor having a higher racial consciousness than that of the supervisee and displaying an active and genuine interest in other cultures, results in the supervisor feeling better equipped to bring up cultural issues in supervision (Inman, 2006; Ladany et al., 1997). In addition these factors foster a culturally competent environment, which in turn creates a safer environment where cultural differences can be explored in supervision.

The degree to which a supervisee will disclose their own personal biases and feelings about working with multicultural clients will depend upon the degree to which the supervisor creates the sense of safety so the supervisee can personally self-disclose (Inman, 2006; Killian, 2001). Having a supervisory relationship that is based in trust and respect is vital to an environment that allows for both the supervisor and supervisee to take risks in the relationship (Killian, 2001). Even in the most trusting of supervision relationships, most supervisees find it very difficult and uncomfortable to share information with supervisors that might put them in an unfavorable light, especially regarding cultural issues (Constantine, 2005; Ladany et al., 1997). There are also limitations to the degree to which supervisees feel they can be understood by supervisors from a different cultural background (Gardner, 2002). Gardner (2002) reported that super-visees were selective in their disclosures, choosing only items that they be-lieved their supervisor could understand. Therefore, supervisors who ex-plore their own personal values, cultural experiences, cultural biases, and stereotypes give the supervisee a model for discussing their own clinical and supervisory struggles within counseling and supervisory relation-ships (Constantine, 2005). Racial and cultural differences between super-visor and supervisee, as well as between supervisee and client, should be acknowledged, and supervisors should be comfortable discussing racial issues with supervisees (Gardner, 2002).

Establishing Clear Goals

While exploration of multicultural issues is critical in a supervisee's abil-ity to develop multicultural competence (Helms & Cook, 1999), the readi-ness of the supervisee to focus on multicultural issues, as well as on their personal cultural style of communication, may directly influence a super-visor's and supervisee's agreement on the tasks and goals of supervision (Inman, 2006, Killian, 2001). For example, while the supervisor may feel it is important for the supervisee to explore their own internalized stereo-types about a client's race or culture, this goal may not be in concert with the supervisee's goal of supervision, or expectation that the supervisor self-discloses first, before they engage in their own personal exploration (Inman, 2006). As a result, conflict and strain may occur in the working al-liance that will need to be addressed openly. Supervisor and supervisee must be in agreement on what the goals and tasks of supervision should be, especially with regard to multicultural issues so that understanding may lead to greater supervision satisfaction.

Case Conceptualization

In addition to addressing personal self-awareness of internalized stereo-types, supervisees need to also be aware of the unique client variables of cultural membership and socialization that affect client problems (Con-stantine & Ladany, 2001). Consequently, the supervisee needs to be able to manage not only their own cultural awareness, but simultaneously inte-grate the client's diversity within their therapeutic relationship (Inman, 2006). The ability to juggle and integrate this information, along with mul-ticultural counseling skills and behaviors, leads to increased competence (Constantine & Ladany, 2001; Inman, 2006).

In order to assist trainees in developing their multicultural case concep-tualization, supervisors will need to have a range of knowledge and skills in working with diverse clients, multicultural sensitivity, and knowledge about the universality and diversity of play in different cultures (Drewes, 2005), as well as the ability to facilitate this learning within supervision. Supervision can become ineffective when the supervisee does not see the supervisor as having these skills (Killian, 2001; Inman, 2006). The supervisor's willingness to be informed by a supervisee who is of another race is especially important as the supervisor models openness, respect, and compassion (Gardner, 2002).

Research findings suggest that trainees may be more prepared academically to work with culturally diverse clients than their supervisors (Constantine, 1997; Duan & Roehlke, 2001). In fact 70 percent of clinical supervisors had not completed a formal course in multicultural counseling, whereas the same percentage of supervisees had done so; supervisees also tended to be more sensitive to racial-cultural issues than their supervisors. Supervisors who are not racially conscious might harm their supervisees and in turn their clients by neglecting racial-cultural issues in conceptualizing the clients' presenting problems and treatment plans (Constantine, 2005). Factors that can also adversely affect the supervisory relationship include "unintentional racism, miscommunication, lack of interpersonal awareness within the supervisory relationship, insensitivity to supervisees' nonverbal cues, undiscussed racial/ethnic issues, gender bias, overemphasis on cultural explanations for psychological difficulties, and an inability to appropriately present questions and responses that elicit valuable information or feedback" (Inman, 2006, p. 74). These factors are even more critical when cross-cultural supervision occurs. Research has shown that supervisees of a different race from their supervisors felt their supervisors were competent if they were knowledgeable; demonstrated good facilitative skills; and displayed compassion, concern, fairness, and honesty, as well as being receptive, dedicated, genuine, humble, empathic, respectful, and humorous (Gardner, 2002).

In summary, in order to help further the supervisory relationship, a collaboration of several components is needed between both the supervisee and supervisor: a mutual agreement as to what the goals of the supervision should be (e.g., exploring the cultural identity of the supervisee, exploring the client's cultural identity within the session); mutual agreement of how this will be achieved in supervision (e.g., watching videotapes and looking for specific cultural issues and responses); and most importantly, a sense of trust, liking, and sharing between the supervisee and supervisor (Bordin, 1983; Inman, 2006). Constantine's (1997) study of multicultural differences in the supervisory process at 22 internship programs found that many of the participants reported that their experience in supervision would have been enhanced if the supervisor had spent more time helping them to process issues surrounding cultural differences in supervision.

Further, in addition to offering guidance and explicit discussion of culture-specific issues, the supervisor's willingness to be vulnerable and share his or her own struggles, along with providing an opportunity for multicultural activities, helps facilitate a culturally responsive supervisory relationship (Fukuyama, 1994; Inman, 2006; Killian, 2001).

The inclusion of role plays, skill practices, modeling, audio- or videotape reviews, along with directive, collaborative, confrontive, supportive, structured, or open-ended supervision that is dependent on the learning needs, style, and personality of the supervisee, helps the supervisee to explore multicultural issues more fully (Gardner, 2002).

CROSS-CULTURAL SUPERVISION

Cross-cultural supervision involves those situations in which the supervisor and supervisee come from different ethnic, cultural, and /or racial backgrounds (Daniels, D'Andrea, & Kim, 1999). Effective cross-cultural supervision requires the supervisor to invite the supervisee to enter into a unique professional relationship wherein both parties agree to work together to discuss their roles and responsibilities in supervision, establish guidelines for giving and receiving feedback in supervision, determine ways together to resolve any potential cultural misunderstandings or disagreements, and encourage each other to discuss the ways in which unintentional forms of racism and ethnocentrism might be manifested in counseling or supervision sessions (Daniels, D'Andrea, & Kim, 1999).

A child or play therapist's willingness to engage a client in a dialogue regarding issues related to race in the therapy session is essential for creating a safe and trusting therapeutic environment. And the therapist-initiated discussions regarding racial issues can facilitate the working alliance and reduce the potential for a therapeutic impasse, premature termination of therapy, or resistance to supervision (Helms & Cook, 1999). But many clinicians are hesitant to initiate discussions of race in therapy for fear of offending. Cross-cultural supervision can also evoke similar reactions and hesitancies. In training situations, it is still taboo to have direct discussions about race and racism that go beneath surface-level explorations (Utsey, Gernat, & Hammar, 2005). In order to find a comfort level that allows for honest and open discussion of race and ethnicity within therapy sessions with a client, the therapist (trainee) needs first to confront his or her own prejudices, assumptions, and biases about other racial or ethnic groups (Pinderhughes, 1989; Utsey, Gernat, & Hammar, 2005). Racial consciousness and the willingness to discuss racial issues are factors that significantly affect cross-racial counseling and supervision (Helms & Cook, 1999). Thus, counselor racial self-awareness is an important prerequisite for developing multicultural competence (Richardson & Molinaro, 1996).

It is important that the supervisee and supervisor try to understand the client's world from the material brought in, both verbally and non-verbally. Unconscious material, such as prejudiced attitudes and feelings, needs to be explored and brought to consciousness in order to understand how it can affect the process of the work (Ryde, 2000). The supervisor and supervisee also need to explore ways in which the relationship with the client is mirrored within the supervisory experience and relationship. Further, the supervisor needs to explore personal reactions and responses within themselves during a supervisory session, and how those feelings may differ from those of the supervisee (Ryde, 2000).

It is important for the supervisor to take the time to initiate discussions on multicultural counseling issues and cross-cultural issues between supervisor and supervisee early in the supervisory process (Daniels, D'Andrea, & Kim, 1999). The supervisor needs to initiate discussion about the supervisor's and supervisee's cultural, ethnic, and racial backgrounds. Such an exploration allows the sharing of values and traditions that may be associated with personal cultural, ethnic, and racial backgrounds that can influence goals in counseling and expectations of supervision. Further, discussion of supervisor and supervisee levels of racial identity development will help in assessing how they may affect the way counseling and supervision is viewed (Daniels, D'Andrea, & Kim, 1999).

DEVELOPMENTAL STAGES FOR CULTURAL SENSITIVITY

It is also important that the supervisor be aware of the supervisee's developmental level (MacDonald, 1997). Lopez and Hernandez (1987) describe four stages in developing culturally sensitive therapists that supervisors should follow. These stages move from the didactic to the experiential, and from the cognitive and objective to the personal and subjective (Porter, 1994).

Stage One

Stage one is structured and didactic, with goals toward reducing defensiveness, building competence and confidence, and allowing time for the supervisor and supervisee to develop a relationship in a nonconfrontational way before more personal or threatening material is brought up (Porter, 1994). Material that could be threatening is presented in an objective, task-oriented manner. Culture should not be over-empha-sized, nor should it be underemployed (Lopez & Hernandez, 1987).

Stage Two

In Stage two, racism, classism, and other oppressions that affect clients' lives, along with sociocultural and acculturation factors, are explored to help in understanding and seeing how these factors are central to the clients' mental health issues and problems (Porter, 1994). The supervisor needs to emphasize the interaction of cultural factors within the larger society. The supervisee is helped to move beyond and away from viewing and labeling symptoms in a "pejorative, pathological context, to seeing them as formerly adaptive solutions to difficult or challenging societal demands" (Porter, 1994, p. 47). "Most White supervisees, as well as some ethnic minority ones, begin exploring these areas more cautiously. Some remain resistant to this perspective, whereas others immerse themselves (Porter, 1994, p. 48). Personal accounts and guided imagery exercises can be powerful in helping to explore the clients' experience.

Stage Three

Stage three is the most personal and difficult stage of supervision as it requires exploring the supervisee's own internalized biases and assumptions of stereotypes and racism toward minority groups, which can further perpetuate racism and affect the therapeutic process. It requires a great deal of trust between the supervisor and supervisee (Porter, 1994). This stage is the most important, especially in cross-cultural supervision, as it is critical that we each confront our own racism and how expectations, goals, and behaviors in therapy can be different for the supervisee and supervisor (Porter, 1994). This stage requires a great deal of self-disclosure, which can be frightening. The therapist/supervisor match is important at this stage, as well as the supervisor having explored his or her own potential racism and biases through self-examination (Porter, 1994).

Stage Four

Stage four requires the supervisor to encourage the supervisee to expand interventions into a social-action perspective allowing for empowerment of the client. Alternatives or additions to the existing individual therapy model using community and group participation are explored (Porter, 1994).

USING PLAY-BASED TECHNIQUES

Through experiential, play-based exercises, the supervisee can begin to explore their personal culture and group identification in a fun, relaxing, and safe way. "Until therapists understand just how their identity and experience are affected by their membership in various cultural groups, it is impossible for them to understand how such memberships affect the lives of their clients" (O'Connor, 2005, p. 568). Play-based techniques can allow exploration of personal culture and group identification, as well as exploration of biases and possible prejudices toward other cultures in a nonthreatening, playful way. In addition, the exploration of the client's culture and group identification can also be modeled by the supervisor and supervisee in a way that will help the supervisee to try out similar techniques within the therapy process.

Use of Sandplay Miniatures

One way to open the dialogue between supervisor and supervisee around personal cultural, ethnic, and racial backgrounds is to utilize miniatures. The supervisor and supervisee each select ten miniatures that best represent their cultural, ethnic, and racial identities. Each person shares what each miniature represents for them. In addition, each person explores and dialogues with the other (1) what worldviews (e.g., values, assumptions, and biases) they may bring to the supervision relationships based on their personal cultural identity, (2) what counseling strengths and limitations contribute to the work with culturally different clients, and (3) what struggles and challenges may be faced in working with culturally different clients based on personal cultural, ethnic, and racial backgrounds (Constantine, 1997).

This same strategy can be used by the supervisee to better understand their client and treatment issues. The supervisee would select ten miniatures representing the cultural, ethnic, and racial aspects impacting their clients' relationship with the supervisee and/or their world. The supervisee could repeat this process for each member of the family. In addition, the supervisee can use this same technique during a therapy session with the client(s) to bring up cross-cultural and multicultural issues.

Personal Symbols

O'Connor (2005) offers another play-based technique to facilitate self-examination by the supervisee, as well as the supervisor. A large sheet of paper is divided into two columns. The first column contains symbols representing the various groups that the supervisee identifies with. The second column contains symbols that represent the groups that others see the supervisee or supervisor as belonging to. The symbols or words should reflect race, ethnicity, gender and gender role, sexual orientation, age, relative physical ability, and religion (O'Connor, 2005). At the top of the column are the symbols of the groups that the supervisee and supervisor feel most positively about, and the ones felt most negatively about are at the bottom of the page.

The following activities were supplied by group members during an experiential workshop in supervision that the author co-facilitated at the 2006 Association for Play Therapy conference.

Group Activity

This activity can be used in group supervision, during the early phase, to help sensitize participants to how the client may feel about disclosing issues to the therapist too soon into the process.

Using small pieces of paper, each group member writes a secret or an issue that is taboo on their piece of paper. It can be one word or a symbol if the person does not want to make up a sentence. Each paper is then folded up by participants and put into a bag. Group members discuss how it felt needing to divulge something uncomfortable so soon into the supervisory process. Parallels and similarities are made to the client who is faced with having to divulge secrets in the beginning of treatment without knowing the therapist.

Each paper is then opened and read out loud. The group again explores how it felt hearing these subjects brought up. Participants explore whether it would have been easier had they known the person before such topics were introduced. The point being made is that the sense of trust needs to be built first before going into secrets or issues that may be taboo to the client or in the client's culture.

Puppets

Having a large basket of puppets helps the supervisee play out scenarios in which they may feel stuck. The supervisee selects one puppet that represents a perspective about the therapist-client situation or in which they may feel stuck in the treatment process. The supervisor explores with the supervisee why they chose that particular puppet, and what attributes may fit the client or client's parent or family.

The supervisee is encouraged to select a puppet that best reflects the supervisee at that moment in the treatment process. What attributes does that puppet have that the supervisee has or does not have? What would the client say about the supervisee's puppet, and what attributes might they give the therapist? The supervisor and supervisee can also select puppets to represent each other and the relationship with each other at that point in time.

The supervisee and supervisor can use the puppets in creating role-plays for practice and mastery in asking clients difficult questions about racial and ethnic identities, or how the supervisee might feel about a given client or the supervisor.

Transitional Object

Multicultural and cross-cultural work is difficult. Newer therapists may feel intimidated, embarrassed, and/or uncomfortable in exploring and overtly discussing racial and ethnic differences between the client and therapist. In order to help lessen the anxiety that may come up in the session as the therapist attempts to tackle these issues, a transitional object can help to offer support. An object or token item, such as a colorful grounding stone or rock, chosen by the supervisor and given to the supervisee as a symbol of support and encouragement, can help serve as such a transitional object. The supervisee can keep it in a pocket and touch it during those moments of worry or fear in facing the client or client's parent/caregiver.

Deep Breathing

Use of deep breathing or guided imagery can generally calm the supervisee. But these methods can also be utilized by the trainee to help relax during supervision and during times that they must confront a client about the care of their child or ask difficult questions about ethnicity and group identification.

Repeatedly practicing deep breathing during supervision, especially during times when the material being discussed is *not* anxiety provoking, helps lead toward mastery. Once mastery is obtained, deep breathing and guided imagery can effectively be used by the therapist in anxiety-provoking sessions with the client. The supervisee can utilize the deep breathing technique to keep calm during stressful sessions. The supervisee in turn can help teach the client and/or parent or guardian deep breathing to help in their stressful moments. In addition, the supervisor should role model deep breathing as an effective way toward therapist self-care.

CONCLUSION

Becoming cross-culturally and multiculturally competent, as a supervisor and supervisee, requires commitment and follow-through along with self-examination and self-disclosure. Supervision needs to be a safe and supportive environment in which both the supervisor and supervisee are able to explore personal culture and understand their view of play in order to be better able to effectively work with children and families of other cultures.

Being an effective, culturally competent therapist does not automatically make a person a culturally competent supervisor. The development of multicultural supervision competence is an on-going, multifaceted, and multilayered process. Such factors as the openness of the supervisor and attention to cultural factors, along with guidance on culture-specific issues, have specifically been determined to be important to a culturally responsive supervisory relationship.

It is important for the supervisor to take the time to initiate discussions on multicultural counseling issues and cross-cultural issues between supervisor and supervisee early in the supervisory process. Modeling by the supervisor and experiential play-based exercises are methods that can be used in individual and group supervision to assist in raising cultural sensitivity and awareness.

REFERENCES

Bernard, J. M., & Goodyear, R. K. (1992). *Fundamentals of clinical supervision.* Boston, MA: Allyn & Bacon.

Bernard, J. M., & Goodyear, R. K. (1998). *Fundamentals of clinical supervision* (2nd ed.). Boston: Allyn & Bacon.

Bordin, E. S. (1983). A working alliance based model of supervision. *Counseling Psychologist, 11,* 35–41.

Constantine, M. G. (1997). Facilitating multicultural competency in counseling supervision: Operationalizing a practical framework. In D. B. Pope-Davis & H. L. Coleman (Eds.), *Multicultural counseling competencies: Assessment, education and training, and supervision* (Vol. 7, 310–24). Thousand Oaks, CA: Sage.

Constantine, M. G. (2005). Culturally competent supervision: Myths, fantasies, and realities. Retrieved September 15, 2005, from www.appic.org/Conference2005/Slides/Madonna.ppt, 1–12.

Constantine, M. G., & Ladany, N. (2001). New visions for defining and assessing multicultural counseling competence. In J. G. Ponterotto, J. M. Casas, L. A. Suzuki, & C. M. Alexander (Eds.), *Handbook of multicultural counseling* (2nd ed., 482–98). Thousand Oaks, CA: Sage.

Daniels, J., D'Andrea, M., & Kim, B. S. K. (1999). Assessing the barriers and challenges of cross-cultural supervision: A case study. *Counselor Education and Supervision 38,* 191–204.

Drewes, A. A. (2005). Play in selected cultures. Diversity and universality. In E. Gil & A. A. Drewes (Eds.) *Cultural issues in play therapy* (26–71). New York: Guilford Press.

Duan, C., & Roehlke, H. (2001). A descriptive "snapshot" of cross-racial supervision in university counseling center internships. *Journal of Multicultural Counseling and Development, 29,* 131–46.

Fong, M. L. (1994). Multicultural issues in supervision. *Eric Digest,* Retrieved October 22, 1995, from www.ericdigests.org/1995-1/supervision.htm.

Fukuyama, M. A. (1994). Critical incidents in multicultural counseling supervision: A phenomenological approach to supervision research. *Counselor Education and Supervision, 34,* 142–51.

Gallon, S., Hausotter, W., & Bryan, M. A. (2005). What happens in good supervision? *Addiction Messenger, 8*(9), 1–5.

Gardner, R. M. (2002). Cross cultural perspectives in supervision. *Western Journal of Black Studies, 26*(2), 98–106.

Garrett, M. T., Border, L. D., Crutchfield, L. B., Torres-Rivera, E., et al. (2001). *Journal of Multicultural Counseling and Development, 29,* 147–58.

Gil, E. (2005). From sensitivity to competence in working across cultures. In E. Gil & A. A. Drewes (Eds.), *Cultural issues in play therapy* (3–25). New York: Guilford Press.

Helms, J. E., & Cook, D. A. (Eds.). (1999). *Using race and culture in counseling and psychotherapy.* Boston: Allyn & Bacon.

Hird, J. S., Cavaleri, C. E., Dulko, J. P., Felice, A. A. D., et al. (2001). Visions and realities: Supervisee perspectives of multicultural supervision. *Journal of Multicultural Counseling and Development, 29,* 114–30.

Hodgkinson, H. L. (1992). *A demographic look at tomorrow.* Washington, DC: Institute for Educational Leadership.

Inman, A. G. (2006). Supervisor multicultural competence and its relation to supervisory process and outcome. *Journal of Marital and Family Therapy, 32*(1), 73–85.

Killiam, K. D. (2001). Differences making a difference: Cross-cultural interactions in supervisory relationships. In T. S. Zimmerman (Ed.), *Integrating gender and culture in family therapy training* (pp. 61–103). New York: Haworth Press.

Ladany, N., Inman, A. G., Constantine, M. G., & Hofheinz, E. W. (1997). Supervisee multicultural case conceptualization ability and self-reported multicultural competence as functions of supervisee racial identity and supervisor focus. *Journal of Counseling Psychology, 44,* 284–93.

Lawless, J. J., Gale, J. E., & Bacigalupe, G. (2001). The discourse of race and culture in family therapy supervision: A conversation analysis. *Contemporary Family Therapy, 23,* 181–97.

Lopez, S., & Hernandez, P. (1987). When culture is considered in the evaluation and treatment of Hispanic patients. *Psychotherapy, 24,* 120–26.

MacDonald, G. (1997). Issues in multi-cultural counseling supervision. *Caring in an age of technology.* Proceedings of the International Conference on Counseling in the 21st century. (6th Beijing, China, May 29–30, 1997), 199–204.

O'Connor, K. (2005). Addressing diversity issues in play therapy. *Professional Psychology, Research and Practice, 36*(5), 566–73.

Pinderhughes, E. (1989). *Understanding race, ethnicity, and power. The key to efficacy in clinical practice.* New York: Free Press.

Porter, N. (1994). Empowering supervisees to empower others: A culturally responsive supervision model. *Hispanic Journal of Behavioral Sciences, 16*(1), 43–56.

Richardson, T. Q., & Molinaro, K. (1996). White counselor self-awareness: A prerequisite for developing multicultural competence. *Journal of Counseling and Development, 74*, 238–42.

Robinson, T. L., & Howard-Hamilton, M. F. (2000). *The convergence of race, ethnicity, and gender: Multiple identities in counseling.* Upper Saddle River, NJ: Merrill.

Ryde, J. (2000). Supervising across difference. *International Journal of Psychotherapy, 5*(1), 37–48.

Sue, D. W., Arredondo, P., & McDavis, R. J. (1992). Multicultural counseling competencies and standards: Individual and organizational development. *Journal of Multicultural Counseling and Development, 20*, 64–68.

Utsey, S. O., Gernat, C. A., & Hammar, L. (2005). Examining white counselor trainees' reactions to racial issues in counseling and supervision dyads. *The Counseling Psychologist, 33*(4), 449–78.

Part II

SUPERVISING SPECIAL POPULATIONS

6

⟨∞⟩

Supervising Counselors Who Work with Special Needs Children

Jody J. Fiorini

Missy, an 11-year-old fifth grader, is referred to the school counselor's office for acting out in class and being a "behavior problem." The teacher reports that she is seldom on task and disrupts the class by speaking out of turn and bothering the children sitting near her. Missy has been diagnosed with attention deficit hyperactivity disorder (ADHD) and a learning disability in reading. When the counselor intern who has been assigned to work with Missy first meets her, she is presented with a girl with a warm smile who simply radiates energy and curiosity. She walks around the office asking about the books and toys on the shelf. She asks who the people are in the pictures on the desk. She asks why the counselor decided to become a counselor. She is so engaging that the session is over before the intern had a chance to "get anywhere" with the session. At the next session, the intern tells Missy that she needs to stay focused so that they can work on the issues for which she was referred. Missy's smile immediately disappears and she says, "Oh, I thought that since you weren't a teacher that maybe you would like me. I didn't know that counselors were teachers too. I'll try to behave better from now on."

The scenario above represents a dilemma that is common for counselors and counselors-in-training who work with children with special needs. Very often the counselor is so focused on meeting the needs of the referral source that the child's needs are overlooked. In the case of Missy, the counselor had an opportunity to emphasize her client's strengths, intelligence, curiosity, and kindness, in order to assist her in being more successful in school. Instead, by focusing on Missy's deficits, communication was shut down.

DEMOGRAPHICS

The number of special needs students identified in the United States is rapidly increasing. Counselors are likely to encounter students with learning disabilities in their caseloads because these students make up 46.2 percent of the school-age population of students with disabilities and 5.9 percent of the overall school population (U.S. Department of Education, 1999). According to the U.S. Department of Education (1999), schools served approximately 2.7 million students with learning disabilities in just the 1997–98 school year alone. According to the Autism Society of America (2005) there has been an estimated 172 percent increase in the incidence of autism since the 1990s. In addition, 3–7 percent of school children are diagnosed with ADHD (Children and Adults with Attention Deficit/Hyperactivity Disorder, 2005).

Since the population of special needs children, particularly those with autism spectrum disorders, is increasing in the United States, it has never been more important for counselors to become knowledgeable and skilled in working with children with disabilities. Better identification practices and screening programs have contributed to earlier identification of children with special needs. As a by-product of this, counselors are able to provide services to children at younger ages. It behooves supervisors of child therapists, then, to become familiar with the common issues that arise for children with special needs and their families as well as the barriers that prevent counselors from best meeting the needs of these individuals.

RISK FACTORS FOR CHILDREN WITH DISABILITIES

Children with disabilities face specific challenges in their lives that can lead to emotional maladjustment (Bowen & Glenn, 1998). One of the most heart-breaking side effects of many disabilities is the social isolation and ostracism that many children experience. Children with special needs often report feeling different and out of place. They may have social skills deficits that interfere with making friends, which may lead to rejection by peers, loneliness, and isolation. These children may be victims of teasing and bullying. They may also be prone to impulsive behavior and may not have the cognitive skills to think through the consequences of their behavior. They may experience delays and difficulties with academic achievement that add to feelings of low self-esteem. In addition, parents of children with special needs often begin a pattern of "doing for" their children, which may squelch the child's sense of self-efficacy and foster dependence. Ironically, counselors can often fall into the same trap of fostering dependency in their child clients with special needs out of a sense of generosity and altruism.

POTENTIAL BARRIERS FOR COUNSELORS
OF SPECIAL NEEDS CHILDREN

In my research (Fiorini, 2001), I have found that many counselors doubt their ability to effectively work with individuals with disabilities. To complicate matters further, counselors also report concerns about their abilities to work with children in general (Duggan & Carlson, 2007). When you add a disability into the mix, counselors may feel that they lack adequate preparation and question whether they are qualified to work with these children. There is evidence to support this notion that counselors are not provided with adequate training in working with individuals with disabilities (Korinek & Prillaman, 1992; Lesbock & Deblassie, 1975; Lombana, 1980; Lusk & Hartshorne, 1985; Tucker, Shepherd, & Hurst, 1986). In one study of school counselors in New York State (Fiorini, 2001), relatively few counselors reported having had any coursework or inservice training in special education or disability. Furthermore, there was a relationship between a counselor's perceived level of adequacy of preparation and the number of activities performed with these students. The better prepared counselors felt, the more activities they performed. Conversely, counselors who did not perceive themselves as having had adequate preparation were less likely to perform an activity.

In addition, the 2001 Council for Accreditation of Counseling and Related Educational Programs (CACREP) standards require that counselor education programs provide counselor-trainees with opportunities to: (a) understand advocacy processes needed to address institutional and social barriers that impede access, equity, and success for clients (Section 2K1g); (b) investigate the counselor trainee's attitudes, beliefs, and understandings related to mental and physical characteristics of clients (Section 2K2b); (c) understand theories of learning, development, and human behavior including an understanding of how disability affects normal and abnormal development (Section 2K3b & c); (d) understand career counseling processes, techniques, and resources including those applicable to specific populations (Section 2K4h); (e) understand how disability impacts assessment and evaluation of individuals (Section 2K7f); and (f) engage in clinical experiences that provide opportunities for students to counsel clients who represent the ethnic and demographic diversity of their community (Section 3K) (Council for Accreditation of Counseling and Related Educational Programs, 2000). Since it seems that counselor-trainees are not being provided with this type of education, supervisors should be prepared to fill in the gaps of knowledge that supervisees may present.

Supervisors need to assist counselors in gaining knowledge and skills in working with this population of children. They need to help counselors confront biases and misinformation that may interfere with their ability to create a working alliance with their clients. They also need to instill in their supervisees a sense of competence in working with children with special needs. The rest of this chapter will provide information that is crucial for supervisors in helping their supervisees work more effectively with special needs children and their families.

WHAT SUPERVISORS NEED TO KNOW

Supervisors of counselors who work with children with special needs need to examine their own strengths and limitations in working with this population. Three areas in particular need to be examined: awareness, knowledge, and skills. Supervisors should engage in a process of self-assessment with regard to their views of disabilities before they will be able to assist their supervisees through the same process.

Self-Assessment—What Are Your Beliefs About Disabilities?

Many common myths about people with disabilities exist in our society. I will examine each of these myths individually and provide examples of each. I invite supervisors to examine their own beliefs with regard to the ideas presented.

Myth 1: Disability=Tragedy

Very often people believe that disability is a tragic event that forever scars and impedes an individual's life. Ironically, it is often our society's focus on being able-bodied, fit, and attractive that truly impairs the self-esteem of an individual with a disability. Counselors who work with children with disabilities must examine their sense of what is "normal." A child who was born deaf knows no other way of living. To them, their experience is not tragic but is the status quo. If a child with a disability encounters a counselor who equates disability with tragedy, they will often feel pitied and misunderstood, which will definitely impede the counseling relationship. Supervisors should help supervisees examine how they have been taught to view disability in their lives. Have they had any personal experience with physical, learning, or mental disabilities? What have they been taught to believe about what it would be like to live with a disability? The supervisor should suggest readings to the counselor that would help him or her examine different perspectives of disability. I would particularly suggest that supervisees read *The Psychological and Social Impact of Disability, Fourth Edition* by Marinelli and Dell Orto (1999) for this purpose.

Myth 2: Individuals with Disabilities Need Specialized Services and Groups

This myth tends to interfere most with a counselor's sense of self-efficacy in working with children with special needs. Although working with children with disabilities may require a counselor to gain knowledge about a particular disability, the skills you would use to work with an individual with a disability are the same skills that you would use with any child. Active listening, play therapy, and art therapy are all approaches that are equally suited to both "typical" and special needs children.

In terms of specialized groups and services, it is my belief that it is important for counselors to help children with disabilities integrate into mainstream society. Children with disabilities often feel different and isolated, so having groups specific to disability, although it may allow children to discuss their unique experiences as people with disabilities, does nothing to integrate them with their nondisabled peers. In my opinion, it is better to refer them for groups and services that deal with their underlying issues such as social skills or loneliness, rather than to create a specific group for special needs children that would only serve to isolate them further from their peers.

Myth 3: Individuals with Disabilities Are Asexual

This may seem like an unusual myth to present in a book about supervising counselors who work with children, but I think it is quite appropriate given the fact that our society views children in general as asexual beings. This is even more the case for children with disabilities. There is an implicit assumption that children and adolescents with disabilities do not have sexual feelings or are not interested in developing intimate relationships. Moreover, individuals with disabilities are often not seen as sexually attractive or "dateable." Imagine the impact this view would have on a child going through puberty. Picture what it might be like to be experiencing all the normal sexual feelings associated with development, body changes, wet dreams, and crushes when the people around you seem to feel that you are incapable of such feelings or worse yet, that those feelings will never be reciprocated. Adults can unknowingly communicate to a child with a disability that they are neither expected nor desired to have normal sexual feelings. For this reason, children with disabilities are often not provided with even the basic sex education that their nondisabled peers receive. This lack of education leaves them particularly vulnerable to sexual exploitation and abuse (Cole, 1991).

Myth 4: All Aspects of a Person's Life Are Affected by Their Disability

This myth is referred to in the disability community as the "spread phenomenon" (Livneh, 1991). This phenomenon occurs when the person's disability is generalized to other, unrelated characteristics such as emotional maladjustment or mental defect. An example of this phenomenon is when a person shouts at a person in a wheelchair or speaks in a patronizing voice and calls a person with a disability sweetie or dear. Imagine if a person like the famous physicist Stephen Hawking had been treated this way. Perhaps the world would never have experienced the benefits of his ingenious discoveries. Counselors need to be careful that they do not succumb to the spread phenomenon and assume that the children with disabilities with whom they work are more impaired than they really are.

Myth 5: People with Disabilities Get a Great Deal of Support

There is a general belief that individuals with disabilities receive a great deal of financial and social support from a variety of agencies. Although there are agencies and foundations out there that support people with disabilities, it has been my experience that individuals with disabilities and their families are largely unaware of the support services that are available. Much of the work I do in working with families of children with disabilities is in helping them explore the different services and support groups offered in their communities. It is important that counselors-in-training and counselors who work with children with disabilities become aware of the resources available within their communities. They should be familiar with the services provided by their state's office of vocational rehabilitation, as well as any local agencies that specialize in assisting children with disabilities. They should also become aware of local and online support groups related to their child's disability. For example, www.ldonline.com is an excellent resource for parents and teachers of children with disabilities as well as the children themselves. There are online chats for each group, shared parenting tips, activities for kids, as well as the latest research in the field of learning disabilities. There are similar Web resources for children with ADHD, autism, Tourette's, and many other disabilities.

Myth 6: Individuals with Disabilities Are Not at Much Risk for Alcohol or Drug Abuse

Like the myth about children with disabilities being asexual, there is also a common assumption that children with disabilities are not at much risk for substance abuse problems. Nothing could be farther from the truth. In fact, individuals with disabilities are at increased risk for alcoholism and substance abuse for a number of reasons (Helwig & Holicky, 1994). First, they may use alcohol as a social lubricant or as a coping mechanism to deal with their feelings of loneliness and isolation. They also might use substances in an effort to alleviate physical pain. It is crucial that the counselor-in-training be aware that children with special needs are at risk for developing alcohol and substance abuse problems so that they can look for potential warning signs and provide prevention activities.

Myth 7: If an Individual with a Disability Is Depressed or Anxious, It Automatically Must Be Related to Their Disability

I often have to remind my supervisees that children with disabilities can be anxious or depressed for reasons that have nothing to do with their disability. For example, imagine that a student with Asperger's syndrome who is going on a school trip across the country suddenly begins to have panic attacks and is concerned about going on the trip. The counselor assumes that the student's disability is the cause of this anxiety, and he or she tries to assure the child that he will have all the support he needs on the trip. After some investigation the counselor learns that the child's parents have been arguing a great deal lately and the child is afraid that if he leaves, his parents will be divorced upon his return. The rule of thumb when children with disabilities present with depression or anxiety is to search for underlying reasons without automatically assuming that the disability is the cause of the symptoms.

Myth 8: Learning Disabilities Only Involve Problems of an Academic Nature

Many people have a faulty notion that learning disabilities only impact a child's ability to perform academically. In truth, however, children with learning disabilities may experience both academic and behavioral problems that could result in a referral to a counselor (Bowen & Glenn, 1998; Thompson & Littrell, 1998). In addition, students with learning disabilities have been shown to be at greater risk for depression, suicide, substance abuse, juvenile delinquency, and victimization (Brier, 1994; Fowler & Tisdale, 1992; McBride & Siegel, 1997; Sabornie, 1994). There are two main reasons why children with learning disabilities are at such risk. The first is that their poor academic performance leads them to feel bad about themselves, which lowers self-esteem and self-efficacy, and raises levels of depression. The second reason is that social skills deficits are often an integral part of the learning disability itself. The same difficulties children have in reading words may also impact their ability to read facial and other nonverbal cues. The social skills deficits of many children with disabilities often lead to their being rejected by their peers, and this increases their sense of loneliness and social ostracism. Counselors need to be aware of the impact that social skills deficits may have on a child's social adjustment.

Myth 9: Counselors and Their Supervisors Are Immune to the Myths Presented Above

All of us are at risk of believing the myths that society perpetuates about individuals with disabilities, and counselors and counseling supervisors are no exception. Supervisors should help their supervisees to examine the myths presented so that they can develop realistic and unbiased notions of disability. To this effect, the following section of the chapter will help supervisors learn how to help their supervisees to self-assess.

HELPING SUPERVISEES SELF-ASSESS

Awareness

The supervisor should first assist their supervisees who work with special needs children to assess their level of awareness about different types of disabilities. They should help them examine their biases and belief systems about physical, learning, and emotional disabilities as outlined in the previous chapter. I engage my supervisees in a series of activities to examine their biases and to help them better understand the experiences of children with disabilities.

- The List: Have your supervisees list every disability they can think of and then have them rank them from easiest to live with to most difficult to live with. Have them examine the reasons behind their rankings. For example, if someone ranks paraplegia as the most difficult to live with and you ask them to examine why they feel that way, they might discover that they hold faulty notions of what people with paraplegia are capable of doing in terms of work and other activities.

- Would You Rather?: Tell supervisees that they have to choose one disability: blindness, deafness, or the loss of the use of their legs. Ask them which they would choose and why. Again, this activity helps them explore their underlying beliefs about disability and gets to some of the myths discussed previously.

Simulation Activities

- Have supervisees write a paragraph with their nondominant hand and ask them to read it aloud. Ask them how it felt to write in such a belabored fashion.
- Have supervisees imagine that they have to go to school where everyone teaches in Greek and all of the books are written in Greek. What would that be like? Now have them imagine doing that 180 days a year for 13 years.
- Ask supervisees to find their way around town or send them on a scavenger hunt where they are not able to use any stairs. Have the final piece of the scavenger hunt be available in a nonaccessible place and then discuss how it feels to experience barriers.

Knowledge

Once supervisees have become more aware of the experiences of children with disabilities, supervisors can help them gain specific knowledge about particular types of disabilities. Counselors should have a working knowledge about the more common disabilities affecting children, such as developmental disabilities, autism, learning disabilities, and ADHD. This can be accomplished by seeking out information from credible sources on the Web and through assigned readings.

Skills

As stated earlier, there are no specific skill sets needed in order to work with children with disabilities. Children are children no matter what their disability status. That said, there are specific counseling modalities that may prove to be more effective with children with special needs, including play therapy, art therapy, and other creative arts therapies such as dance and music. There have been several books written about using play therapy and art therapy with children with disabilities. I would recommend *Creative Play Activities for Children with Disabilities: A Resource Book for Teachers and Parents* by Rappaport-Morris and Schultz (1998), and *Art for All the Children: Approaches to Art Therapy for Children with Disabilities* by Anderson (1992).

CONSULTING WITH PARENTS OF
CHILDREN WITH DISABILITIES

Very seldom will a counselor work only with a child with a disability. Often they will also engage the parents of the child in the counseling process as well. This provides the counselor with a wonderful opportunity to help the child by assisting the parents in dealing with their issues related to raising a child with special needs. Supervisors can help their supervisees understand the pressures that these parents face and assist them in developing ways to help parents cope. Specifically, supervisors can help supervisees gain skills in helping parents examine their biases; in assessing parents' emotions, cognitions, and behaviors with respect to raising their special needs child; and in helping parents gain knowledge and confidence in meeting the needs of their child with a disability. Ironically, supervisors will be assisting counselors in facilitating the same self-assessment process that they themselves went through in supervision with parents, and this is the key to a successful consulting relationship.

It is critical that supervisees understand the stages of the grief cycle that many parents experience when they raise a child with special needs. This cycle ranges from when parents receive the initial diagnosis to when they come to an acceptance of their child's disability (Healey, 1996).

Receiving the Initial Diagnosis

Supervisees need to understand the impact of how the initial diagnosis was relayed to the parent. How the information was relayed sets the stage for how the parent will cope with their child's disability. Often the parent will receive a diagnosis from a medical professional who may or may not be trained to provide this information in a hopeful manner. The following scenarios will better clarify the importance of this issue.

Scenario 1: Dr. Lacks-a-lot

Denise, a mother of two, just had a baby girl in a local hospital. Her baby was immediately transported to a regional teaching hospital before Denise even had a chance to see her. After a brief stay in the hospital, Denise and her husband rush 150 miles to see their baby. All through her stay in the hospital, Denise had been worried sick about what was wrong with her baby. No one at the hospital would give her any straight answers. Upon arrival at the hospital, Denise and her husband demand to see their child. Instead they are ushered to a waiting area where they wait for two and a half hours for the specialist to arrive. Dr. Lacks-a-lot enters the room and proceeds to talk in jargon about the child's condition that Denise and her husband cannot understand. He ends his speech by saying, "I'm not a believer in false hope. The bottom line is that this baby will never smile, never react to you, or even know you are there. With any luck, she won't live very long."

Scenario 2: Dr. Nice-Guy

Denise is allowed to hold her baby immediately after giving birth. It is immediately apparent that there is something seriously wrong with the child. She is covered from head to toe in hair. Her hands and feet are webbed. One ear is not fully formed. The nurse explains that the baby needs to be taken to the regional hospital for diagnosis and treatment by a team of specialists. She reassures Denise and her husband that their daughter will be in the best of hands and that as soon as Denise is physically able, she will be able to join her baby. She tells her not to panic and helps Denise in arranging care for her two small children. When Denise and her husband arrive at the regional hospital, they are immediately taken to the neonatal ICU to see their child. The doctor joins them and explains the diagnosis to them as best he can in layman's terms. He says, "The baby has a very rare condition. I know she looks a bit odd to you right now, but she really is a cute little sweetie with that covering of fur. Now, let me put your mind at rest about some things. We can treat the hirsuteness, or hairiness, with medication and other topical treatments. Her hands and feet can be repaired with cosmetic surgery to a point where you would never know there had been anything wrong. We can fix the appearance of her ear, but she will never have any hearing on that side. That's not that big a deal though; lots of people live full healthy lives with only one good ear. The more difficult news, however, is that she does have some cardiac problems that will require surgery to repair. It will probably require a series of surgeries to get your baby to a completely healthy state. With her condition, however, there is a good chance that she might also experience severe cognitive and developmental delays. In other words, she may not be the perfect child you always imagined, but she is still a beautiful baby who has a great life ahead of her with a family who loves her." Dr. Nice-Guy then gives Denise the number of a woman in Australia whose child has the same disorder. This woman runs a website for families of children with this particular condition, and they get together once a year to exchange notes and provide support for one another. Denise picks up her baby and begins to make cooing sounds at her. She turns to her husband and says, "Isn't she beautiful?"

The previous scenarios illustrate the importance of how the diagnosis is delivered to the parent. Unfortunately, Scenario 1 is a true story of a mother I worked with in counseling. She came to me feeling hopeless. Her husband had left her, and she was feeling guilty and inadequate as a mother. I worked with her to gain knowledge about her child's condition, to establish a bond with her child, to help her get in contact with other parents of children with her child's disorder, and to work through her feelings of guilt and shame. Eventually, she and her husband reunited and when she left counseling, she gave me a family portrait that she had just had professionally taken. Apparently her son and daughter had fought over who was going to hold the beautiful furry baby who sat front and center on Mom's lap in the picture.

Stages in the Grief Cycle

The stages that people go through in the grief process are adaptable for parents of children with disabilities as well (Healey, 1996). In order to illustrate the stages of this cycle in a meaningful way, I will share my experience of when my daughter was diagnosed with Tourette's syndrome when she was eight years old.

Utter Shock!

I was an educational consultant for the Learning Disabilities Association when I attended a day-long conference on working with children with Tourette's syndrome. I can distinctly remember how I became increasingly numb as I listened to the speaker describe the symptoms of Tourette's. I quickly began to recognize that the rapid eye blinking, throat clearing, and scratching behaviors that my daughter engaged in were possible symptoms of Tourette's. My anxiety became worse when the speaker described the obsessive-compulsive features of the disorder and the escalating tantrums that accompany this disorder. Just that morning my daughter had fought with me because her pants were not tight enough (the same pants she had worn two days prior without incident) and that her socks didn't "feel right." Her frustration often escalated to screaming, sobbing, and behaviors that seemed to exceed those warranted by the circumstances. As the day wore on, I became more and more dissociated, and I now recognize this as the first stage in the grief process—shock.

Denial: Not My Child!

I quickly moved into the second stage of the grief process—denial. I went home and convinced myself that I had overreacted to the information presented at the conference. I did not want to think about the possibility that there could be something wrong with my child. As time went on, however, I could not ignore the evidence that was right in front of me as I watched my daughter tic repeatedly. Eventually, I told my husband what I suspected, and he went through his own denial process, basically telling me that I was overreacting and that there was nothing wrong. At this point I decided to seek medical help. I took my daughter to her pediatrician, who referred us to a neurologist who specialized in tic disorders. My daughter was then officially diagnosed with Tourette's syndrome, and all of the denial just slid away.

Guilt: It's My Fault!

With shock and denial out of the way, I now began to feel guilt about the fact that I had not understood my daughter's condition before. What kind of disability specialist cannot see obvious signs of a disorder in her own child? What kind of mother tells her child with tics to "stop blinking so much"? I was filled with self-reproach and blame at this stage.

Shame: Don't Tell Anyone!

At the same time that I was feeling guilty, I was also feeling a great deal of shame. I did not want to let anyone know that my daughter was not perfect. I did not want my boss to doubt my abilities to work with people with disabilities because I was so inept that I could not even see a disability in my own child. I felt like a complete fraud at work, and I eventually quit my job because I felt that I could not possibly help other parents when I couldn't even help myself.

Fear: What If She Gets Picked On?

I next moved into a stage of fear. I could only picture the worst-case scenarios with regard to my daughter. She would tic uncontrollably in school and would be subject to endless ridicule. At this stage, parents often begin to isolate their children in an effort to "protect" them. Their own fear can easily be transmitted to their child at this stage and can stunt the child's emotional growth.

Loss/Sadness: She Will Never Be Normal.

I also felt a huge sense of loss at this point. I pictured her walking down the aisle at her wedding with an uncontrollable tic. Then I reasoned that that would not happen since she would probably never have a date. I grieved the real loss of no longer having the perfectly "normal" child I had once thought I had. Worse yet, I grieved all sorts of potential imaginary losses that were built on my hopes and dreams for my child.

Anger: Why Didn't Someone See This?

I next switched to feelings of anger. Why didn't her teachers see this? Why didn't the doctors diagnose it earlier? Why would God do this to a child? I was particularly angry with myself, and I often took it out on my husband.

Acceptance: She's Still My Baby!

Finally, one day I sat and looked at my daughter playing and realized that she was still the same child she always was. She was smart, beautiful, social, talented, and most of all, happy! I learned to look at my child again from a more realistic perspective. She didn't even know she had a disorder—she was just normal. One day she came home and told me that a boy in her class was telling her to stop blinking her eyes all the time because it was "freaking him out." When I asked how she responded she said, "I told him, they're tics. I can't help it and you're just going to have to live with it." At this point I knew that my baby would be just fine.

Parent Support

I have spent a great deal of time talking about the parents of children with special needs because their reactions have a great impact on how the child copes with their disability. Parents need to come to grips with their reactions to their child's diagnosis before they can begin to help their child. It is important for counselors and their supervisors to understand the grief cycle so that they can assess the messages that a child may be receiving about their disability. If a parent is still in the fear stage, for example, it is likely that the child may be feeling smothered and overprotected. It is important to note that the grief cycle is not linear; it is cyclical. Each new developmental stage may bring a parent back to a previous stage of adjustment to their child's disability. For example, a parent may be doing just fine with his or her child's disability until it comes time to enter kindergarten. If the parent is fearful that the child will be ostracized in school, the child may develop school phobia in response to the parent's fears. Likewise, other developmental rites of passage such as dating or staying overnight at a friend's house may reawaken fears and inadequacies in a parent. A counselor should assess parents in terms of their emotions, cognitions, and behaviors. Throughout the adjustment process parents are likely to feel many differing emotions, and each emotion accompanies a set of thoughts and behaviors.

- Emotion: Fear
- Thought: My child will be hurt
- Behavior: Overprotection

By helping parents come to terms with their child's disability, you ultimately help the child cope.

Helping Parents Reach a Level of Acceptance

Gaining Knowledge

Parents will want to learn as much about their child's disability as they can. In the initial stages they may become overwhelmed by all that they are reading and hearing (Naseef, 2002). A counselor can help parents by encouraging them to take it slow. Supervisors can help their supervisees with this process by knowing what resources are available in their area and helping the supervisee and parents in sifting through all the material available, and then critically evaluating the information. Counselors should also have a thorough understanding of the disability laws such as IDEA, Section 504, and the ADA. Supervisors should help their supervisees to understand a child's rights under the law so they can help families advocate for their children and teach the child to self-advocate.

Gaining Perspective

Counselors should help parents remember that their child is not their disorder (Packer, 1998). This process can be facilitated by helping them rediscover all that they love about their child. Have them introduce you to their child descriptively and/or literally. Counselors should also help parents realize that not all behaviors are directly related to the disability.

Renewing Spirituality/Finding Meaning

It is important for counselors of children with special needs to understand that their child's disability may have shaken the very foundation of a parent's spiritual beliefs. They may ask, "Why me?" They may be angry with God. They may feel that they are being punished for their sins. The counselor should help parents explore their feelings and find meaning in their child's experience.

Finding Support

Often the best thing you can do for a child with a disability is to help their parents find support. This can be done by encouraging parents to engage in parent support groups, to rekindle or develop friendships, to make use of respite care, to enhance their relationship with their spouse, and to engage in Internet support groups.

Helping Others

Many parents of children with disabilities become strong advocates and resources for other parents whose children are newly diagnosed. This helps them find meaning in their child's disability and to give back to their community. The best thing you can do when counseling parents of children with disabilities is to be empathic and just listen. A counselor should let parents feel free to share their secrets with you ("I am ashamed when my son acts like a freak in public") without fear of judgment. It is also important to continually remind them that taking care of themselves *IS* taking care of their child!

CONCLUSION

It is my hope that this chapter has provided supervisors of counselors who work with children with special needs with the tools they need to assist their supervisees in assisting their clients and their families. It is imperative that counselors-in-training, counselors, and their supervisors gain the awareness, knowledge, and skills that they need in order to be effective advocates for their child clients who have disabilities.

REFERENCES

Anderson, F. E. (1992). *Art for all the children: Approaches to art therapy for children with disabilities* (2nd ed.). Springfield, IL: C. C. Thomas.

Autism Society of America. (2005). Autism facts. Retrieved April 1, 2007, from www.autism.org.

Bowen, M. L., & Glenn, E. E. (1998). Counseling interventions for students who have mild disabilities. *Professional School Counseling, 2*, 16–25.

Bradley, C., & Fiorini, J. (1999). Evaluation of counseling practicum: National study of programs accredited by CACREP. *Counselor Education and Supervision, 39*, 110–19.

Brier, N. (1994). Targeted treatment for adjudicated youth with learning disabilities: Effects on recidivism. *Journal of Learning Disabilities, 27*, 215–22.

Children and Adults with Attention Deficit/Hyperactivity Disorder. (2005). The disorder named AD/HD–CHADD Fact Sheet #1. Retrieved April 1, 2007, from www.chadd.org.

Cole, S. (1991). Facing the challenges of sexual abuse in persons with disabilities. In R. P. Marinelli & A. E. Dell Orto, *The psychological and social impact of disability* (3rd ed.). New York: Springer Publishing.

Council for Accreditation of Counseling and Related Educational Programs. (2000). *The 2001 standards.* Alexandria, VA: Council for Accreditation of Counseling and Related Educational Programs.

Duggan, S. H., & Carlson, L. A. (2007). *Critical incidents in counseling children.* Alexandria, VA: American Counseling Association.

Fiorini, J. (2001). An investigation into the school counselor's role with students with learning disabilities. (Doctoral dissertation, Syracuse University, 2001) *Dissertation Abstracts International, 62.* 06A.

Fowler, R., & Tisdale, P. (1992). Special education students as a high-risk group for substance abuse: Teachers' perceptions. *The School Counselor, 40,* 103–8.

Healey, W. (1996). Helping parents deal with the fact that their child has a disability. Retrieved April 1, 2007, from www.ldonline.org/ld_indepth/teaching _techniques/helping_parents.htm.

Helwig, A. A., & Holicky, R. (1994). Substance abuse in persons with disabilities: Treatment considerations. *Journal of Counseling and Development, 72,* 227–33.

Korinek, L., & Prillaman, D. (1992). Counselors and exceptional students: Preparation versus practice. *Counselor Education and Supervision, 32,* 3–11.

Lesbock, M. S., & Deblassie, R. R. (1975). The school counselor's role in special education. *Counselor Education and Supervision, 15,* 128–34.

Livneh, H. (1991). On the origins of negative attitudes toward people with disabilities. In R. P. Marinelli & A. E. Dell Orto. (1999). *The psychological and social impact of disability* (3rd ed.). New York: Springer Publishing.

Lombana, J. H. (1980). Guidance of handicapped students: Counselor in-service needs. *Counselor Education and Supervision, 20,* 269–75.

Lusk, P., & Hartshorne, T. (1985). *Counselor adequacy in special education.* (Report # CG 020 362) ERIC Document Reproduction Service # ED 289 096.

Marinelli, R. P., & Dell Orto, A. E. (1999). *The psychological and social impact of disability* (4th ed.). New York: Springer Publishing.

McBride, H. E., & Siegel, L. S. (1997). Learning disabilities and adolescent suicide. *Journal of Learning Disabilities, 30,* 652–59.

Naseef, R. (2002). Counseling parents of young children with disabilities. Retrieved March 28, 2004 from www.pbrookes.com/email/archive/august02/august 02EC2.htm.

Packer, L. E. (1998). Social and educational resources for patients with Tourette Syndrome. *Neurologic Clinics of North America 1997, 15,* 457–71.

Rappaport-Morris, L., & Schultz, L. (1998). *Creative play activities for children with disabilities: A resource book for teachers and parents.* Champaign, IL: Human Kinetics Publishers.

Sabornie, E. J. (1994). Social-affective characteristics in early adolescents identified as learning disabled and nondisabled. *Learning Disability Quarterly, 17,* 268–79.

Thompson, R., & Littrell, J. M. (1998). Brief counseling for students with learning disabilities. *Professional School Counseling, 2,* 60–67.

Tucker, R., Shepherd, J., & Hurst, J. (1986). Training school counselors to work with students with handicapping conditions. *Counselor Education and Supervision, 26,* 55–60.

U.S. Department of Education, National Center for Education Statistics. (1999). Children 0 to 21 served in federally supported programs for the disabled by type of disability: 1976–77 to 1997–98. *Digest for Educational Statistics 1999.* Washington, DC: U.S. Government Printing Office.

7

⌒⌒⌒

The Supervision Process

Working with Traumatized Children in an Outpatient Mental Health Clinic

Susan Hansen and Judith M. Dagirmanjian

This chapter focuses on the play therapy supervisory process as it pertains to working with traumatized children and families in the authors' outpatient clinic setting. We provide an overview of the treatment setting, population served, child supervision process, and the rationale for the use of play therapy techniques in supervision. We identify dynamics that impact treatment effectiveness and use case examples to illustrate the processes that occur within the supervision relationship, including discharging emotion, reducing psychic defensiveness, and realigning with the self. Play therapy interventions will be described that support the exploration of these three processes.

The clinical supervision process within the field of play therapy is meant to provide a learning environment for processing individual professional struggles so that introspection and insight can support clinical growth. The challenges we all face as clinicians stem from our personal experiences and the interfacing of those experiences with the particular population we serve. Supervision can be a powerful tool to process these challenges and acknowledge the successes that invigorate the clinical work. In addition, focus in supervision is to buffer against the vicarious trauma that often accompanies clinical work with traumatized children.

OUTPATIENT CLINIC SETTING

Outpatient mental health clinics have been established in communities across the United States to serve children and families in need of mental health services. Meeting the needs of these communities has been a daunting task, as current epidemiological studies (Brandenburg, Friedman, & Silver, 1990; Costello, Messner, Bird, Cohen, & Reinherz, 1998; Lavigne et al., 1996; Reinherz, Giaconia, Lefkowitz, Pakiz, & Frost, 1993) estimate that 18 to 22 percent of American children and adolescents suffer from serious difficulty in psychosocial functioning at any given time, and that 5–8 percent of these children have problems severe enough to qualify as a mental illness. . . . These percentages translate into over four million young people in the United States who are currently in need of mental health services and treatment (as cited in Dore, 2005, p. 149).

Despite the vast need for services, "Recent [U.S. Department of Health and Human Services, 1999] figures indicate that only about one in five children who need mental health services actually receive them" (Dore, 2005, p. 19). Needless to say, outpatient clinics have attempted to restructure their settings to meet the specific needs of their communities. The structure of outpatient clinics may vary, but the mission is similar in that outpatient clinics seek to provide therapy services to children and families in the most cost-efficient and effective manner possible within the context of their communities. During the past 20 years, the field of child treatment has grown exponentially in terms of the creation of treatment models designed to address specific mental health issues (Dore, 2005). Given the shifts in the child treatment field, our clinic has worked to develop programs that serve children in the context of their family and within their community. An additional focus of the treatment we provide is on collaborating with the child service system to maintain children within the community setting. Bronfenbrenner (1979) introduced the social-ecology model of human development and provided a greater understanding of how children function within a larger social context, including their family environments, peer groups, schools, and neighborhoods. "Each level of the social ecology plays a key role in some aspects of healthy child development, and as such, may serve an important recovery function when the child is exposed to traumatic stress" (Saxe, Ellis, & Kaplow, 2007, p. 71). As our clinic seeks to provide effective treatment to traumatized children, understanding how children relate to their larger environments and identifying the strengths and weaknesses of those environments are of great importance.

POPULATION: CHILDREN IMPACTED BY TRAUMA

In our clinic setting, the authors serve a disproportionate number of children with histories of trauma. As we studied our child service delivery system in the last several years, we learned that a large percentage of the children referred to our services (anywhere from 50 to 90 percent, depending on the program they were involved in) were struggling with dysregulated, chaotic family systems associated with abuse, neglect, and/or trauma. Despite the fact that, "only about a third of abused and neglected children in clinical settings meet diagnostic criteria for [posttraumatic stress disorder] PTSD" (van der Kolk, 2002, p. 131), many of the children in our clinic struggle with either the full spectrum of PTSD symptoms or a range of emotional and behavioral dysregulation symptoms. We have come to understand that,

> Traumatic stress . . . is about survival-in-the-moment. . . . The survival circuits are the means by which the brain processes stimuli that are potentially life-threatening and translates this perception into life-sustaining responses. In traumatic stress, there are fundamental problems with this type of processing, and responses become highly maladaptive. (Saxe et al., 2007, p. 25)

In addition, a child's attachment history either serves to build resilience through a solid interpersonal connection or serves to become a risk factor for the later difficulties in adapting to environments surrounding that child. "The quality of earliest interpersonal relationships sculpts the brain's survival circuits to make the child more or less able to regulate emotion when faced with a stress" (Saxe et al., 2007, p. 44). In order to understand the impact of abuse and neglect on children's behavior, we must look at their attachment patterns, emotions, and overall functioning capacity. Our clinic continues to explore treatment options to increase the efficacy of our child service system. At the same time, we recognize the need to focus more attention on effectively supporting the clinical staff who are impacted by the trauma experienced by our client population. Play therapy has become fully integrated into our clinic setting as a treatment tool, and its application to the supervision process is a natural progression for further exploration.

DYNAMICS IN CHILD SUPERVISION

"Supervision is viewed as a collaborative effort to which both parties can and do learn from each other. Mutual empathy, particularly around the anxiety-ridden areas of experience, is seen as one of the more important facilitative elements of both supervision and therapy" (Wells, Trad, & Alves, 2003, pp. 21–22).

The supervisor-supervisee relationship is of paramount importance to successful clinical treatment with clients who have experienced trauma. Supervision of child therapy clinicians requires a wide range of skills and a full perspective on the unique issues that child therapists inevitably encounter. Kadushin and Harkness (2002) state, "supervision of psychotherapy with children, from infancy to age 18, is strikingly distinct from supervision of therapy with adults. Child therapy demands different knowledge, evokes intense emotions in supervisees, and requires engagement with many social systems" (as cited in Neill, 2006, p. 7). The child client does not enter into the treatment relationship alone, but rather with the involvement of parents, foster parents, caregivers, and other formal community systems working with the child. This involvement requires great energy on the part of the clinician, as well as sophisticated negotiation skills to remain aligned with all members of the child's "system."

TRANSFERENCE AND COUNTERTRANSFERENCE

An effective supervisory relationship supports the identification of dynamics involved in transference, countertransference, vicarious trauma, parallel process, and cultural issues. These dynamics are at the core of clinical practice as they each relate to the relationships created in the therapeutic process and are the mechanisms through which growth and change occur. Play therapy interventions that support the exploration of these dynamics will be introduced.

The identification of the countertransferential process is particularly complicated when working with children. There is an inherent vulnerability in children who attend therapy that often elicits a sense of increased responsibility on the part of the clinician. An effective supervisor will support the process of identifying this sense of responsibility and managing the countertransference that follows. Janet Mattinson (1975) states that the clinician's "psychological skin needs to be sensitive enough to pick up some of the psychic difficulties of his client but it needs to be firm enough around his own being to be able to distinguish between what belongs to him and what is, in fact, some feeling he has introjected from the client" (as cited in Kahn, 1979, p. 522). Child therapy clinicians must create "psychological skin" to help buffer the impact of the trauma work and to inform them of the difference between the child's experience and the clinician's experience of the treatment. According to Gil and Rubin (2005), "traditional, adult-oriented, verbal therapies for addressing countertransference may not be optimal for those involved in the treatment of children and adolescents, and for those using play therapy in particular, because play therapy is not exclusively dependent on the verbal elements of traditional therapy, that is, discussion, inquiry, and interpretation" (p. 88). Given this, the use of play therapy interventions can be effective in increasing our understanding of the clinician's own countertransference and supporting the processing of feelings and beliefs that accompany working with child clients.

VICARIOUS TRAUMA

Vicarious trauma is another powerful dynamic within the field of child therapy. "Just as trauma alters its victims, therapists who work with victims may find themselves permanently altered by the experience" (McCann & Pearlman, 1990, p. 144). According to McCann & Pearlman (1990), "Persons who work with victims may experience profound psychological effects, effects that can be disruptive and painful for the helper and can persist for months or years after work with the traumatized persons. We term this process, 'vicarious traumatization.'" (p. 133). In addition, McCann & Pearlman (1990) have identified that there can be a "long-term alteration in the therapist's own cognitive schemas, or beliefs, expectations, and assumptions about self and others," (p. 132) when working with survivors of trauma. Play therapy techniques introduced into the supervisory process can support greater insight into the degree to which the clinician is experiencing shifting cognitions based on the therapy work with this vulnerable population.

PARALLEL PROCESS

The parallel process within therapy focuses on the concept that there is a concurrent dynamic occurring within supervision that reflects and shapes the direction of the therapy process itself. "The concept of the parallel process refers to the simultaneous emergence of similar emotional difficulties in the relationship between the social worker and client, social worker and supervisor, and postulates a link between these two relationships, whereby emotions generated in one are acted out in the other" (Kahn, 1979, p. 521). If this is true, then the supervisory relationship is the most important vehicle to support the movement of the therapeutic process. When supervision provides safety, structure, and clarity, the treatment process will follow a similar course. Within clinical practice, the most important aspect of developing a treatment plan is the formulation of a clear conceptualization of the dynamics that create the symptoms leading to the referral for services. When the clinician is able to utilize supervision to filter out her own internal struggles and dynamics, as well as recognize the parallel process, she is more likely to formulate a clear, concise conceptualization. Play therapy interventions can support greater awareness of how the parallel process evolves within the supervisory and therapy relationships.

CULTURAL DIVERSITY

In our clinic setting, there is a commitment to create an environment for staff and clients that recognizes and values the cultural diversity of the population we serve. Cultural differences in race, ethnicity, gender, religious affiliation, and sexual orientation between the organization and its staff, clinicians and their clients, and supervisors and supervisees need to be acknowledged and used to support effective clinical treatment. Although the research on clinical supervision from a cross-cultural perspective is not that extensive, greater attention is being given to deepening our understanding of how the supervisory relationship is impacted by cultural differences between supervisors and supervisees.

Wells et al.'s (2003) relational model of supervision takes into account the importance of both the supervisor and the clinician being aware of their own cultural perspectives, appreciating individual and cultural differences, and being open to understanding the meaning clients attach to events and behaviors. A supervisory structure and process should be created in which the impact on therapy outcomes of culturally influenced values, perceptions, and historical experiences of supervisors, supervisees, and clients can be discussed and explored. The supervisor can support the clinician in identifying differences between the clinician and the client's cultural backgrounds and enhance the clinician's capacity to integrate cultural factors into all aspects of the therapy process. These differences may include culturally based parenting practices, gender roles, behavioral expectations, meanings attached to the trauma, and beliefs around the value of therapy. The supervisor's "sensitivity and perspective is especially critical with trauma survivors who tend to misinterpret their differences as defects and often look to others to interpret their experiences for them" (Wells et al., 2003, p. 22). An inquiry into the impact of cultural factors on assessment, case conceptualization, development of treatment goals, decisions around play therapy interventions, and the therapist's countertransference process can be an enriching experience for the supervisory process.

PLAY THERAPY RATIONALE

Play is a medium that is naturally engaging to children as well as adults. Play builds rapport between children and clinicians, and also facilitates effective treatment. The Association for Play Therapy (2001) defines play therapy as "the systematic use of a theoretical model to establish an interpersonal process wherein trained play therapists use the therapeutic powers of play to help clients prevent or resolve psychosocial difficulties and achieve optimal growth and development" (p. 20). Play is symbolic and metaphoric in nature. "Metaphoric thought can create new meanings by relating images in different ways and suggest new directions for creative action" (Pearce, 1992, p. 155). As clinicians in the play therapy field begin to delineate the specific aspects of effective play therapy, researchers are making progress in conducting more empirically based studies and comprehensive data analyses to determine the clinical utility and efficacy of play (Reddy, Files-Hall, & Schaefer, 2005). A summary follows of the most recent data that is beginning to validate what play therapists have known intuitively for many years.

In 2001, Ray, Bratton, Rhine, & Jones (as cited in Ray, 2006, p. 137) identified the small size inherent in play therapy studies, which results in poor generalizability as particularly challenging for researchers. To address this limitation, Ray (2006) states that psychotherapy has relied on meta-analytic methodology to determine the effectiveness and efficacy of specific treatment models combining results from individual studies in order to produce an overall effect size. In 2006, Ray summarized the two meta-analytic studies (LeBlanc & Ritchie, 1999; Ray, Bratton, Rhine, & Jones, 2001) that examined the effectiveness of play therapy with children. LeBlanc and Ritchie's (1999) meta-analysis included 42 experimental studies comprised of 166 individual outcome measures from 1947 to 1997. In these studies, play therapy resulted in an overall positive effect size of .66 SD, indicating a moderate treatment effect of play therapy with children 12 years and younger. In a later publication (2001), LeBlanc and Ritchie (as cited in Ray, 2006) reported that the benefit of play therapy appears to increase when parents are involved in their child's treatment and the duration of treatment is sustained over time.

Ray (2006) reported that an even larger meta-analysis on play therapy outcomes was conducted by Ray et al. (2001), and further detailed by Bratton, et al. (2005). This meta-analysis was based on data collected from 93 experimental studies, from 1942 to 2000, the results indicated that children receiving play therapy interventions performed .80 SD above children who did not receive play therapy. Like the earlier conclusions, this more recent analysis also correlated parent participation in the treatment and optimal treatment duration with a beneficial treatment effect. Further results also found that, "Play therapy has been demonstrated to improve the self-concepts of children, decrease anxious behaviors, lessen externalizing and internalizing problem behaviors, and increase social adjustment" (Ray, 2006, pp. 152–53).

For the first time, Reddy et al. (2006) bring together in a single text a comprehensive overview of empirically validated play interventions for children. This text adds an important dimension to the play therapy field as agencies are requiring more evidence-based treatment approaches to link effective treatment with funding.

Play therapy can be a powerful intervention for children who have experienced trauma by helping them access, process, and integrate traumatic material in a manner that leads to appropriate resolution. We have come to understand that traumatic events are often stored in a disjointed, dissociated manner, which can impact the ability to recall and retell the story in an accurate, complete format. The emotional components of the event are often not integrated with the more cognitive components of the event, thereby making it difficult for the child or adolescent to verbally communicate about the experience. This same difficulty is not present when one engages a child in play therapy. Play therapy provides an avenue for the child or adolescent to engage in a natural, fulfilling activity while at the same time access unconscious material that otherwise may remain defended against and hidden.

The symptom profile of traumatized children is varied and includes cognitive and perceptual alterations, emotional and behavioral adaptations, as well as physiological, organic changes that all adapt well to the use of play therapy. Play allows a creative process to unfold and is the foundation of future concrete and formal thinking processes that are crucial to a child's development. In our clinic setting we seek to utilize recent trauma theory and play therapy research to inform our clinical practice.

INTEGRATION OF PLAY THERAPY TECHNIQUES INTO THE SUPERVISION PROCESS

As we have learned more about the population we serve, we have also had to re-evaluate the tools we use to support our clinical staff. The beneficial aspects of play realized within the therapy process are also experienced within clinical supervision. We contend that a series of internal processes must be brought forth in the context of supervision. The awareness of these processes, including discharging emotion, reducing psychic defensiveness, and realigning with the self, allows for a greater level of

Table 7.1. Supervisory Processes

Process/Meaning	Allows For
Discharge of Emotions	
Release of intense emotions induced by traumatic material from the client's experience	• Insight into the clinician's own process • Management of countertransference • Awareness of vicarious trauma impact
Reduction of Psychic Defensiveness	
Mitigate resistance through more flexible use of defenses	• Quick entry into the unconscious • Engagement of right-brain, creative processes • Easier access to internal processes • Increased tolerance for feedback
Realignment with the Self	
Clarification of internal experience through heightened awareness of the self	• Increased attunement to self • Groundedness • Centering in the present moment

competency in the clinical work. Increased insight results in clearer conceptualization directing all aspects of the treatment process. We have identified three primary processes, as shown in Table 7.1.

DISCHARGE OF EMOTIONS

Clinicians inevitably experience their own emotions as part of the clinical process. It is imperative that supervisors address with supervisees the impact of expending ongoing and intense emotional energy so they can better understand, validate, and empathize with their client's experience of trauma (McCann & Pearlman, 1990). In supervision, the clinician must be afforded the opportunity to identify issues of countertransference and vicarious trauma as she gains insight into how she is impacted by the clinical process. Intense emotional reactions are a sign that the clinician is struggling to manage the material presented by the client during the therapy session. No trauma clinician is exempt from this experience. This is not a sign of incompetence or weakness, but rather an indicator that supervision is necessary. Clinicians who work in the field of trauma require considerable support from their supervisors around the phenomenon of burn-out, which Wells, et al. (2003) describes as the result of clinicians "over-extending, over-promising, or over-identifying" (p. 33) with their clients. Helping clinicians acknowledge and respect their personal and professional limits, as well as engaging them in frequent discussion around appropriate boundaries, self care, and self protection, is an essential part of mitigating the impact of burn-out.

The following case examples demonstrate how the clinician's feelings and the personal meaning the clinician attaches to the client's experience impact the treatment. The internal experience of the clinician influences treatment decisions, including both the development of the case formulation and who the clinician chooses to involve in the therapy process.

Case Example 1

Angelina, a six-year-old client was referred to Maria, a novice clinician, following disclosure of chronic sexual abuse perpetrated by her stepfather, who has been living in the home for the past two years. Child welfare officials have been notified, and legal activity is under way. Maria describes Angelina as a "beautiful, fragile" child with little capacity to make eye contact or engage verbally, while also conveying a sense of longing for support and connection. Angelina follows prompts to engage in directed activities yet exhibits little initiative and looks to the clinician for continuous approval and guidance. Intermittently she begins to cry and becomes inconsolable, asking to leave the session. In supervision, Maria appears preoccupied with protecting and rescuing Angelina while directing her energy toward blaming Angelina's mother. She attempts to justify her refusal to involve Angelina's mother in any treatment intervention by concluding that the mother is toxic and unable to meet Angelina's needs in any way.

Supervision Overview

During supervision, it became clear that Maria was angry with Angelina's mother for failing to protect her daughter from abuse that occurred over a third of her life. Maria saw Angelina as "beautiful" and special, and she felt invested in protecting this suffering child. As Angelina cried and attempted to leave the session, Maria's feelings of incompetence and hopelessness increased. She wanted to help this child yet felt inadequate and insufficiently trained to do so. Maria focused on the attachment she was attempting to make to Angelina through directive play therapy activities. As Angelina became more symptomatic during sessions, Maria became more verbal to her supervisor about wanting to isolate Angelina from her mother. Maria began to pathologize the mother and unconsciously conveyed judgment. As Maria struggled to help this child, her own feelings of anger and incompetence were projected onto Angelina's mother, and the treatment formulation was tainted by these feelings. Play therapy interventions in supervision were supportive to Maria in helping her gain insight and greater understanding of her countertransferential process.

Supervision Intervention

The supervisor might utilize the following play therapy tools:

- Feelings Imagery:
  - Draw an "image" of how you see Angelina's mother
  - Draw an "image" of yourself as a clinician at this point in time

Both of these drawings would elicit a visual representation of Maria's countertransference and her perception of herself as an effective clinician. According to Rubin (1984), the "therapist can also use her own artwork as an aid to self-understanding, in addition to helping the patient" (p. 58). Gil and Rubin (2005) have suggested the terms "countertransference play" (p. 93) and "countertransference art" (p. 94) and the use of these strategies to increase self-awareness and enhance supervision. Imagery allows for the projection of unconscious material without the pressure of creating a literal depiction of the object. This creative process evokes greater understanding of the clinician's internal experience.

REDUCTION OF PSYCHIC DEFENSIVENESS

Unlike play in the treatment process, play in supervision is focused on specific personal challenges for the clinician. In this way, play in supervision is used to illuminate the clinician's struggle and help the clinician bring forth unconscious material that may be impacting the clinician's capacity to provide a corrective experience for the client. Mishne (1986) has stated that, "Defense is a term used to describe struggles of the ego, unconsciously employed, to protect the self against perceived danger. The threat of recognition or conscious awareness of repressed wishes or impulses causes anxiety and guilt and must be avoided" (p. 348). As material is presented in therapy, clinicians are vulnerable to utilize defenses to attempt to ward off a variety of impulses and emotions. Similar to play in therapy, play in supervision has the potential to lower the resistance of the clinician by connecting the clinician to her internal process in a nonthreatening manner. Unconscious material can be brought to the surface with less effort as play and art elicit conflicts that might otherwise be more challenging for the clinician to verbally admit, have insight into, or tolerate.

The following case example illustrates how a clinician's inability to tolerate a child's anger activates her defenses and interferes with her ability to conceptualize the case. The clinician's failure to place the child's behavior within a context and explore its etiology renders her ineffective.

Case Example 2

Kathy, a clinician, has little empathy for a an eight-year-old boy, Luke, who exhibits externalizing, violent behaviors including head banging, biting, and hitting. In session, Luke recently directed his aggressive impulses toward Kathy by throwing a chair across the play therapy room. He has intermittently engaged in these externalized, aggressive behaviors since the age of five following his removal from his parents' custody after disclosing physical abuse by both parents. He is now in his fourth foster home after several foster placement disruptions due to uncontrollable behavior. Kathy has resorted to pathologizing him in her supervision and has little belief in the Luke's capacity to change.

Supervision Overview

As Kathy discussed this case, it became evident to her supervisor that she lacked a conceptual understanding of the dynamics leading to Luke's externalization of problematic behaviors. Kathy had been unable to capture the etiology of Luke's behavior, and instead resorted to blaming him for the intolerable expression of his rage. As the supervisor became attuned to this dynamic, Kathy increased the intensity and rigidity of her responses and projected this blame onto the supervisor as well. Through the use of play therapy interventions, the supervisor engaged Kathy in a nonverbal representation of this internal conflict. This experience allowed her to reduce defensiveness, identify her own triggers, and connect to underlying personal issues that she might have had difficulty exploring in a conscious way.

Supervision Intervention

The supervisor might utilize the following play therapy tools:

- Defense Imagery:
  - Draw an image of a person standing guard over a fortress. Represent the fortress and all the individuals and objects in the fortress. Be careful to include all people and things that might need to be within the confines of the fortress.

This play therapy tool is similar to Gil and Rubin's (2005) directive approach to countertransference art, in which the supervisor may request that the clinician draw a troubling session or one in which feeling remnants are left behind. The use of metaphor and symbolism provides a measure of distance from the unconscious conflict thereby allowing easier access to the defended material.

- Boundary Representation:
  - Within a sand tray, create two distinct representations. Divide the representations with a physical barrier from available materials. In one portion of the tray, create an image of yourself, and in the other portion, represent the world around you.

This tool will help assess the permeability of the clinician's boundaries to generate constructive dialogue between supervisor and supervisee. It is important to utilize supervision as a way of continuously monitoring the impact of the clinical work on the clinician.

SELF-ATTUNEMENT/REALIGNMENT WITH "THE SELF"

A clinician's ability to be truly present and "in the moment" as she works to engage and treat a child is of paramount importance. In order to maintain a clear, focused presence, the clinician must monitor her own sense of attunement and alignment with the "self" in order to make the necessary connection to her child client. Attunement may best be expressed as a communication "dance" in which the clinician and the client attempt to read the cues of one another and respond based on the understanding of those cues. Of course, the more attuned one is to oneself, the more attuned one can be to others. Siegel (1999) describes the concept of attunement with reference to children as follows, "the developing mind uses the states of an attachment figure in order to help organize the functioning of its own states. . . . The sensitivity to signals and attunement between child and parent, or between patient and therapist, involves the intermittent alignment of states of mind" (p. 70). As clinicians become more attuned to themselves and to the cues of their child clients, they become more effective change agents.

The process of becoming more connected to the self and thereby enhancing attunement with the client is supported by the use of the creative process. Winnicott (1971) stated, "It is in playing and only in playing that the individual child or adult is able to be creative and to use the whole personality, and it is only in being creative that the individual discovers the self" (p. 54). For Winnicott, the search for the self could only be successful if creativity were present.

The following case example demonstrates the need for the clinician to be grounded and attuned to herself and her clients. Therapy requires the clinician to understand her own internal experience as she seeks to help support enhanced functioning in others.

Case Example 3

A school social worker refers Cameron for therapy to an outpatient clinic after discovering her in the girl's locker room in the act of cutting. After the initial school-based crisis assessment, it was determined she did not require hospitalization. In the first outpatient session with Dan, her clinician, Cameron is mute and physically agitated. She stares off into the corner of the room and does not respond to direct questions. Dan continues to request details regarding the incident at school, what precipitated this self-injurious behavior, and information about her history of cutting. As he attempts to delve further, Cameron becomes even less responsive. In supervision, Dan makes the case that Cameron's needs cannot be met at the outpatient level since she is incapable of engaging in verbal dialogue with him around her self-injurious behavior.

Supervision Overview

In supervision, a novice supervisor identified that a parallel process was occurring between her and Dan as she realized her own hesitation around assigning such a "risky" case to Dan. The supervisor's own internal process and anxiety around supervising a high-risk case had prevented her from attuning to Dan's needs. The supervisor realized that safety had not been created and, therefore, Dan had been unable to learn and enhance his skills around attunement to his client. The parallel process of misalignment had led Dan to focus on gathering facts and trying to "get Cameron to talk" rather than helping her engage. It was clear that just as Cameron was disconnected from her own experiences and had difficulty remaining grounded, Dan and his supervisor were also not attuned to themselves or to one another. Play therapy interventions were used to help Dan build skills to attune to himself and become grounded when he was triggered by a client's intense emotion or trauma history. The supervisor was able to help Dan communicate a need for increased safety in the supervisory relationship.

Supervision Intervention

The supervisor might utilize the following play therapy tools:

- Attune to the Environment
  - Sit in silence and notice the environment. Identify five sensory experiences noticed within the room by naming sounds, sensations, or thoughts.
- Sand Environment

○ Create an environment in the sand that depicts a safe space where attunement can occur. Include all objects necessary to support this image.
• Attunement Visualization
  ○ Create an internal representation of an environment that depicts attunement. Include all objects or images that symbolize all required elements. Once completed, draw this image to create an externalized representation.

These tools will support greater insight into the clinician's level of attunement and facilitate a dialogue between supervisor and supervisee to enhance safety within the supervision.

GROUP THERAPY SUPERVISION SEMINAR

The supervision processes discussed within this chapter are specific to individual supervisory relationships. Nearly all discussion in the field of supervision focuses on the effective use of the individual supervisor-supervisee relationship. However, the authors believe a group therapy supervision seminar is a valuable, adjunctive resource for play therapists. Despite its value, it is not a substitute for individual supervision. In a group supervision model, several clinicians participate in a forum, which provides education about play therapy, as well as a safe process in which all participants can experience play therapy for themselves. This forum has the potential to be a powerful tool to provide supervision to a number of people together and gather the wealth of experience among all those involved. A group supervision model offers clinicians an opportunity to share case conceptualizations, provide and receive feedback, expand thinking around possible interventions, manage vicarious trauma, and experience first hand the power of play as a treatment modality.

CONCLUSION

This chapter has focused on the utilization of play therapy interventions in supervision of child therapy clinicians working in an outpatient clinic setting. We have identified dynamics and internal processes that impact treatment effectiveness and provided case examples to illustrate how play therapy can support professional growth and personal insight. We believe that more attention is needed in the study of how the supervision process can be enhanced through the use of play. As we have learned more about the efficacy of play in child trauma treatment, the next logical area of exploration is how play can enhance supervision. This chapter has outlined a way to apply play therapy interventions and deepen the clinician's awareness of internal experiences that influence all aspects of treatment.

REFERENCES

Association for Play Therapy. (2001, June). Play therapy. *Association for Play Therapy newsletter, 20,* 20.

Brandenburg, N. A., Friendman, R. M., & Silver, S. E. (1990). The epidemiology of childhood psychiatric disorders: Prevalence findings from recent studies. *Journal of the American Academy of Child and Adolescent Psychiatry, 29,* 76–83.

Bratton, S. C., Ray, D., Rhine, T., & Jones, L. (2005). The efficacy of play therapy with children: A meta-analytic review of treatment outcomes. *Professional Psychology, 36*(4), 376–90.

Bronfenbrenner, U. (1979). *The ecology of human development.* Cambridge, MA: Harvard University Press.

Costello, E. J., Messer, S. C., Bird, H. R., Cohen, P., & Reinherz, H. Z. (1998). The prevalence of serious emotional disturbance: A re-analysis of community studies. *Journal of Child and Family Studies, 7*(4), 411–32.

Dore, M. M. (2005). Child and adolescent mental health. In G. P. Mallon & P. M. Hess (Eds.), *Child welfare for the twenty-first century* (148–72). New York: Columbia University Press.

Gil, E., & Rubin, L. (2005). Countertransference play: Informing and enhancing therapist self-awareness through play. *International Journal of Play Therapy, 14*(2), 87–102.

Kadushin, A., & Harkness, D. (2002). *Supervision in social work.* New York: Columbia University Press.

Kahn, E. M. (1979). The parallel process in social work treatment and supervision. *Social Casework: The Journal of Contemporary Social Work, 60*(9), 520–28.

Lavigne, J. V., Gibbons, R. D., Christoffel, K. K., Arend, R., Rosenbaum, D., & Binns, H. (1996). Prevalence rates and correlates of psychiatric disorders among preschool children. *Journal of the American Academy of Child and Adolescent Psychiatry, 35,* 204–14.

LeBlanc, M., & Ritchie, M. (1999). Predictors of play therapy outcomes. *International Journal of Play Therapy, 8*(2), 19–34.

Mattison, J. (1975). *Reflection process in casework supervision.* Research Publications Service.

McCann, L. & Pearlman, L. A. (1990). Vicarious traumatization: A framework for understanding the psychological effects of working with victims. *Journal of Traumatic Stress, 3*(1), 131–49.

Mishne, J. M. (1986). *Clinical work with adolescents.* New York: Free Press.

Neill, T. K. (2006). *Helping others help children: Clinical supervision of child psychotherapy.* Washington, DC: American Psychological Association.

Pearce, J. C. (1992). *Evolution's end: Claiming the potential of our intelligence*. San Francisco: HarperCollins Publishers.

Ray, D. C. (2006). Evidence-based play therapy. In C. E. Schaefer & H. G. Madison (Eds.), *Contemporary play therapy: Theory, research and practice* (136–57). New York: Guilford Press.

Ray, D., Bratton, S., Rhine, T., & Jones, L. (2001). The effectiveness of play therapy: Responding to the critics. *International Journal of Play Therapy, 10*(1), 85–108.

Reddy, L. A., Files-Hall, T. M., & Schaefer, C. (2005). Announcing empirically based play interventions for children. In L. A. Reddy, T. M. Files-Hall, & C. E. Schaeffer (Eds.), *Empirically based play interventions for children*. Washington, DC: American Psychological Association.

Reinherz, H. Z., Giaconia, R. M., Lefkowitz, E. S., Pakiz, B., & Frost, A. K. (1993). Prevalence of psychiatric disorders in community population of older adolescents. *Journal of American Academy of Child and Adolescent Psychiatry, 32,* 369–77.

Rubin, J. A. (1984). *The art of art therapy*. New York: Brunner/Mazel, Inc.

Saxe, G. N., Ellis, B. H., & Kaplow, J. B. (2007). *Collaborative treatment of traumatized children and teens: The trauma systems therapy approach*. New York: The Guilford Press.

Siegel, D. J. (1999). *The developing mind: Toward a neurobiology of interpersonal experience*. New York: The Guilford Press.

van der Kolk, B. A. (2002). Assessment and treatment of complex PTSD. In R. Yehuda (Ed.), *Treating trauma survivors with PTSD* (127–56). Washington, DC: American Psychiatric Publishing, Inc.

Webb, N. B. (1989). Supervision of child therapy: Analyzing therapeutic impasses and monitoring countertransference. *The Clinical Supervisor, 7*(4), 61–76.

Wells, M., Trad, A., & Alves, M. (2003) Training beginning supervisors working with new trauma therapists: A relational model of supervision. *Journal of College Student Psychotherapy, 17*(3), 19–39.

Winnicott, D. W. (1971). *Playing and reality*. London: Routledge Publications.

8

❦

Supervision of Play Therapists Working with Aggressive Children

David A. Crenshaw

Working with aggressive children in the play therapy room tends to be one of the most vexing and often anxiety-producing challenges faced by play therapists. Children with variable, tenuous impulse controls and deficient affect regulation skills are easily triggered into episodes that can quickly escalate and spin out of control. Probably no other challenge a play therapist faces, with the possible exception of sexualized behavior in the playroom, depends on the play therapist's ability to stay centered, calm, and firmly able to establish limits quickly. If the play therapist is anxious, frightened, or angered by the child's threatening behavior, the situation can be ignited as explosively as throwing fuel on a fire.

APPRECIATING COMPLEXITY IN UNDERSTANDING THE AGGRESSION OF CHILDREN

Effective play therapy intervention with young aggressive children needs to be grounded in a solid understanding of the vast developmental and developmental psychopathology literature that identifies the multiple and interacting determinants of childhood aggression. The play therapist needs to appreciate the complexity of etiological factors and not be quick to pounce on single determinants that often lead to inadequate treatment planning. Like heart disease, childhood aggression does not have a single cause. Rather it is a result of a complex interaction between

129

genetic, biological (including molecular and neurobiological factors), psychological, family, social, and cultural influences.

Gender differences are also important. Substantial gender differences in the prevalence of physical aggression are observed at seventeen months of age, with 5 percent of boys but only 1 percent of girls manifesting physically aggressive behaviors on a frequent basis (Baillargeon, Zoccolillo, Keenan, et al., 2007). The quality of attachment that children experience with parenting figures is a contributing factor. In six-year-old children, boys with disorganized attachment and children with ambivalent attachment reported a higher level of externalizing problems than did secure children (Moss, Smolla, Guerra, et al., 2006). Interestingly, these same researchers found that disorganized attached children also reported a higher level of internalizing problems than secure children. Severe marital conflict and harsh maternal parenting have been found to be direct pathways linking to child aggressive-disruptive behavior at home and school (Erath and Bierman, 2006).

In a study that shows that fathers do matter, it was found that father support was a key factor in mitigating aggression in the preschool classroom among Asian children (Ang, 2006). This finding adds to a gradually expanding research base documenting the benefits of fatherly support across various cross-cultural settings.

Adding to the complex threads of the tapestry influencing aggressive behavior in children is the finding that a behaviorally uninhibited temperament, callous-unemotional features, and harsh parenting have been associated with specific patterns of aggressive behavior in older children and adolescents (Kimonis, Frick, Boris, et al., 2006). Another study of preschool boys found that boys with hyperactive behavior problems showed higher rates of aggressive, noncompliant, nonsocial behaviors and lower rates of prosocial behavior and peer acceptance than boys in the comparison group (Keown and Woodward, 2006). Cumulative risk factors are crucial in influencing aggression in children. Studies at the Research Institute for Addictions in Buffalo, New York, reveal that children in families with high cumulative risk scores—reflective of high parental depression, antisocial behavior, negative affect during play, difficult child temperament, marital conflict, fathers' limited education, and hours spent in child care—had higher levels of aggression at 18 months than children in low-risk families (Edwards, Eiden, Colder, & Leonard, 2006). These associations were moderated by child gender. Boys had higher levels of aggressive behavior at all ages than girls, regardless of group status.

Empathy is perhaps the most important of pro-social skills, and it plays an especially crucial role with respect to moderating the development of aggression in children. When children in kindergarten and first grade were studied, the results indicated that as compared to low-empathic peers, more empathic children were reported to exhibit greater prosocial behavior and less aggression and social withdrawal (Findlay, Girardi, & Coplan, 2006). Adding still more layers of complexity, in a study of extremely aggressive children with a minimum of two years' history of this behavior, a link between the serotonin transporter (5-HTT) gene and childhood aggression was found (Beitchman, Baldassarra, Mik, et al., 2006). The investigators noted that this is the first study to report a significant association between the 5-HTTLPR gene and childhood aggression.

In another important study, cocaine exposure, male gender, and a high-risk environment were all predictive of aggressive behavior at five years (Bendersky, Bennett, and Lewis, 2006). These researchers observed that the group of boys exposed to high environmental risk is most likely to show continued aggression over time.

Keep in mind that the above is not a comprehensive literature review. On the contrary it only covers a few of the most recent studies on aggression in children, but the brief review points to the multiplicity of factors contributing to the aggression that play therapists see in the playroom. It is important to remember, as Jerome Kagan (1998) emphasized in a lecture at the 1998 Psychotherapy Networker Conference in Washington, DC, entitled, "How We Become Who We Are," that even the most aggressive children are not aggressive all the time. We can't really talk about aggressive behavior in children without the context and the specifiers. Some children are aggressive at school but not at home or vice versa. Some children attack their siblings but not other children. The context is very important and needs to be spelled out.

Sociocultural influences are difficult to study in psychological laboratories or to use with randomized controlled experiments, yet these are crucial influences on the development of aggression in some children. Growing up in extreme poverty and suffering devaluation due to class, race, gender, or heterosexual bias, or exposure to violence, crime, or abuse, especially on a chronic basis, can inflict deep wounds on the psyche (Crenshaw & Hardy, 2005; Crenshaw & Garbarino, 2007; Crenshaw & Mordock, 2005a; Crenshaw & Mordock, 2005b; Crenshaw & Mordock, 2007; Garbarino, 1995, 1999; Hardy & Laszloffy, 2005). Sociocultural trauma arguably is the least studied of all forms of trauma impacting children. The wounds to the soul of the child caused by the assaults on his or her dignity lead inevitably to both profound sorrow and rage. Kenneth Dodge (2006) at Duke University has studied the social maps that aggressive children develop as a result of their exposure to the world and their early experience. It only makes sense for children to develop maps that adults are reliable and to be trusted if children have been treated in a loving and caring manner. If that is not their experience, their social maps will develop accordingly: "people are not to be trusted"; "hurt before they hurt you."

Many of the children encountered in play therapy who display aggressive behavior have developed such social maps early on as a means of survival.

A CASE STUDY IN HUMILITY

In our work with aggressive children of wounded spirit, we are taught lessons in humility every day. Sometimes we think we really understand a child, only to find out that there is so much more we need to appreciate. Carlos is a good example. I was supervising a doctoral psychology intern who was working with Carlos. One day in the classroom, his teacher turned around and thought he noticed that Carlos had thrown an eraser at another child. His teacher reprimanded Carlos, who immediately protested that he didn't do it. Certainly, such denials and insistence that the child has been wrongly accused are commonplace, but what was different about this situation, was the intensity of Carlos's reaction. He quickly escalated to the point that it was necessary to remove him from the classroom and take him to the crisis room, while all during this time Carlos was yelling at the top of his lungs: "You don't believe me!" "You don't believe me!" Most of the well-intentioned teaching and crisis intervention staff who intervened with Carlos at the time of the incident assumed it was just another case of a kid erupting in rage without any reasonable provocation. These assumptions, however, can block the path to a deeper understanding of a child like Carlos.

Over a period of time while following up this incident, the astute and persistent intern was eventually able through empathic listening to enable Carlos to tell his story. It was a lesson in humility that the intern and I will never forget. It taught us in a dramatic way about the triggering of trauma and trauma re-enactment. Carlos, who was ten at the time, was able to tell his therapist that shortly after he was born in Haiti, his mother gave him to a friend to take care of him temporarily, but his mother never came back. Carlos was raised by the woman who was his mother's friend, but whom he thought was his mother. When he was eight years old his biological mother showed up one day at his elementary school with a lawyer and all the proper legal papers confirming that she was the mother of the child and insisted that Carlos leave with her. Carlos protested because he didn't know this woman and fought vigorously as he was dragged kicking and screaming into the mother's car, all the while shouting, "You don't believe me!" "She is not my mother!"

Within a few days he and his biological mother were on a plane headed for the United States, and he never saw again the woman who had raised him—the woman whom he thought was his mother. We should never presume we know what drives the aggressive behavior of children. How many stories like Carlos might there be that kids have not been able to tell us? We don't always take the time to listen, probe, and explore for the real reasons they behave the way they do. The social maps that Carlos had developed made sense in terms of his unique life experiences. It was absolutely vital that adults believe him because his not being believed at a moment of desperate pleading is etched in his mind and memory vividly. Shortly after reaching the United States, he ran away from his biological mother's house and was placed in the foster care system, and when he ran away from several of his foster homes, he was eventually placed at our residential treatment center. I will never forget Carlos and the valuable lesson that he taught. There is always so much more to see and hear if we are willing to look and listen deeply.

ASSESSMENT OF THE SUPERVISORY RELATIONSHIP

While a therapeutic relationship is not the same as a supervisory relationship, the quality of relationship between supervisor and supervisee is as critical as it is in a therapeutic relationship for the experience to be productive. Assessment of the quality of the relationship needs to be a collaborative process. The supervisor and the play therapist supervisee should be equally free to explore concerns about issues related to comfort, openness of communication, goals of the supervision, the supervision process and content, the roles of each, and methods of formal evaluation. The latter issues need to be spelled out explicitly in the beginning of the supervision and need to be reviewed and updated as the supervision proceeds.

Supervisors will of course bring their own individual style to the supervisory relationship, and each supervisee will likewise enter into the collaborative relationship with their idiosyncratic gifts, qualities, strengths, and weaknesses. In my work I always place great importance on the safety of the supervisory relationship established by clear boundaries, expectations, support, and empathy that enables the supervisee to feel safe in "not knowing." If the trainee feels they must hide what they don't know, this will greatly constrain their learning opportunities. I believe that establishing such a supervisory climate is just as important as establishing a "safe place" in therapy (Havens, 1989). In no way does such emphasis on creating a warm, safe supervisory climate preclude a challenging style of supervision. In fact, it makes it more likely that such challenging supervision will be conducive to learning because the foundation of trust and openness in communication has already been established.

ISSUES OF COUNTERTRANSFERENCE

Conflicts about Limit Setting

In work with aggressive children, perhaps one of the most crucial capacities in the therapist is the ability to set limits when needed in a calm, firm, decisive, but nonpunitive manner. When done so in this manner, most children prone to aggressive acting-out respond and even welcome the adult taking charge because it reduces their anxiety. If they feel that the adult is not strong and competent enough to set limits or maintain structure and safety in the playroom, their anxiety escalates and often their behavior spirals out of control. Some play therapists have a natural, calm, and confident way of setting and maintaining needed limits in the playroom, and others struggle, usually related to unresolved conflicts and issues related to discipline in their original families. The origin of such conflicts is a matter clearly to be taken up in their personal therapy, but skills in setting the necessary limits to maintain safety and a sense of security with the therapist is an important focus of supervision for play therapists working with children who act out aggressively or in a sexualized manner in the playroom. Some therapists allow the child to escalate too far before imposing limits. Others overcompensate by too quickly imposing limits and stifling children's opportunities to work with anger in their play dramas for fear it will get out of control. The child senses the therapist's anxiety about this issue, and this in turn increases the child's anxiety and creates a vicious circle.

Projective Communication

The work with an aggressive child is fraught with potential countertransference land mines that can be stepped on even when the therapist is deeply committed to helping the child. Aggressive kids are provocative, sometimes threatening, occasionally dangerous and violent, and love to push the envelope and relentlessly test limits and the therapist. One of the most important insights that I learned from my years of psychoanalytic supervision with the late Walter Bonime, MD, senior training psychoanalyst at New York Medical College, is that no matter how frustrated, discouraged, angry, hopeless, or impotent the therapist is, it can't begin to match the depth of the same feelings in the child.

The superlative clinical work at the Tavistock Clinic in London with severely deprived and aggressive children in the early 1980s culminated in a book (Boston & Szur, 1983) based on seminars at the clinic. It focused on how to help such challenging children in therapy. These clinicians described the important phenomenon of *projective communication*. They defined countertransference as a term that refers to the response of a therapist who is receptive to the transferred feelings of the patient that can therefore be used in understanding the patient's state of mind. In psychoanalytic writings, countertransference often refers only to the therapist's inappropriate responses to the patient, i.e., those that are connected with the therapist's own private preoccupations and are not related to the patient at all (pp. 133–34).

These psychoanalytic clinicians in the tradition of the British Object Relations School, which included Bion, Winnicott, and Klein, used the concept of projective communication to gain a portal of entry into the child's inner world that could only be revealed by projecting the unbearable feelings onto the therapist. By examining the emotional impact of such projections and "containing" them rather than responding in personal ways (reflecting instead of reacting) to the child's provocative and often aggressive behavior, therapists were able to gain valuable insight into the deeper roots driving the aggressive acting-out behavior of the child.

Even experienced teachers, childcare workers, and therapists on occasion react in a personal or even retaliatory way to a child's aggression because these children in spite of our best intentions are highly skilled "at drawing blood." Whether working with these children as a play therapist, a teacher, a social worker, or childcare worker, there is no more valuable time that can be spent than in examining one's feelings and reactions and to do it often, preferably in the context of a supportive supervisory relationship. This is the most valuable of all therapeutic activities. (Freud is reported to have engaged in such self-examination every day when he had finished seeing his patients.) Unfortunately for most therapists, it does not receive the time and attention it deserves because of the pressure to deliver clinical services at a pace that mitigates against such quiet reflection, adequate supervision, or frequent consultation with colleagues. Those play therapists that do have ready access to regular and dependable supervision with someone experienced and skilled in play therapy are quite fortunate.

THE INVISIBLE WOUNDS OF THE THERAPIST

Therapists working with highly wounded children, manifested often in aggression and rage toward the therapist, may well be carrying invisible emotional wounds of their own. Therapists are not exempt from the quirks, unresolved grief, and sometimes trauma issues that plague other human beings. Therapists can be wounded as well as their clients. It is incumbent, however, on the therapist to undertake their own healing prior to attempting to heal others. The emotional demands on the therapist working with aggressive children are great, and the more severe the aggression, the more taxing it can be. As a result, therapists need to commit to their own therapy, to work toward resolving issues that would otherwise leave them vulnerable if the invisible wounds of the child were to trigger the invisible wounds of the therapist. The secret of healing the wounds of aggressive children is embedded in the ability to be committed to these children whole-heartedly without hinging one's own self-worth or self-definition on what comes back either negative or positive. One moment they may scream at you that they "hate your guts," and the next moment ask you if you will take them home and adopt them. Neither should unhinge the balanced, grounded, and seasoned therapist who views both the extreme negative and the undying professions of love as stemming from the emotional deprivation that many of these children have suffered.

EMOTIONAL AVAILABILITY WITHOUT LOSS OF OBJECTIVITY

I once supervised a very bright and empathic young clinician who worked in our residential treatment program. She told me one day that when she first began the work with the children in the treatment center, she read their life histories. She confronted the descriptions of the horrifying events that many had suffered in their young lives, and she was deeply emotionally moved. She found these stories extremely painful to absorb. This clinician said to me after working in the program for a year that she was distressed because when she read these stories and confronted the traumatic events in their life histories, she no longer had the strong emotional reaction that she did in the beginning. She felt she had "hardened" her emotional responsiveness not as a conscious choice, but as an adaptation to encountering this degree of horror and trauma in the lives of the children. She expressed worry to me that this would make her less emotionally available to the children when they were ready to tell their stories.

This young clinician eloquently described the challenge facing people who work with children who have been severely abused and traumatized. Our emotional responsiveness is absolutely essential in order for us to be a healing instrument in the lives of these children. But every clinician and direct care worker has his or her limits. They can easily reach the place where they rightly feel that they just can't hear one more horror story. This is where balance in our lives becomes essential.

Commitment to life-long learning is critical. I have made it a practice throughout my career to seek out regular supervision from a clinician that I deeply respect and still do so today after 38 years in the field. I also believe that for someone doing this work, their own personal therapy is extremely helpful, as previously stated. I think a therapist who avails him or herself of personal therapy will be able to more easily work with the reactions stirred up in him or her and reduce the chance that this will create problems in the therapeutic relationship. Each helper will need to find the right combination that keeps them emotionally alive and energized and still able to find the work rewarding. Balance is essential since the work otherwise can be emotionally depleting. We need to cherish our family and personal relationships; exercise, nutrition, and rest are all important. Doing fun things, being playful, nourishing a sense of humor, cultivating a wide range of interests, and finding creative outlets are all ways to assist in achieving such vital balance.

PLAYFUL TOOLS IN SUPERVISION OF PLAY THERAPISTS

The Heartfelt Feelings Strategy

Gil and Rubin's (2005) descriptions of some excellent play, drawing, and symbol strategies in dealing with countertransference issues have inspired me to develop similar tools. The *heartfelt feelings strategy* (HFS) builds on the work of other clinicians who have developed similar strategies most notably (Goodyear-Brown, 2002; Kaduson, personal communication, 2006; Lowenstein, 2006; Riviere, 2005). Many other therapists, including play, sandplay, and art therapists, have for many years used the heart shape in a variety of ways for therapeutic purposes. Some of these other approaches are spelled out in detail in previous writing (Crenshaw, 2006a) and are beyond the scope of this chapter. The feature of the HFS that most distinguishes it from all the other similar strategies using the heart shape in play, art, sandplay, and family therapy is that in both the HFS (Crenshaw, 2006a) and the heartfelt feelings coloring card strategy (HFCCS) (Crenshaw, 2006a), I emphasize two core domains: the expressive and the relational. The expressive component offers structured therapeutic practice in identifying, labeling, and expressing feelings—a key skill in affect regulation and for developing social competence. Schore (1994; 2003a; 2003b) has demonstrated that affect dysregulation is central to nearly all forms of psychopathology, so therapeutic interventions that address this crucial deficit will have wide application across the psychodiagnostic spectrum.

The relational component consists of structured exploration of the heartfelt feelings in connection with key attachment figures and other important persons in children's interpersonal world. Obviously our most heartfelt emotions do not develop in a vacuum. They develop in a relational context. Our most strongly felt emotions tend to be elicited in relation to the key attachment figures in our lives. Witness the outpouring of some of the most intense emotions human beings are capable of displaying when an attachment bond is broken, such as in separation or divorce or, in the case of a child, abandonment by or death of a parent. In the HFS the relational is accomplished in two ways. Typically, I ask the children to color the heart in relation to a very specific relational issue, such as, "Color in the heart according to how you felt when Daddy got mad and left the house last night." The second way this is emphasized in the HFS is in the list of follow-up questions. Some of the questions are related to the Expressive (E) component such as, "Which feeling was the strongest?" Or "What feeling is the hardest for you to express?" Another group of follow-up questions, however, are specifically focused on Relational (R) issues such as, "Who in the family would agree with your choice of the emotion that is expressed the least in the family?" or, "What emotion is most uncomfortable for you to express, and who else in the family is uncomfortable expressing that same emotion?" The social context is critical. In the HFCCS the cards are divided into two succinct sets, the expressive and the relational, to once again emphasize these two key components.

The HFS is a tool that can be used in supervision to explore countertransference feelings and issues. The typical way that I use it in supervision is in relation to difficult cases, often with aggressive children and noncompliant families. I ask the therapist I am supervising to color in the heart by picking a color for each feeling in proportion to the strength of that feeling in relation to feelings about the therapy with that particular child or family. The tool can be used as an ongoing self-monitoring process at the beginning, and in middle stages and then again toward the end of therapy, or it can be employed when the therapist feels "stuck" or when either therapist or supervisor notes a disproportionate emotional response to the client. Often therapist supervisees are astonished when they apportion their feelings according to intensity of such feelings and sometimes are surprised by an emotion they depict in the heart of which they were not previously aware. This can lead to useful reflection, a meaningful exchange with the supervisor, and in some cases becomes "grist for the mill" in their personal therapy. If, for example, anger predominates in their depiction of their heartfelt feelings and in exploring what evokes such anger in working with this child, they discover that the trigger is the child's refusal to expose any vulnerability or dependency needs, it may lead the therapist, in personal therapy, to explore the need to be needed by the child. Many young and inexperienced therapists fall prey to the need to prove their adequacy and skills as a beginning therapist and become enraged when the child does not cooperate or make progress. This can become a self-reinforcing disruptive process since the pressure the therapist feels to prove their competence is experienced by the child and interferes with the natural pace that is healing for the client.

The Heartfelt Feelings Coloring Cards Strategy

The HFCCS is a variation of the HFS. The HFCCS uses greeting cards in child therapy with the heart shape on the cover of the card and instructions on the inside of the card divided into two main categories: expressive and relational. The various therapeutic strategies describing the instructions for using these cards are spelled out in detail in a therapy manual (Crenshaw, 2006a). For the purposes of exploring countertransference issues, however, a strategy that I have found useful entails using the relational cards and asking the supervisee to draw an image in the heart on the card that comes to mind when they think of their most troubling therapy case; more often than not it is an aggressive child who is always testing limits or provokes anxiety and anguish in the therapist. The image could be anything that comes to mind for the therapist, but in some cases it is a picture of the child or the child and the therapist in some kind of struggle with each other. In one case, the image drawn by the therapist was of her pushing a heavy rock up a hill, expressing her exhaustion and utter frustration in her efforts to help a seven-year-old boy who made a practice of thwarting her efforts. In the latter instance it became clear that the image of pushing the heavy rock up the hill was related to far more than her frustration with this particular child. It was related to depression she had been battling, and this image was the jumpstart she needed to seek her own therapy to address her mood disorder. The next step with the HFCCS relational cards is to write a note on the inside of the card (produced in the form of greeting cards) to the child or the family. Sometimes I alter the instructions and ask them to write a note to the supervisor summarizing their feelings as symbolized in the image they drew within the heart.

Like with the HFS, the HFCCS is a tool to enrich the dialogue between supervisor and supervisee about countertransference issues that arise in therapy with children, but particularly may be useful when treating aggressive children since the therapy with these youngsters is often fraught with anxiety and can place an emotional strain on the therapist. Several of the therapists that I have used the HFS and HFCCS with in supervision have continued to use it as a self-monitoring tool in working with their own reactions in therapy with a wide variety of clinical cases.

The Symbol Association Therapy Strategies

My most recent work, inspired by Gil's (2003) use of the individual play genogram, is with the therapeutic use of symbols. The background and development of the symbol association therapy strategies (SATS) is described elsewhere (Crenshaw, 2006b). For the purposes of working with countertransference issues in supervision with particular application to play therapy with aggressive children, I have developed a special variation of the

SATS. As with the HFS and HFCCS, the SATS has an expressive and a relational component. The expressive component consists of evocative words that have been shown in a range of empirical studies in experimental psychology, particularly in the study of cognition, perception, and memory to have either negative or positive emotional valence. In other words they are emotionally significant or evocative as compared to neutral words. In the expressive strategies of the SATS the client is instructed to pick from a collection of miniatures (symbols) the best match for each of the seventy-five evocative word categories. This tool combines the evocative power of image or symbol with the empirically determined emotional significance of these particular words. Thirty-seven of them have negative and thirty-eight have a positive emotional valence. In the relational component of these strategies the client does a symbol-sorting task with relational categories that encompass the three primary relational domains of the child's life: family, school, and peers. These strategies, like so much of my recent work, are designed with the modest goal of creating a portal of entry to access the inner world of the child. Like Hughes (2006), I don't believe we can afford to ignore either the inner life of the child nor the child's relational world. Creating dialogue focused on these central aspects of the child's inner and relational world is the focus of all three of the above groups of strategies. None of these strategies are intended to be a stand-alone approach to therapy but rather can be integrated into a wide range of therapy and theoretical orientations.

The specific application that I have developed to deal with countertransference issues and other issues in supervision entails the use of a symbol-sorting task with the word categories as given in Figure 8.1.

The four word categories are printed on laminated category boards and are included in the SATS KIT and placed in front of the supervisee. The supervisee is then invited to select from a collection of miniatures the symbols they wish to place on each of the categories to represent their work with a particular child, family, and supervisor, as well as select one or more symbols to represent the self as therapist.

Sandplay therapists have long used symbols and appreciated their therapeutic application based on Jungian theories (Jung, 1960) and the pioneering work of Lowenfeld (1939; 1979) and Kalff (1971; 1980). I have admired greatly the work of contemporary sandplay therapists such as Allen (1988), Carey (1998), DeDomenico, (1999) and Green (2004; 2006) to name just a few. But I did not fully appreciate the therapeutic power of symbol until I was introduced to Gil's work with the Individual Play Genogram (2003) and Gil and Rubin's (2005) use of various play strategies in the examination of countertransference issues in play therapy. Having been trained (Bonime, 1962; 1989) in a culturalist psychoanalytic tradition,

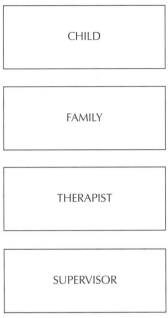

Figure 8.1.   Word Categories for the Symbol-Sorting Task.

I do not approach the meaning of symbols in the way that is typical of Jungian-trained therapists. I approach it rather in a collaborative way with the client with no assumptions about universal or collective meaning of the symbols (Crenshaw, 2006a). When the supervisee has accomplished the symbol-sorting task above, it is laid out in front of both the supervisor and supervisee and together in a collaborative process they can pursue the meaning it has for that particular supervisee. The supervisee can use this same tool to self-monitor and self-examine their therapeutic reactions with any of their ongoing cases if they so choose.

CONCLUSION

Children aggressively acting out in the playroom typically place great strain on the play therapist. The issues of danger, threat, safety, and possible damage to the therapeutic relationship all are fraught with anxiety for the therapist, particularly those relatively inexperienced with this population. The art of limit setting with aggressive children in the playroom is one of the most important skills to learn in supervision and is typically not taught in graduate courses. Many children prone to aggressive behavior have been repeatedly judged and viewed as simply "bad kids," and many believe it themselves. Often they test therapists to see whether they can make them give up on them like many adults in their lives already. They do not know how to handle warm, tender, and caring feelings, and these can be just as disorganizing to the child as rage. The mindset of the therapist is a crucial healing ingredient. In order for the play therapist to approach these children who often are viewed as unlikable with a compassionate therapeutic attitude, it is essential that the play therapist have an appreciation and understanding of the complexities of the etiology of aggression in children. Otherwise they may unwittingly further the devaluing and stigmatizing process of simply viewing these kids as "bad."

Some of the key countertransference issues in working with aggressive children are outlined and discussed in this chapter. The use of play and symbol activities, along with drawing and symbol strategies, to explore countertransference issues and the relationship between the supervisee and supervisor can be useful in the supervision process. Perhaps the most important effort we can make in preparing to work with the aggressive acting out of children is the work we do with ourselves.

REFERENCES

Allen, J. (1988). *Inscapes of the child's world: Jungian counseling in schools and clinics.* Dallas: Spring Publications.

Ang, R. P. (2006). Fathers do matter: Evidence from an Asian school-based aggressive sample. *American Journal of Family Therapy, 34,* 79–93.

Baillargeon, R. H., Zoccolillo, M., Keenan, K., Côté, S., et al. (2007). Gender differences in physical aggression: A prospective population-based survey of children before and after 2 years of age. *Developmental Psychology, 43,* 13–26.

Beitchman, J. H., Baldassarra, L., Mik, H., De Luca, V., et al. (2006). Serotonin transporter polymorphisms and persistent, pervasive childhood aggression. *American Journal of Psychiatry, 163,* 1103–5.

Bendersky, M., Bennett, D., & Lewis, M. (2006). Aggression at age 5 as a function of prenatal exposure to cocaine, gender, and environmental risk. *Journal of Pediatric Psychology, 31,* 71–84.

Bonime, W. (1962). *The clinical use of dreams.* New York: Basic Books.

Bonime, W. (1989). *Collaborative psychoanalysis: Anxiety, depression, dreams, and personality change.* Rutherford, NJ: Fairleigh Dickinson Press.

Boston, M., & Szur, R. (Eds.). (1983). *Psychotherapy with severely deprived children.* London: Routledge & Kegan Paul.

Carey, L. (1998). *Sand play therapy with children and families.* Northvale, NJ: Jason Aronson.

Crenshaw, D. A. (2006a). *The heartfelt feelings strategies.* Rhinebeck, NY: Rhinebeck Child and Family Center Publications.

Crenshaw, D. A. (2006a). *Healing paths to a child's soul.* Lanham, MD: Jason Aronson.

Crenshaw, D. A. (2007a). Heartfelt feelings. *Play Therapy: Magazine of the British Association of Play Therapists, 48,* 12–17.

Crenshaw, D. A. (2007b). *Heartfelt feelings coloring card series (HFCCS) clinical manual.* Rhinebeck, NY: Rhinebeck Child and Family Center Publications.

Crenshaw, D. A. & Garbarino, J. (2007). The hidden dimensions: Profound sorrow and buried human potential in violent youth. *Journal of Humanistic Psychology, 47,* 160–74.

Crenshaw, D.A. & Hardy, K. V. (2005). Understanding and treating the aggression of traumatized children in out-of-home care. In N. Boyd-Webb, (Ed.), *Working with traumatized youth in child welfare* (171–95). New York: Guilford.

Crenshaw, D. A. & Mordock, J. M. (2005a). *A handbook of play therapy with aggressive children.* Lanham, MD: Rowman & Littlefield.

Crenshaw, D. A. & Mordock, J. M. (2005b). *Understanding and treating the aggression of children: Fawns in gorilla suits.* Lanham, MD: Rowman & Littlefield.

Crenshaw, D. A. & Mordock, J. M. (2007). Lessons learned from "fawns in gorilla suits." *Residential Treatment for Children and Youth, 22*(4), 33–47.

DeDomenico, G. (1999). Group sand tray-worldplay: New dimensions in sandplay therapy. In D. Sweeney & L. Homeyer (Eds.), *The handbook of group play therapy: How to do it, how it works, whom it's best for* (215–33). San Francisco: Jossey-Bass Publishers.

Dodge, K. A. (2006). Translational science in action: Hostile attributional style and the development of aggressive behavior problems. *Development and Psychopathology, 18,* 791–814.

Edwards, E. P., Eiden, R. D., Colder, C., & Leonard, K. E. (2006). The development of aggression in 18 to 48 month old children of alcoholic parents. *Journal of Abnormal Child Psychology, 34,* 409–23.

Erath, S. A., & Bierman, K. L. (2006). Aggressive marital conflict, maternal harsh punishment, and child aggressive-disruptive behavior: Evidence for direct and mediated relations. *Journal of Family Psychology, 20,* 217–26.

Findlay, L. C., Girardi, A., & Coplan, R. J. (2006). Links between empathy, social behavior, and social understanding in early childhood. *Early Childhood Research Quarterly, 21,* 347–59.

Garbarino, J. (1995). *Raising children in socially toxic environments.* San Francisco: Jossey-Bass.

———. (1999). *Lost boys: Why our sons turn violent and how we can save them.* New York: Anchor Books.

Gil, E. (2003). Play genograms. In C. F. Sori and L. L. Hecker (Eds.), *The therapist's notebook for children and adolescents: Homework, handouts, and activities for use in psychotherapy* (49–56). New York: Haworth Press.

Gil, E., & Rubin, L. (2005). Countertransference play: Informing and enhancing therapist self-awareness through play. *Journal of Play Therapy, 14,* 87–102.

Goodyear-Brown, P. (2002). *Digging for buried treasure.* Antioch, TN: P. Goodyear-Brown.

Green, E. J. (2004). Activating the self-healing archetype: Spontaneous drawings with children affected by sexual abuse. *Association for Play Therapy Newsletter, 23,* 19–20.

Green, E. J. (2006). Jungian play therapy: Activating the self-healing archetype in children affected by sexual abuse. *Louisiana Journal of Counseling, 8,* 1–11.

Hardy, K. V., & Laszloffy, T. (2005). *Teens who hurt: Clinical interventions to break the cycle of adolescent violence.* New York: Guilford Press.

Havens, L. (1989). *A safe place.* Cambridge, MA: Harvard University Press.

Hughes, D. A. (2006). *Building the bonds of attachment: Awakening love in deeply troubled children* (2nd ed.). Lanham, MD: Jason Aronson.

Jung, C. G. (1960). *Man and his symbols.* New York: Dell.

Kagan, J. (1998, March). How we become who we are. A presentation at the 1998 Psychotherapy Networker Symposium. Washington, DC.

Kalff, D. M. (1971). *Sandplay: A mirror of the psyche.* San Francisco: Browser Press.

Kalff, D. M. (1980). *Sandplay: A psychotherapeutic approach to the psyche.* Boston: Siglo Press.

Keown, L. J., & Woodward, L. J. (2006). Preschool boys with pervasive hyperactivity: Early peer functioning and mother-child relationship influences. *Social Development, 15,* 23–45.

Kimonis, E. R., Frick, P. J., Boris, N. W., Smyke, A. T., et al. (2006). Callous-unemotional features, behavioral inhibition, and parenting: Independent predictors of aggression in a high-risk preschool sample. *Journal of Child and Family Studies, 15,* 745–56.

Lowenfeld, M. (1939). The world pictures of children: A method of recording and studying them. *British Journal of Medical Psychology, 18,* 65–101.

Lowenfeld, M. (1979). *The World Technique.* London: George Allen and Unwin.

Lowenstein, L. (2006). *Creative interventions for bereaved children.* Toronto: Champion Press.

Moss, E., Smolla, N., Guerra, I., Mazzarello, T., et al. (2006). Attachment and self-reported internalizing and externalizing behavior problems in a school period. *Canadian Journal of Behavioural Science, 38,* 142–57.

Riviere, S. (2005). Play therapy to engage adolescents. In L. Gallo-Lopez & C. E. Schaefer (Eds.) *Play therapy with adolescents* (121–42). Lanham, MD: Rowman & Littlefield.

Schore, A. N. (1994). *Affect regulation and the origin of the self: The neurobiology of emotional development.* Hillsdale, NJ: Erlbaum.

Schore, A. N. (2003a). *Affect dysregulation and disorders of the self.* New York: Norton.

Schore, A. N. (2003b). *Affect regulation and the repair of the self.* New York: Norton.

RESOURCES

The Heartfelt Feelings Coloring Cards for the HFCCS can be obtained from the Coloring Card Company: www.coloringcardcompany.com. Telephone 908-237-2500 or e-mail@coloringcardcompany.com.

The SATS Basic Symbol Kit can be obtained from The Self Esteem Shop (www.self esteemshop.com/). Telephone 800-251-8336.

9

⌀

Supervising Filial Therapy

Louise Guerney

Since the essence of filial therapy (FT) is the employment of parents or other adults significant in the lives of child clients (e.g., foster parents, teachers) to serve as play therapists for the children, filial therapists themselves are responsible not only for instructing the parents in child-centered play therapy (CCPT)—the model of play therapy used in FT—but also for providing ongoing supervision of the parents' play sessions. The filial therapist also assumes responsibility for the conduct of the FT group, whatever its nature, a family, or an assembly of several families. (Private practitioners most often see one parent or one couple with their one or two children rather than working with a group.) So the work of the filial therapist is multidimensional and demanding as well as very rewarding.

A higher level of supervision is also required for filial therapists. Filial therapists must receive supervision of their execution of the method by more experienced practitioners of FT. The FT supervisor must provide feedback and processing on three dimensions—conduct of the session, instruction of parents, and the supervision provided to parents. The supervisor of the filial therapist must be very mindful of his or her relationship with the supervisee and their respective roles. In the next sections, I will discuss the details of these multilevel supervision processes, starting with the FT supervision of parents themselves. In order to make clear the context of the supervision of parents, I will give some description of the way in which they are trained to serve as therapists for their children.

INSTRUCTION IN CHILD-CENTERED PLAY THERAPY

The method of play therapy taught to parents is traditional CCPT, classical Axline (1969). At the time of the intake when FT is recommended, the rationale for CCPT and why it would be expected to be helpful for a child are presented. Once the FT sessions begin, the filial therapist reviews this information and explains the principles of CCPT play.

For the next few sessions, depending on the number of children included, parents observe play sessions conducted by the filial therapist and have ample opportunity to ask questions about why the therapist responds as he or she does. They also ask about the responses of their children. The therapist provides the appropriate labels for the responses used in the session and relates them to the child's behavior. Responses are woven into the broader principles so that parents can see how both relate.

Teaching parents new ways to relate to their children, even though they understand that the play session task is a limited, therapeutic one and not a new way to parent 24 hours a day, does create some dissonance for them. This must be addressed at the emotional level as well as the cognitive. The filial therapist must express empathy toward the parents' feelings about these issues. The empathic responses take priority over the instructive or cognitive responses at all times. Generally, the pattern is to deal first with the feelings behind the issue raised, then move on to information or whatever else would apply at the cognitive level (Andronico, Fidler, Guerney, & Guerney, 1967; Guerney & Stover, 1971).

Case Example

A mother has observed her child playing with the therapist for the first time. The child has said very little but has asked for a few directions.

Mother: He seemed kind of uncomfortable in there. Why wouldn't you get him started on something instead of just waiting for him to do it? He asked you what he should do.

Therapist: You are not sure that it was really the most helpful way to go. I said, "You are really not sure what you'd like to do in here right now. You are thinking it might be easier if I told you what to do. (Pause) In this special playtime, you are the one who gets to decide what you will do."

Therapist (switching now to instruction): That would be reflecting his feelings and then providing some structuring; which tells him again that this is his time to decide what to do. Remember, we always reflect the feelings *first*. Then we add any information or rule we need to tell the filial children.

Mother: But suppose he is too unsure what to do. Maybe he needs a little start and that would get him going.

Therapist: You are worried that a child might really get stuck and you and the child would *stay* uncomfortable. Then that would really be unpleasant for everybody.

Mother: Sure, he would expect me to give him a suggestion. That is what I would do at home.

Therapist: It's kind of strange not doing the same things you would normally do for you and your child. You're not sure how that will feel. It might feel too strange.

Mother: It might.

Therapist (sensing parent is finishing up becomes more instructive): This is a special time, with very different conditions from home, which your child already recognized. He just doesn't know what they mean for him yet. This situation is geared to give the child every opportunity possible for self-expression, to lead the way in the direction that his feelings and thoughts lead him. It is from going in his direction that he can work out his feelings and positive changes can take place. That is what this therapy is based on. If *we* lead the way, as we so often must in real life, the child loses that opportunity. It might be a little uncomfortable for him at first, and most of all YOU too, but it will pay off in terms of the child gaining a sense of self-competence and not needing to resist doing what you tell him to do, as he now does at home. He has a set time every week to take charge when it is appropriate. It does seem to work out that way for most families. He did get started eventually. I expect that the next time, it will be a lot easier for him. It was also a new situation with the observation booth and everything.

In addition to observing play sessions with their children, parents learn the skills of the play therapist by role-playing with the therapist and each other and enact mock play sessions before they attempt to play therapeutically with their own children.

PARENT PLAY SESSIONS

At this point in the FT process, the filial therapist's supervisory skills are most exercised. There are two phases to the parents' play session component: Phase one: labeled parent practice or demonstration sessions held at the treatment site. Phase two: sessions held at their homes.

Phase One

These are the first sessions (usually two) when the parents play directly face-to-face with their own children. The practice with play therapy skills has not been in live demonstrations except for mock play sessions with adults.

This phase brings a lot of performance anxiety for parents, particularly if they are not being seen individually. The therapist must be a super keen observer of both child and parent responses in the play session, an expert at providing empirically oriented feedback, and a master of reinforcement "for all things great and small" that parents do that are related positively to the model. The therapist must bear in mind that first attempts are likely to be minimal and adjust feedback accordingly. Reinforcement is lavish without exceeding boundaries of genuineness. There is no parent too sophisticated or too lacking in self-esteem to accept positive reinforcement for even weak performances. Fortunately, the identification that the therapist feels with the parents' struggles to master the methods, and the parents' delight and their children's delight with the experience, makes it easier for the therapist to enjoy the experience with the parent, even when corrective feedback is also in order. In FT, we use a three-step system of giving feedback. First, a positive feedback statement is made. Next, corrective feedback is given if needed (for beginning parents it is nearly always needed), and the third step is the strongest of the positive feedback statements that can be genuinely given. This has the effect of leaving the supervisee with a general feeling of success even though corrective feedback may have been necessary. The corrective feedback is always in terms of what behavior would be better to use next time and never personalized, for example, how the supervisee should think or feel. This system of reinforcement, coupled with great attention to their feelings, leaves parents feeling that each practice has been a step in the right direction.

Over the years, we have worked out methods of ameliorating parent anxiety about this beginning phase. These sessions are shorter than later sessions. If a parent says, "I really don't think I could play 15 minutes" (the usual demonstration session length), we will shorten it to 10. We will also allow the most hesitant group member to be the last in the group to play. Our stance is that without the parent feeling up to the task, we do not help the child. Of course, we ascertain through empathic exchanges with the parents how much adjustment they really require versus simply experiencing the normal performance jitters.

To the author's knowledge, there have been no issues of countertransference between FT therapists and parents. The educational format, with the emphasis on empathizing with the parents, and the support to make the process one that permits the pace to be within the parents' management seems to prevent this. Group members relate comfortably to each other. The groups are really like small classes with the focus on the children, unless parents want to have some attention on themselves in processing the concepts and feelings. Parents also learn to emulate the filial therapist in empathizing and become extremely supportive of each other. These constructive attitudes between group and leader permit energy to be expended totally on the work of therapy with the children and the positive benefits that has for parents (Andronico et al., 1967).

Phase Two

The second phase of parent play sessions follows the demonstration sessions and usually does not entail as much detailed feedback on technique of conducting the play session. Home sessions are now being held in the typical FT program. Private practitioners sometimes do not have parents conduct play sessions at home but prefer to have the parents play in their offices as the main agenda of the therapy session, followed by feedback and processing.

Home Play Sessions

When home sessions are held, the format of the filial meeting with the therapist changes. Time is needed for short structured reports on the home sessions and/or the showing of a tape or a DVD made of the home play session by the parent, as is often more common today. These are all seen by those present and processed. Because the therapy session is now held outside of the therapy site, attention more naturally turns to the world outside and there is more discussion of things at home in addition to the home therapy session. All of this is responded to in the same empathic and instructive style used throughout FT.

Demonstration sessions continue to be held at the treatment site so that the filial therapist can monitor the parents' continuing use of the CCPT skills and the behavior of the child. Comparisons are frequently made between the play of the child in the treatment site demonstration sessions and those held at home, since they sometimes follow different themes. If both parents or two other adults from the same family are playing with one or more children, comparison of the pairings are made and discussed. These differences may have significance for the adults. Deep feelings may emerge at these points, and the filial therapist may for a short time become a therapist to one or more of the adults.

Case Example

> *Mother:* When she plays with her father, she always wants to play a nice constructive game and just have a lot of fun. When she plays with me, she plays out angry people—puppets or dolls or something—and never seems to want to play something nice. Is she mad at me? Does she blame me for her problems? At home, she is nasty to us both as well as to her brother. I could see how she can change in the play session but why not with me too?

Therapist: It is distressing to see your daughter behaving in a pleasant way with her father, a way you'd like her to be, and not playing the same nice way with you. You can't help but wonder why.

Mother: Yes, she used to be a "daddy's girl" when she was little, but she isn't anymore. I think that it all goes back to the birth of her little brother. I think she never got over having to share us with him. But we try so hard to treat her so that she feels special. She's our little girl. And all of that. And sometimes I actually feel guilty that we don't give enough to her brother. He's so much easier going. It's just easier to pay more attention to her because she makes so much of everything.

Therapist: The patterns that you see in family life still persist in spite of the play sessions. You see some positive movement when she plays with her dad but not in your play sessions. She still seems to be on the warpath when she plays with you. You would like to see it being more even and, of course, to see some change at home.

Mother: Yes, I know now that I am not such a bad mother, but she is still mad with a capital M.

Other group member, Mrs. Y: It's probably good that she is working out her anger in the play session. I'll bet she'll start being less annoyed with you in real life after a few more sessions just like my Julie has done.

Therapist: Susie may need more time to work out her feelings with you, Mrs. X, than with your husband. She couldn't find a better way to do it than in the play session. Do you think that that could happen as it did with Mrs. Y and Julie?

Mother: Well, I'm not giving up hope. We didn't get anywhere with a behavioral program, and I do think she is actually a little better at home. I just feel really bad that she chooses me to keep up her nastiness with.

Therapist: So it is perhaps not such a bleak picture overall. You feel you can hang in there. You would just feel much better about it if she did not express so much anger when she played with you.

Mother: Yeah. I think that is it.

Therapist: Children take different lengths of time to work out their angry feelings in play therapy. As we see in the group, it is very variable. And interestingly, they sometimes work them out differently with one adult compared to the other. I would dare say that if she had only one parent to play with her that she would be continuing to be angry with whichever parent it happened to be. She has some anger in her, and it is going to need to be worked out. Her pleasant side is there too. Why she chooses to display that with her dad, we will not know. That is not important here, although very interesting. We deal here with what we see and how that is affecting the child and the parent, and we don't worry too much about why. Ours is a "here and now approach" as we have mentioned a number of times before when you all have wondered about how your children developed some behavior in real life or in play. We deal with interactions we observe, and that is the most productive. We will see how it goes. If Susie does not get past the angry phase for many more sessions, we will then need to re-evaluate.

In instances such as that described above, the filial therapist does not spend a lot of time on the parent's personal concerns, not because they are not important, but because they are not the primary items on the FT agenda. If passing attention such as that just illustrated would not be sufficient for the parent's expressed emotional needs, the therapist would invite the parent to have a private talk with him/her at a different time. Or if the filial therapist were not a personal, adult counselor as well as a play therapist, he or she would see that a connection with a counselor were made. FT focuses on parents' feelings to facilitate the process of learning and providing play sessions for the children and enhancing the parent-child relationship and not on personal therapy. This is important for therapists to remember and a place where the supervisor of the filial therapist frequently needs to provide redirection. It would be very easy for a counseling professional to be drawn into a lengthy discussion about the above mother's possible feelings of rivalry with her husband about the daughter's feelings and perhaps about broader issues and feelings about her own competence in comparison with her husband, Electra complexes, and so forth. This could turn into personal therapy that might be of great benefit but is a side track for FT. Studies have shown that parents make gains in personal adjustment without this type of personal therapy as a result of conducting FT in the way it is being described here (Guerney & Stover, 1971).

FILIAL THERAPIST'S SUPERVISORY ROLE IN FINAL STAGES OF FILIAL THERAPY

Home sessions usually continue for six to ten weeks. The focus continues to shift more and more from the play session per se in most cases to life in the family and the outside environment. Discussion and instruction, always with empathic understanding, are conducted with the parents in relation to appropriate transfer of CCPT skills to situations outside the play room. Empathic responding, limit setting, and structuring skills are directly transferable, and extensive discussions and practice, role-playing, and other forms of instruction are needed here to help parents in making these transfers. The filial therapist must continue using both dynamic and didactic skills but, by this time, parents are generally quite open to the concepts and are looking for help in application and offering fewer challenges.

In a group, other members join in with the filial therapist so that there is general group support for this task.

Management of a group can become the most challenging task for the filial therapist at this time since nearly everyone wants to talk and has stories to relate. Keeping opportunities for fair time distribution among all willing participants becomes a challenge, and the FT supervisor often can be helpful in monitoring this process and providing assistance in helping the filial therapist with an overzealous or overconsuming parent.

DVDs of the parent meetings are extremely valuable for supervision purposes. No filial therapist can remember the flow of conversation or the details of exchanges with such accuracy that all nuances of possible significance in group interaction can be observed and remembered. We encouraged FT therapists to watch these for their own education and self-supervision. We like to watch recordings of FT sessions together with the filial therapist when providing supervision and stop the recording at points we or the therapist consider important to discuss.

THE SUPERVISING FILIAL THERAPIST

As can be seen from the above description of the magnitude of the task of the filial therapist, the supervising filial therapist is indeed a *super*visor of a really high order. This role requires a background of understanding and experience in CCPT and FT. In supervising groups, it is extremely helpful if the supervisor has had experience in working with adults in group formats. Actually, adult education backgrounds are more useful than ones in group therapy, since the group goals do not include therapy of individuals or the dynamics of individuals relating to other co-group members. It is learning in a group, with a focus on feelings in order to help facilitate mastery of the play therapy, they are attempting to offer their children and, along the way, to gain insight into their relationship with their children. Parents are the primary providers. They are family members, participants in a family service delivery model, partnering with a professional who values what they will offer and tries to make the process intellectually and emotionally manageable for them. A teaching orientation on the part of the FT proves much more compatible with this model. Those who have prepared for teaching at any level and expanded their education with counseling skills more easily step into this role. However, psychologists (all of the original developers are psychologists, social workers, and other mental health professionals) are quite able to learn and perform as first-rate FT supervisors after experience with the model and a lot of feedback from someone more experienced.

Tasks of the Supervising Filial Therapist

The FT supervisor focuses on the filial therapist when observing a live or recorded session. Feedback is given on all therapist responses and the context in which they were made. If time becomes limited, only those sections that offered a challenge or were deemed less appropriate by the supervisor need to be discussed. The supervisor should be looking for patterns that fall short of the standard and help the filial therapist devise better ways of dealing with such situations. The supervisor of the therapist follows the three-step feedback pattern used with the parents and deals with them empathically, should any issues be expressed. Instruction can also be offered in a mini-exchange like a role-play if the supervisor and therapist think that would serve as an example for another similar situation that would be likely to occur in the future.

The tone of the FT supervisor and filial therapist meeting is always collegial. If there is any disagreement about what actually took place with a parent, the supervisor defers to the filial therapist, on the grounds that he or she was on the actual scene, which does always provide a few more cues than can be observed even on a good DVD or videotape.

The most common failing of filial therapists to which the supervising FT must attend is providing instruction to parents about demonstration play sessions in too much detail. Only the most salient points should be dealt with at one time, until ultimately the finer points have been covered.

First, group time management can be a problem if time is not divided to meet the needs of individual group members so that some are left with less time available to them than would be desirable.

Second, getting drawn too deeply into personal issues of parents that are not related in a clear way to their ability to relate to their child or to conduct a quality therapeutic play session can be problematic. It is easy when parents seem anxious about an issue of some sort, like a conflict with an adult family member not involved in FT, to provide therapeutic responses much longer than the FT model really is structured to do. If this happens in a group, it is especially inappropriate because other group members are not involved and can tolerate this kind of exchange for a limited time only. But, the primary reason for not allowing parents' personal issues to take over the agenda is that the goal of shepherding the parent through the FT process is disrupted. At such times, it can happen that even play sessions at the treatment site are given short shrift. The child's needs are the focus, and the parent as service deliverer rather than client is the first item on the FT agenda. We all know that such therapeutic discussions can be great help to a parent, maybe even critical, but the context of an educationally oriented, child-focused program is not the time and place for it. The FT therapist has to monitor this carefully and know when such issues need to be referred to another time.

Third, the absolutely most common error is forgetting to first deal with feelings in a meaningful way before moving on to an instructive point. It seems that the filial therapist is so eager to have the parents learn the skills that they jump into addressing the skill issue, overlooking the underlying feeling issue that should always be dealt with first, even if the feeling is only a minor one, e.g., confusion. Supervisors frequently role-play these instances as a corrective re-run of the scenario. However, they are in turn very careful to deal with the feelings of the therapist in the process of reviewing and suggesting improved ways for future sessions. The model in FT is to have the pattern of empathically oriented instruction carried up and down the hierarchy. It parallels what parents are doing for their children in the play session (sans the instruction component in CCPT). The filial therapist aims to address parent feelings along with instructional content, and the supervisor does the same. It is this element that reduces countertransference at all levels. Even with the supervision of the filial therapists, it is at almost zero. If one is genuinely empathic with a supervisee, it is difficult to create negative reactions.

There was a group a few years back that "ganged up on me"—they had obviously gotten together when I wasn't present to bring up the subject. The elected spokesperson said, "There is one thing wrong. You never tell us what we are doing wrong. We feel we ought to know."

The gentle tone of the corrective feedback nested between the two positive feedback segments covered up the perception that they were wrong. The wording, which always follows this pattern, is very effective in helping supervisees modify behavior without generating a feeling that they have made mistakes—certainty not things that would make them "wrong doers."

Case Example

> *Therapist to mother:* Mary, that was really a fun session. Billy had a great time blowing those bubbles and tossing them all over the room, even on you a few times. You were laughing with him and seemed to enjoy it too.
>
> *Mother:* I didn't know what to do when he wanted to blow them into my face. I know they don't burn, but I just didn't like the idea.
>
> *Therapist:* It makes it hard to deal with the child's feelings when you are not sure of your own. Now that you are removed from the pressure of the moment, how do you wish you had responded? Do you think that you would be more comfortable if you set a limit on bubbles in your face?
>
> *Mother:* Well, I guess I would, but I don't like to have too many limits. After all, it really doesn't hurt anything.

Therapist: You want to be free and easy but you are not really sure you can come across as sincere about it.

Mother: That is it. If I am wincing and turning away, he will know I am really not liking it and maybe he'll do it more, just to get my dander up. You know how he is.

Therapist: You can see that if you are not truly "with him," which we have talked a lot about being important in this kind of special play, that it might show and awaken other feelings, not the friendly ones the play started with.

Mother: Yes, that could happen, and I think does happen at home sometimes.

Therapist: You know that "double messages can be confusing" and even annoying so you would like to avoid those.

Therapist: So, how do you think you might want to handle it if it came up again? Do you think your feelings could be different a different day? We want to be with the child and also not violate our own feelings since it will probably be picked up by the child if we do.

Mother: I think I would set a limit if I am feeling uncomfortable.

Therapist: And to play the old song again: What feeling message would you give to Billy first?

Mother: Billy, it's a lot of fun blowing those bubbles in my face. That is the one place where I really feel that I can't let you blow them.

Therapist: Great. You reflected his feeling and made it clear what the limit would be. You have really sorted out this conflict very well. You know now where you want to go, how to get there, and you see how sending two messages at once to Billy can have a negative effect on his behavior other places too. Excellent!

Mother: Yes, it was more fun than previous sessions. I wasn't sure what to do before. It made me a little nervous.

The filial therapist supervisor can work with a single therapist or up to three or four therapists, depending on time and circumstances. When working with multiple therapists, because of time restrictions, the therapist supervisor usually asks therapists to select for showing areas that were troubleshot, especially illustrative of some point, or examples of something that was especially successful—generally a parent breakthrough in conducting a play session or in expressing an insight in the discussion.

Generally, it is helpful to look at some videotape footage, or at least have the therapist explain the preceding and following sequence after the section observed. In this way, the supervisor gets the complete circle of events and their effects on all involved.

Filial Supervisors' Contribution to the Process

Case Example

An experienced FT supervisor was supervising a competent filial therapist who was conducting a FT group with a mother in it who could not
get along with her 10-year-old daughter. They constantly fought, and the
daughter was quite negativistic. This greatly disturbed the mother because the child had been adopted because, after bearing two boys, the
mother really wanted a girl and went to a great deal of trouble and expense to adopt her. Nothing was supposed to be wrong; it should have
been the way she dreamed of it being. The mother learned to conduct adequate play sessions but frequently had a problem setting and enforcing
limits. This seemed to be due more to denial that limits were in order than
because she did not understand the rules that were part of a CCPT session. In one session, the daughter threw a bean bag at the mother's head.
In denial, the mother said, "You wanted me to have that." When she
threw it a second time at the mother's head, the mother said, "You RE-
ALLY wanted me to have that bean bag."

The filial therapist, honoring, with the group members, that a limit was
definitely violated, went over again how to set limits so that the mother
could do a better job next time. The filial therapist was so distressed that
the mother did not know how to do that at this point in the therapy that
she was very focused on the instruction. She failed to address the
mother's feelings about the child's motivation and her reaction to it.

This was loud and clear to the supervisor, who worked with the therapist to re-focus first on the mother's feelings and then instruction. The
supervisor advised that the FT therapist simply point out what really
happened in the playroom and not do anything confrontational about
her denials. This would have caused defensiveness. As you will see in
the next scenario, this behavioral notation worked. Since problem areas
tend to recur in play sessions and not get resolved until feelings are adequately addressed, the situation arose again, although with a rag doll.
This time, per the help of the supervisor, the filial therapist first addressed the feelings of the parent in believing that the child was just
throwing the object aimlessly about when it hit the mother with words
to this effect:

Therapist: It was a shock when Z hit you with the rag doll. You just wouldn't
expect Z to hit you with something even in a play session.

Mother: Well, no, I'm not sure she really meant to do it.

Therapist: You think it could have been an accident. However, she did have to
make a special point of placing it to aim it at you, I think. It seems like last

time she did the same thing with the beanbags. I'm wondering if these incidents are as accidental as they might seem.

Mother: Well, she does give me a hard time but never hits me. Of course, this is a play time and she knows it.

Therapist: You think Z might see this as a different situation with different rules and might behave somewhat differently.

Mother: It is possible, I guess. But why would she want to throw something at me? She knows that I love her. I am nicer to her than I am the boys—which they remind me of. They think she is spoiled.

Therapist: So it is hard for you to see that kind of feeling going on in Z yet it does seem to appear in the play sessions. You don't like to think she could have any negative feelings toward you. You don't have them toward her.

The mother begins crying and tells the group how it is very important that there be no negative feelings because she was a specially acquired child, just what she wanted, and it has to be good.

The therapist suggests that she and the mother have a special counseling session later in the week to deal with this in greater depth since it is too important to be dealt with in the short time available in the group.

The mother agrees and faces up to child's hostility and her own reaction to the loss of the "dream relationship." Play sessions immediately stop with attacks on the mother when she permits herself to set limits. In the personal counseling session, in addition to dealing with this long unexpressed feeling, the therapist stresses the value of limits in real life for the child, practicing how to use them in the play session so that the child feels the security of some boundaries. Rather than making her daughter love her more, she was making her daughter feel less protected when she failed to set rules for her. After having her feelings explored and accepted, the mother was able to hear this as she had not been able to hear it in a traditional parent education class she had previously taken, which was simply instructive.

CONCLUSION

While there is no empirical data on the effectiveness of the supervision methods described in this chapter, a lot of data shows the effectiveness of FT (Bratton, Ray, Rhine, & Jones, 2005; VanFleet, Ryan, & Smith, 2005) with many populations of great diversity. Of course, the concept of parent inclusion is the unique and crucial key element in FT. However, the methodological "infrastructure" successfully makes the concept work. Analogously, a bridge could have a perfect design but without well-executed supports and other infrastructure elements, it will not be functional for long. FT has been in existence for some 40 years now, having been first introduced in 1964 by Bernard Guerney (1964). The same methodology, more refined and fine tuned, has supported the concept all of these years. This system of teaching and supervision is the core of the methodology, and keeps FT the viable, enduring approach it has remained.

REFERENCES

Andronico, M. P., Fidler, J., Guerney, B. G., Jr., & Guerney, L. (1967). The combination of didactic and dynamic elements in filial therapy. *International Journal of Group Psychotherapy, 17,* 10–17.

Axline, V. M. (1969). *Play therapy* (Rev. ed.). New York: Ballantine Books.

Bratton, S., Ray, D., Rhine, T., & Jones, L. (2005). The efficacy of play therapy with children: A meta-analytic review of the outcome research. *Professional Psychology: Research and Practice, 36*(4), 376–90.

Guerney, B. G., Jr. (1964). Filial therapy: Description and rationale. *Journal of Consulting Psychology, 28*(4), 303–10.

Guerney, B. G., Jr., Guerney, L., & Stover, L. (1972). Facilitative therapist attitudes in training parents as psychotherapeutic agents. *The Family Coordinator, 21*(3), 275–78.

Guerney, B. G., Jr., & Stover, L. (1971). *Filial therapy: Final report on NIMH grant 1826401.* Silver Spring, MD: NIRE/IDEALS.

VanFleet, R., Ryan, S. D., & Smith, S. K. (2005). Filial therapy: A critical review. In L. A. Reddy, T. M. Files-Hall, & C. E. Schaefer (Eds.), *Empirically based play interventions for children.* Washington, DC: American Psychological Association.

materials in an imaginative way. She also mentioned that she was raised in a frugal family, and that wasting materials was considered disrespectful in her house. Jamie concluded, "Maybe I was a little jealous that Garret and Justin could be so carefree when it's not something I've ever experienced."

In this case, the supervisor used two main skills. The first was to provide techniques of experience such as scheduling of sessions, limiting materials in the playroom, and gaining assistance in cleaning. The second skill was the simple act of listening beyond the supervisee's words to the level of emotion motivating an intense reaction and speed to set limits. Once the supervisor confronted the supervisee's level of emotion with reflection, the supervisee was able to explore her own motives and develop a stronger sense of acceptance.

Matching and Timing

Because so much interaction is taking place in a group play therapy session, therapists often find it challenging to maintain a matched level of responsiveness and energy. New group play therapists will especially find themselves a "beat behind" the level of interaction between children, challenging their ability to be immediate in session. This issue usually dissipates with experience as therapists learn to respond to more pressing interactions and less to general activity. Supervisors can assist in professional growth by reviewing such moments in video recordings of sessions and discussion of responses.

Supervision Case Study

Still new to group play therapy, Jamie showed her recorded session with Garret and Justin in supervision. Kim, her supervisor, noticed that despite the high level of energy in the session, Jamie stayed quiet, seemingly overwhelmed. Kim mentioned this observation to Jamie.

Kim: There's so much going on in the room yet you seem really quiet.

Jamie: I felt so overpowered by them. They were so loud and active that I could not focus. . . . I was just thinking, "What is going on?"

Kim: It's like watching a movie where so much is happening and you just can't keep up. Each minute you're trying to figure out what happened in the previous minute. I just want you to know this is typical of therapists who are new to group play therapy. It takes time to develop a sense of comfort with the level of activity.

By reflecting Jamie's struggle and providing a sense of normalcy to the situation, Kim attempted to connect to Jamie's emotional level. Secondly,

Kim suggested that the two watch the video again, but this time muted in order to focus on the children's play without being distracted by the sounds. Together, Jamie and Kim made reflections to the play while they watched the silent tape. Jamie was able to focus on the nonverbal expressions of the children and come up with more accurate responses. She was also able to acknowledge a pattern of the children's behaviors that she was not aware of during the session. The purpose of this exercise was to help Jamie practice being more "in the moment" with the children and transfer this skill to the session.

Limit Setting

In all play therapy (from our experience), limit setting is the most discussed issue in supervision. Not surprisingly, limit setting in group play therapy is a typical focus of supervision. The presence of more children inspires more concerns regarding the need for limits and how to set those limits. Typical questions involving limit setting of group play therapists include, "Is this behavior okay in group play therapy versus individual play therapy?" "How far do I allow them to go when I see that we're headed for a limit?" "How much responsibility do I turn over to them to solve the problem versus set the limit for them?" "When there is more than one, how do I enforce the limit?" etc. There is no right answer to any of these questions, and they are usually addressed on a case-by-case basis. The basic underlying message from the therapist to the supervisor is, "I'm scared things are going to get out of control and become nontherapeutic. How do I keep that from happening?" If a supervisor can help the therapist explore the underlying message of concern, this will help the therapist to make future case-by-case decisions involving limits. Limit setting in group play therapy requires quickness of response from the therapist because activity moves at such a rapid rate and the possibility of harm to another is greater. Supervision is helpful when the supervisor and supervisee can brainstorm possible scenarios and find the best solutions.

Supervision Case Study

In triadic supervision (supervisor with two supervisees), Christian, a supervisee, expressed her frustration and overwhelmed feeling with her very first group play therapy session.

> *Christian:* In group, everything was happening double and triple speed than in an individual session. When a limit was necessary, I was thinking of alternatives in my mind. But it took so long for me to come up with the alterna-

tives that the situation was already over and the children were moving on to different play. It was too late.

Ben, her supervisor, noticing the other supervisee nodding with Christian's remarks: It seems that these feelings ring bells and resonate with both of you.

Susan: Yeah, I just don't feel like I can keep up and before I know it, they are saying mean things to each other or trying to fight.

Christian: Sometimes, I'm not sure if what I'm doing is even therapeutic. They might be better off with another therapist.

The supervisees continued to share feelings of inadequacy, disappointment, feeling overwhelmed, and fear of being out of control. Because rapid judgment and responses of a group play therapist are often improved with experience, Ben decided to do role play with Christian. Ben and Susan played the roles of children and played out multiple possible scenarios that would require limit setting, and Christian was asked to respond as a therapist.

In the next supervision, Christian reported that she was less tense and feeling more comfortable with the group play therapy session because she felt that she had some "stored alternatives" from the role play practices. Christian also mentioned that feeling more capable and confident allowed her to be more vulnerable in the session.

Christian said, "One time, I was not able to come up with alternatives when I set a limit. It used to be my biggest fear. But instead of being frozen, I was able to be genuine and tell the children that I was not sure what could be glued in addition to paper. Then, one child in the group came up with an idea of putting glue on Play-Doh! Not only did he stop putting glue on puppets, but also he was able to come up with an alternative by himself. He was so proud of himself about the solution. It was the best outcome."

Philosophy Challenges

The issue of limit setting is directly related to the therapist's belief in the self-directed nature of children. There is no greater laboratory for experimenting with the question of a need for guidance for children versus a belief in their ability to positively self-direct their behavior than the group play therapy room. For child-centered play therapists, this is an especially salient issue. Many child-centered play therapists embrace the belief that children have the ability to direct their behavior to positive outcomes, specifically in individual play therapy. However, in group play therapy, when a play therapist is forced to step between two children physically engaging in a fight, this belief system is challenged. The therapist must make the decision regarding the need for the introduction of a problem-solving method or the continued allowance of such aggression (while still stepping in when physical aggression is pursued) until the children tap into their positive nature and develop coping skills from an internal sense of doing what moves them toward self-actualization. In supervision of group play therapy, the supervisor is offered the opportunity to help the therapist explore and clarify belief systems about children that help the therapist become a stronger, more effective agent for change.

Supervision Case Study

Laura, a supervisee, shared a significant concern regarding an incident in her recent play therapy group session. Laura recounted that there had been constant fights and arguments in every session and that she felt the sessions have not been therapeutic. According to Laura, one of her group members, nine-year-old Jordan, wanted to be in charge in the session and became intensely irritated when the other group member, seven-year-old Gabriel, did not follow Jordan's plan. Due to his speech impairment, Gabriel did not talk often. Instead, Gabriel expressed his frustration and anger toward Jordan by throwing toys at him. When Gabriel threw the toy, Jordan exacted revenge by making fun of and mocking Gabriel's speech.

In the video-recorded session, Nancy, the supervisor, observed that Laura set limits appropriately, stayed neutral, and reflected Jordan's and Gabriel's feelings accurately.

> *Nancy:* It seems like you are really staying with them at an equal rate and you've set several limits in a quick manner that appeared to keep things from escalating.

> *Laura:* But I feel like what I have been doing is not enough to make the situation better. I used to believe that children are capable of moving toward something positive by themselves. But this group has been shaking my belief. I started thinking that some children may need some teaching or guidance to change the direction that they are taking in order to have positive changes. Maybe that should be my role. I feel the session is stagnant.

Nancy acknowledged Laura's feeling of being lost and her doubt regarding her beliefs. Nancy helped Laura revisit her own general philosophy of working with people, such as human nature, process of personality change, and role of relationship. In order to take action in a concrete way in the session, Nancy believed that Laura needed to re-examine her belief system about children because it is imperative for therapists to conceptualize and then respond in an internally consistent way so that there is consistency and credibility to the therapy. In this process, Laura embraced her initial belief in the self-actualizing tendency that is innate in children, and the healing power of the relationship that reduced her need to bring problem-solving or teaching methods into the session.

Once Laura concluded that she would prefer to act from a child-centered philosophy, Nancy suggested that Laura reconsider group selection of members. Due to his aggressive need for control, Jordan's sense of insecurity seemed intensified in a group play therapy setting. Individual play therapy for Jordan seemed a more appropriate intervention at this time. In addition, although the chronological age difference between Jordan and Gabriel was within two years (an acceptable guideline for group play therapy), the developmental age of Gabriel seemed below an average seven-year-old boy, which increased developmental differences between Jordan and Gabriel. The success of group play therapy may well be related to the careful consideration of selecting group members.

Note that, alternatively, this is often the situation where a therapist might embrace a belief that children are in need of guidance by the therapist and make a decision to integrate problem solving into the play session. If this is the case, the supervisor might have helped the supervisee integrate problem-solving methods for this particular group before moving to a rearrangement of the group.

Role of Therapists

When therapists choose to become play therapists, they are often attracted to the idea of serving as a therapeutic agent of change for a child. Play therapists often develop intimate relationships with their individual clients because the children allow therapists, and sometimes only the therapist, to see their whole world. In group play therapy, the modality relies on the presence and interaction of other children who will serve as change agents for each child. Often, the therapist will "take a back seat" to the group of children in the expression and development of new coping skills. Although the group play therapist serves a critical role in providing the environment and facilitating group members' interactions, direct interaction and involvement is limited as compared to individual play therapy. In supervision, we have found that some therapists are disappointed in this role and prefer to have the more intimate connection provided in individual play therapy. When this issue arises, supervisors can help their supervisees explore their personal needs and motivations being fulfilled in play therapy and how these needs might by negatively affecting their abilities as play therapists.

Supervision Case Study

A school counselor, Amy, has been conducting group play therapy with two third-grade students, Maria and Stacy, for two months. Maria exhibits high anxiety and seldom talks in class. Stacy has just moved to the area a month ago, and she has been struggling with making friends. At the beginning, both Maria and Stacy engaged in individual play. They avoided any contact with each other, but sought interactions with Amy independently. Amy was patient with the process, reflecting the feeling that both of them were curious about each other but feeling nervous about playing together. Amy was feeling competent. After one month, both Maria and Stacy began to demonstrate positive interactions with each other, expressing their needs and setting limits on or with each other. It was evidenced that the group dynamics were evolving encouragingly.

Contrary to the progress of the group, Amy started addressing her feeling of incompetence in a triadic supervision. She also mentioned her plan to add a new group member to Maria and Stacy's group.

> *Amy:* Sometimes, I am even not sure if they are aware that I am there with them. So I feel it is pointless to make responses to them. I feel ignored.

> *Kate (another supervisee):* The group seems to be working well. They are developing more mutual help and support of each other. That's great. It sounds like you felt more effective when they were more dependent on you.

Amy acknowledged that she had a strong need to be needed and that she honestly felt disappointed that she was no longer directly involved in the children's play. Kate linked Amy's feeling of being inadequate and her feeling of not being needed in a group play therapy, and also she confronted Amy regarding a possible hidden motivation behind her idea of adding a new child.

Steven, the supervisor, mentioned a parallel process of the two groups. Similarly to Maria and Stacy in group play therapy, Amy and Kate were inner directed and taking more responsibilities toward an issue presented by Amy, and they were able to create meaningful interactions without Steven's direct involvement in the process. Amy was able to redefine her role as a group play therapist through her own experience in supervision.

Control Issues

The need for control is perhaps one of the more dangerous personality needs embraced by play therapists. If a play therapist has a strong need for control, this might be somewhat challenged by individual play therapy but it will be greatly challenged in group play therapy. When a play therapist displays a need to control the setting, the interaction, and the play of the child so that it is directed to the outcome desired by the therapist, play therapy can be negatively affected by disallowing the child to move toward a more helpful direction identified by the child. In group play therapy, children will directly challenge this need for control through their play, activity level, breaking of limits, attitude toward the therapist, and other destructive behaviors that place the focus of therapy on "winning." Ultimately, when a therapist actively engages with a child to establish control, everyone loses and the therapeutic process ceases to be therapeutic. Although limits are essential to the play therapy process, limits are set as necessary to enhance therapeutic process for the child, not to establish control over the child by the therapist. In supervision, we have encountered many play therapists whose issues of control were revealed in the group process and impacted their ability to be effective. In these cases, supervision required a direct confrontation of the issue, hopefully acknowledged and accepted by the therapist. Upon recognition of the issue as a problem, supervision entailed discussion of personal conflicts surrounding the issue of control and exploration by the therapist on their ability to directly deal with their needs in the context of their professional goals. This exploration is usually followed by the therapist's participation in personal therapy, a continued awareness of the experiences that initiate the need, or, occasionally, an awareness that play therapy might not be a compatible match for the therapist's personality.

Supervision Case Study

Judy has been conducting group play therapy with eight-year-old Mike and seven-year-old Sam. Both were originally referred by their parents for their defiant behaviors. Both Mike and Sam have been engaging in play with a theme of power and control by playing a "cop game" in which one becomes a criminal and the other becomes a policeman. One day, neither Mike nor Sam wanted to be a criminal, and they came up with an idea of having Judy take the role. Judy was very hesitant to take the part, and often she did not follow what the children asked her to do. One day, Mike and Sam decided to put her in a "jail" behind a puppet theater and sentenced her to 1,000 years of imprisonment. She was reluctant to stay behind the puppet theater and ceased to make any responses to Mike and Sam's play. After a while, Judy suddenly stood up saying, "I choose not to be in jail," and she went back to her chair.

In a triadic supervision, Judy expressed that she did not like to play the role of a prisoner and that she felt stupid. She also mentioned that she thought that it would be therapeutic for the children to compromise by taking a role they did not want. Her supervisor, Carol, sensed that Judy's strong need to be in charge and her fear of being vulnerable in the session were inhibiting the therapeutic process in the group. However, Carol was concerned, due to Judy's lack of awareness of this personality need, with rupturing her relationship with Judy by directly confronting her need to be in control in a session. Instead in a separate supervision session, Carol introduced the concept of the four Adlerian personality priorities, identified as superiority, control, pleasing, and comfort (Holden, 2000) to the supervisees and had them explore how their choice of personality priority was affecting their lives.

Judy quickly identified control as her primary personality priority and mentioned that it was not surprising to her. She said that her leadership skill was one of her strengths and that she liked to be a decision maker, having others follow her lead. She acknowledged her frustration and dissatisfaction with play therapy because of the egalitarian relationship with children and the perceived role of the therapist as follower when children needed leadership. She began to question her choice as a play therapist and expressed frustration with her facilitation of adult therapy also. Carol asked to have an individual supervision session with Judy where she suggested that Judy explore these important professional issues in personal therapy to help Judy decide where she would professionally progress most successfully. After being able to explore such questions in a supportive environment, Judy was open to the suggestion of therapy and pursued the option immediately.

CONCLUSION

Group play therapy requires a level of commitment to children and to the process of play beyond what is required in individual play therapy. Slavson (1999) emphasized this point in his warning statement, "The anxiety stimulated by the presence of other children and the support they give one another in their hostility toward the adult include hyperactivity and destructiveness seldom encountered in the play of one child" (p. 25). Hence, the group play therapy supervisor needs to be experienced not only in group play therapy, but in the facilitation of the anxiety related to the supervisee and how best to process this anxiety for successful outcomes. A mix of techniques and abilities to increase awareness in the supervisee as well as educate them in the process of group play therapy will help to extend the effectiveness of supervision. The supervisor's skill in active listening to observe the intentions and motivations behind the words used by supervisees is perhaps the most essential skill available to the supervisor. Group play therapists will often focus on concrete, observable activities among children and resist exploring the personal fac-

11

༼ᨏ༽

Enhancing Role Play Activities in Play Therapy Supervision Groups

Sandra B. Frick-Helms

R ole play is frequently used to facilitate supervisee skill practice. The role play supervision method described in this chapter focuses on supervision of client- or child-centered play therapy, but can be adapted for most other play therapy theoretical frameworks. Role play is defined by O'Donnell and Shaver (1990) as "a dramatic technique in which individuals improvise behaviors that illustrate acts expected of persons involved in defined situations." They add "role-play simulations are learning situations in which learners take on the role-profiles of specific characters in a contrived educational game. As a result of playing out roles in a role-play simulation, learners are expected to acquire the intended learning outcomes as well as make learning enjoyable."

Role play has been used as a teaching technique at all levels of education (Bailey & Watson, 1998; Brandt & Bateman, 2006; Cutler & Hay, 2000; Gray, Wykes, & Gournay, 2003; Hardoff & Schonmann, 2001; Kofoed, 2006; Out & Lafreniere, 2001; Sander, Stevenson, King, & Coates, 2000). It has been used to enhance children's oral and written achievements (Cook, 2000; Good & Robertson, 2003); to teach counseling (Larson, Clark, Wesely, Koraleski, Daniels, & Smith, 1999); civic participation (Smith, 2004); ecology (Bailey & Watson, 1998; Hillcox, 2006); evolution, geography (Cutler & Hay, 2000); physics (Kofoed, 2006); political science and history (Ip & Linser, 2001; Vincent & Shepherd, 1998); science (Hodson & Reid, 1988); and social work, and to evaluate teachers (Alkin & Christie, 2002) and civic participation (Smith, 2004).

Role play has been used at least since the 1960s in professional/vocational education, including economics, law, international relations, medicine, and the military (Vincent & Shepherd, 1998), as well as business (Mercado, 2000; Sadler-Smith & Riding, 1999). One of the major educational uses for role play has been in professional education of medical students and physicians, in teaching communication skills (Hardoff & Schonman, 2001; Rollnick, Kinnersley, & Butler, 2002); cultural competency (Loudon & Anderson, et al., 1999); genitourinary medicine (Knowles, Kinchington, Erwin, & Peters, 2001); sexual history taking (FitzGerald, Crowley, Greenhouse, & Rrobert, 2003); and violence screening skills. Role play has also been used to teach nurses and nursing students cultural competence (Shearer, 2003); medication management (Gray, Wykes, & Gournay, 2003); communication skills in mental health (Lam, Kuipers, & Leff, 1993; Minghella & Benson, 1995); and to teach nursing assistants how to work with elderly patients (Pillemer & Hudson, 1993). Role play has also been used as a method for training caretakers of mentally retarded patients (Harper & Wadsworth, 1992) and in the education of veterinary medicine students (Brandt & Bateman, 2006).

Role play has been used in a variety of clinical and research situations including to assess parent-child interactions (Anderson, English, & Hedrick, 2006); to increase parenting effectiveness (Forgatch, Bullock, & Patterson, 2004); to modify attitudes toward teen pregnancy and teen parenting (Out & Lafreniere, 2001); to intervene with families reported or at risk for child abuse or neglect (Lutzker, Bigelow, Doctor, & Kessler, 1998); in breast and cervical cancer education (Hurd, Muti, Erwin, & Womack, 2003); in AIDS education; and with alcoholics (Monti, Rohsenow, & Hutchison, 2000).

In mental health situations, role play has been used with children with social phobia (Alfano, Beidel, & Turner, 2006; Beidel, Turner, & Morris, 1999); children exposed to urban violence (Ceballo, Ramirez, Maltese, & Bautista, 2006); students with emotional/behavioral disorders (Chen, 2006); and depressed adolescents (Marcotte, 1997). It has also been used to investigate associations between sexual abuse history and HIV-related attitudes and behaviors of adolescents with a psychiatric disorder (Brown, Kessel, Lourie, & Ford, 1997) and with schizophrenic patients (Ihnen, Penn, Corrigan, & Martin, 1998; Penn, Kohlmaier, & Corrigan, 2000).

Role play has also been used in war games (Johnson, McDermott, Barrett, & Cowden, 2006); to investigate management styles and managers' leadership effectiveness (Korabik, Baril, & Watson, 1993); to teach gun-safety skills to children (Himle, Miltenberger, Gatheridge, & Flessner, 2004); to forecast business decisions (Green, 2002); and to facilitate teamwork in airplane cockpits.

NECESSARY CRITERIA FOR EFFECTIVE ROLE PLAY

There are certain criteria that role play exercises should meet in order to be effective. The role player must imagine what it is like to *be* the role being played. When a supervisee role-plays a play therapist, the supervisee considers what a play therapist would look like, how a play therapist (in a play therapy situation) would act, and other aspects that are to the supervisee uniquely *play therapist*. This means that the way a supervisee role-plays a play therapist is based upon what the supervisee (cognitively) knows and believes about play therapists. In order to translate these cognitions into the actual role play, the supervisee must actively and carefully consider characteristics that match his or her perception of play therapists while mentally discarding characteristics that do not match that perception.

The supervisee must also imagine what *other* individuals know and believe about play therapists and try to match his or her role play to these beliefs. This criterion helps to ensure that the supervisee's concepts about the role to be played (which were learned in more structured situations) are in accord with generally accepted practice. A reasonable scenario must be set up in which the role play occurs. The situation should involve some idea of where a play therapist would be found, what a play therapist's environment would look and be like, and what other individuals (actors) would be involved in a scenario with a play therapist. Even if actual props are not used, the role player should role-play the use of props that are typical to the role being played in the situation.

An effective role play requires the role player to carefully reflect on what he or she knows and believes and on what others know and believe about the role that is played. The word "reflect" is chosen deliberately. If the word *reflect* is used in relation to a mirror, it is defined as *giving back* or *showing* an image of whatever is being reflected by the mirror. In role playing, the role player must give back or show a representation of what the role player knows and believes about the role being played, about what others know and believe about the role being played, and about the context in which the role would be played. This reflecting process actively involves the learner in what he or she is role-playing. When a learner is actively involved in learning about concepts and behaviors, what is learned is retained longer and more accurately than when a learner is provided the concepts and behaviors in a passive mode such as in a lecture or a reading assignment (Chen, 2006; Kolb, 1984; Vincent & Shepherd, 1998).

Role playing that involves more than one role player (or actor) also requires planning, usually in advance of the actual role play. If one supervisee is role-playing a play therapist setting a limit and another supervisee is role-playing a child, they may plan in advance how the child will go about breaking a limit. In addition to what the various actors would say to each other, the supervisees might plan what real or imagined objects will be used and under what conditions their use would be limited (e.g., if the play therapist allows balls to be thrown but does not allow other playroom objects to be thrown). In order for this planning to be effective in facilitating the role play, the various actors must work co-operatively with each other. So role playing also involves learning the kinds of interactions that might facilitate the role play. Even with advanced planning, most role plays require improvisation by the various actors. As the role play progresses, one actor will say or do something for which the other actor will not be totally prepared. Because the second role player has carefully considered the different criteria for role play, he or she should be able to respond to the first role player within the context of the role play. This need for improvisation within the prescribed role and context is much of what makes role play an active learning experience. As the individual role-plays different variations of his or her role of child client, the individual role-playing the play therapist gets practice in meeting different criteria for fulfilling his or her prescribed role.

One might ask, why can't the individual learn as much about the role by watching a movie or TV show dramatizing the roles, interactions, and context involved in the role play? When people watch a movie or TV show, they are passive. They watch the role behaviors of actors in the dramatization without having to choose how to react to those behaviors. In role play, the role players *actively* interact, making choices about how to act and react according to their knowledge and perception about what is appropriate to their role.

Reisman and Reibordy's (1993) description of role play between therapist and child is adapted here to describe role play in supervision groups. The supervisor "demonstrates the desired role behaviors of play therapist" first "while the (supervisee) either observes or plays another role in the scenario." The supervisee would then be asked to "assume a role that requires performing some of the desired behaviors" (p. 96). Kelly's (1955) "fixed role therapy" provides a basis for having an individual pretend to be someone else. In the present case, the supervisee is role-playing the therapist as modeled by the supervisor.

Having the role player share his or her feelings about thoughts and feelings during the role play allows the supervisor to resolve inaccurate perceptions. For example, a supervisee may believe being silent is more therapeutic in some client-centered situations than empathically reflecting what the role-played child is doing and/or saying. When the supervisor notes the supervisee engaging in periods of silent nonresponding, the supervisor can ask the supervisee about the periods of silence, correct the inaccurate belief, and immediately have the supervisee role-play according to the corrected belief. Without role play, the supervisor may not have found out the inaccurate belief. Also, when the supervisor comments this way on the role-played behaviors, supervisees are made more aware of their own perceptions than they might have been if there had been no role play.

Supervisees who are learning new concepts and skills often feel nervous and uncomfortable when they first attempt to carry out the learned concepts and skills. According to Beebe and Risi (1993), "role playing, which can be an effective technique for a variety of conditions may not only encourage problem solving skills, but can also bridge the gap between the artificial environment and *in vivo* . . . situations" (p. 381). By assigning role-play scenarios to each member of a supervision group, the supervisor provides supervisees with a safe arena for trying out new knowledge and skills. Beebe and Risi (1993) also recommend that learning techniques such as role play should be "individualized to suit the strengths and weaknesses" (p. 395) of the role player. If there is a particular area that the supervisee is having difficulty performing, the supervisor can assign role-play scenarios that emphasize the area (Fox, Dunlap, & Powell, 2002).

Just as role play may seem silly or embarrassing to children and adolescents, role play can be difficult for supervisees. According to Bergin, Eckstein, Manns, and Wallingford (2001), role play makes learning difficulties obvious; not all students enjoy learning in public. Many supervisees feel embarrassed or inadequate when asked to role-play, especially if the role play is in front of a group. Role play can be introduced in a way that facilitates supervisee skill. Role play situations that involve concrete, easily described behaviors help decrease feelings of embarrassment or inadequacy and facilitate supervisees' ability to grasp the basic skills. If a supervisee falters when he or she perceives a "mistake" was made, the supervisor can watch for the next *acceptable* response and acknowledge that response by (empathically) whispering something like, "You did that!" This empathic acknowledgement should have the same effect of encouraging continued performance as child-centered methods tend to have on children in child-centered play therapy. The supervisor can also provide the supervisee with additional opportunities for success by having the role-played child do something very obvious, such as building a block tower and getting visibly mad when it falls. When another *acceptable*, "correct" response is given, the supervisor is again able to acknowledge the "correct" response. As role play continues over the course of one or more supervision sessions, the supervisor can "play out" specific problem behaviors or, in groups, specify problem behaviors to be role-played by the child character.

ENHANCING THE LEARNING VALUE OF ROLE PLAY

While teaching a yearlong seminar in child-centered play therapy, I discovered a useful way to enhance the process of learning through role play. Each student was required to role-play at least once as a child and once as a play therapist. The remaining members of the seminar were instructed to observe and take notes on the role-played sessions. They were told that, at the end of each role play, they would be asked to make at least one comment on a positive therapist behavior and at least one suggestion for improving the behaviors of the play therapist. At the end of the seminar, students filled out evaluations. One of the items on the evaluation form asked students to name the "one learning activity that was most valuable" to them. The overwhelming majority of students responded "role play." I have continued to use this activity in seminars and in one three-credit graduate course. "Role play" has continued to be the most frequent response to the item asking for the most valuable learning activity.

THE ROLE PLAY SUPERVISION PROCESS

Initiating the Role Play Activity

When introducing role play to supervision groups, I usually begin by role-playing the therapist myself. According to Frey, Hirschstein, and Guzzo (2000), teachers can model strategies so that students with difficulties can see what the strategies look like in context. I ask for a volunteer to role-play the child but will assign a group member if there are no volunteers. I am careful to provide an accurate and competent model because students (or supervisees) tend to find models who "behave in a manner consistent to the values they teach" more meaningful than listening to the educators lecture about those same values (Curwin & Mendler, 2000). This initial role play usually lasts no longer than five minutes.

Using the same procedure as before to obtain a supervisee role player, I role-play a child while a supervisee role-plays a child-centered play therapist. Other group members are asked to observe the role play and comment upon it in the same manner as before. In addition, they are asked to be prepared to comment upon one positive child-centered behavior they saw the play therapist role player use and one suggestion for a way in which the individual role-playing the play therapist can improve his or her use of client-centered techniques.

The supervision group can then be split into pairs to practice. Initially, this may just be an arbitrary pairing. Later the pairs may be chosen according to which supervisee desires to role-play a scenario that has taken place with one of their clients. Each supervisee takes a turn at role-playing the child and role-playing the play therapist. Early role-play scenarios may involve simple, easily performed skills and (role-played) "children" who behave well; usually last no longer than five minutes; and may focus on only one of the basic child-centered play therapy skills (being nondirective, empathic responding, using unconditional positive regard, and being genuine or congruent). This allows supervisees to focus attention on learning each skill separately before trying to put them all together. After these initial role plays, supervisees can begin role-playing longer contrived scenarios or events from actual sessions they have had with child clients.

Analyzing Role Play Scenarios

At the completion of each supervisee role play, I discuss the role play with the supervision group members. I ask the supervisee who role-played the child and the supervisee who role-played the play therapist to comment on how it felt to *be* the child or therapist. This tends to normalize the situation for supervision group members because it allows supervisees to know that their feelings about role playing are shared by others. For the supervisee who is first to role-play the play therapist, I note that it is difficult to be the first member of a group to participate in role play. Commenting on the difficulty of being first acknowledges that individual's contribution and probable feelings about the contribution. This is in keeping with the child-centered play therapy theoretical framework, as it (empathically) reflects the individual's probable feelings in an (unconditionally positively regarding) accepting way. Often, I add child-centered responses such as "you did that" or "even though you were nervous, you were able to do that." Using child-centered responses as a basis for comments models appropriate wording of child-centered responses and tends to establish a positive learning set. By having supervisees relate personal feelings, learning is taken out of the passive mode of just hearing or seeing the information and becomes more active.

Supervisor Commentary

After each role play, I model the kind of verbal feedback that should be most useful to the therapist role player, as well as appropriate use of client-centered skills. I start by commenting on a positive therapist behavior. Then each member of the supervision group comments verbally on the role player's performance.

Group Commentary

I ask supervision group members to comment on what they saw and heard in each role play, framing their comments so they relate to the theoretical framework of child-centered play therapy. Simply commenting on what was seen is a relatively passive learning activity. Using child-centered theory as a basis for comments requires supervisees to attend to the role-play scenarios while thinking about how the content of those scenarios meets or doesn't meet criteria for appropriate child-centered play therapy. Being required to comment verbally using previously taught material is in accord with one of the basic laws of learning: *repetition* (Glaser, 2000; Shanks, 1995; Shuell, 1986). I respond to each supervisee comment with a child-centered (genuine, nondirective, empathic, and unconditionally with positive regard) statement such as "it sounds as if this was something you would do also." I also find and comment upon at least one positive (or correct) aspect of each supervisee comment to further establish a positive learning set.

Positive therapist behaviors are communicated in a first round, and suggestions for improvement are communicated in a second round. Hearing verbal comments from me and their seminar peers gives each play therapist role player immediate feedback. Hearing comments on positive therapist behaviors before suggestions for improvement helps to establish a positive learning set for the role players and the students commenting. Research has shown that naturally occurring social reinforcers, "such as praise, attention, and positive feedback" are among the most effective ways to "encourage new behaviors in different settings" (Elksnin & Elksnin, 1998). At the end of the seminar session, each observer submits written positive comments and suggestions for improvement to me as shown in figure 11.1.

Observing a role play and being required to evaluate it according to specified criteria is an active approach to learning. The supervisee has to watch the activity, while actively keeping the evaluation criteria in mind and actively choosing from among those criteria to complete the activity. Telling supervisees they will be required to comment verbally and in writing on child-centered play therapy skills that had previ-

Name of individual writing comments: _____

Name of individual role playing the therapist: _____

General comments regarding CCPT role play: "I thought you were brave to go first."

At least one positive comment on role play performance: "When you raised your hand like the child raised hers, you used nonverbal empathy."

At least one suggestion for improvement on role play performance: "Every time she asked a question, you didn't say *anything.*"

Figure 11.1. Written Role Play Comment Form - Student.

ously been taught helps ensure that supervisees will be mentally engaged in the process of critically evaluating child-centered play therapy skills. After each supervisee has participated in role play, I tally the written comments submitted and provide the anonymous result to each student at a later date. An example of this tally is shown in figure 11.2.

Since I began including this way of using role play, supervision group members appear more comfortable with commenting on the role plays and the actual demonstration (live and videotaped) play sessions with children. Additionally, they tend to make longer, more specific comments. When one group member makes a comment, other group members will nod and contribute additional information, often the type of information I might have made to expand on a comment to make it more specific.

There are some areas that tend to be commented upon over and over again by students and supervisees. Many supervisees comment that, after role-playing a child client, they have a better appreciation of how affirming it can be to a child to be responded to with unconditional positive regard in a nondirective, genuine, and empathic manner. A frequent question resulting from the role plays is how often to respond to the role-played child. Beginning client-centered play therapists sometimes tend to be afraid that children might think the play therapist is copying them or making fun of them if they give frequent reflections. I assure the supervisees that the majority of children do not have difficulty with client-centered responses; in fact many children tend to enjoy them and feel affirmed by them. I also remind them that the theoretical framework for client-centered play therapy provides the basis for responding to children who complain about frequent responding (Frick-Helms, 2002a). Another area that raises a lot of questions is limit setting. Concerns here tend to center around the possibility that children will spend entire sessions

Comments on these summaries are verbatim as they were written by your classmates. Additional comments (in italics) are added when it appears that further explanation would be helpful to the individual being evaluated.

Name of individual role playing the therapist: _____

Positive comments on your role play performance: "When you raised your hand like the child raised hers, you used nonverbal empathy." "Worded limit to show UPR [unconditional positive regard]." "Avoided naming the toy soldier." *This maintains being nondirective.* "When you said, 'You've noticed I talk different during special play time,' in response to the child's 'why are you talking funny,' you allowed the child to decide what to do about empathic responding."

Suggestions for improvement on your role play performance: "Every time she asked a question, you didn't say anything." *Silence may convey that certain behaviors (talking) of the child are more desirable than others (silence), thus violating UPR. Can reflect questions by rephrasing as a statement, e.g. "you want to know why I talk this way."* "When she ran around, laughing, you said, 'you're running around and laughing. You could have added a feeling reflection, e.g., 'you're happy'."

Additional comments and suggestions from supervisor: *By staying in one spot while the child rapidly circled the playroom, you respected her need to explore and allowed her to become comfortable, to gradually adjust to the setting, and get closer to you at her own pace.*

Figure 11.2.   Written Role Play Comment Form - Faculty.

testing and breaking limits. I try to assure the supervisees that, with most children, this does not become an issue. The very nature of client-centered play therapy tends to make limit testing and limit breaking less likely, and the procedure for dealing with limits tested and/or broken helps assure the child that her/his concerns will be addressed (Frick-Helms, 2002b).

I have continued to use this activity in seminars and in a graduate course. "Role play" has continued to be the most frequent response to the item asking for the "most valuable learning activity." Obviously, the information presented in this chapter is not the result of a carefully constructed survey. This might be a question for future research. This method of facilitating supervision group member role play has been beneficial to me and to the supervision group members who have been involved. An example of a short role play and comments from supervisees and supervisor can be seen in appendix 11.A, with additional comments in appendix 11.B.

Appendix 11A.   Role Play Script and Comments from Supervisees and Supervisor

Role-Played Child	*Role-Played Play Therapist*
Standing with therapist.	The therapist walks the client into the playroom and states to the client, "This is the playroom. You can do almost anything you want in the playroom. If you have any questions, ask."
Walks slowly into the playroom and looks curiously around the room. Responds "okay," with uncertain facial expression and soft tone of voice. Standing next to play therapist (not facing her), no eye contact.	Watches child look around, facial expression neutral. "You are looking around the playroom to see what you want to play with." Tone of voice is matter-of-fact. Moves from position to face child about 36 inches away. Crouches down to about the child's eye level.
Continues to look around the playroom, facial expression of mild curiosity.	"You see what you want to play with."
"Yes." Soft, but agreeing tone of voice. Turns back to play therapist while looking at the watercolor paints on the table in the middle of the playroom, facial expression uncertain. Walks to paints, still with back turned.	Watches. No verbalizations.
Squares shoulders, picks up brush and jar of paints. Turns to face play therapist and says, in assertive tone, "I want to play with this!"	"You want to play with that," while pointing to the paints. Voice is matter-of-fact.
Trying very hard to open paint jar. Look of fierce concentration directed at paint jar, bent over with muscles straining, face "screwed up" in intense concentration. After about one full minute, succeeds. Looks at play therapist with exultant facial expression. "I did it!" in pleased tone and louder voice.	With similar voice tone and volume, "You did it!"
"Yes I did!" in extremely pleased tone of voice and with satisfied facial expression.	No actions; no verbalizations.

Appendix 11.B.   Comments from Supervisees and Supervisor

Sample Positive Comments from Supervisees Regarding Role Play Script:

- "Appropriate (structuring) opening statement."
- "Phrase, 'You can do almost anything you want in the playroom,' in opening statement is appropriately nondirective."
- "When you moved to be 36 inches away from her, you were giving her appropriate space. This contributes to unconditional positive regard because it lets the child decide whether to move closer."
- "When she got the paint jar open and said 'I did it!' your response of 'You did it!' matched her tone and volume—good empathy."

Sample Suggestions for Improvement from Supervisees Regarding Role Play Script:

- "In your opening statement, you said, 'If you have any questions, ask.' This makes the statement directive. You could say 'If you have any questions, you can ask,' to be less directive."
- "In the beginning of the session, when you said, 'You are looking around the playroom to see what you want to play with,' I don't think you matched her feelings. I thought she looked unsure of herself and maybe wasn't even thinking about what to play with. You could have given a feeling response like, 'You're not sure about what to do,' which might be more empathic."
- "You didn't reflect when she was trying so hard to get the top off the paint jar. You could have said, 'You're working really hard to get the top off.'"

Sample Suggestions for Improvement from Supervisor Regarding Role Play Script:

- "Concentrate on noticing how her body postures and facial expressions reveal feelings, and try reflecting these feelings with simple statements, e.g., 'You're really pleased that you did that by yourself.'"
- "Try to give verbal responses to non-verbal behaviors of the child in addition to the child's verbalizations. By keeping silent when she is silent, you could inadvertently violate the core condition of unconditional positive regard by giving the impression you approve of her more when she speaks. A good rule of thumb is to give a verbal response every 15 to 20 seconds."

REFERENCES

Alfano, C. A., Beidel, D. C., & Turner, S. M. (2006). Cognitive correlates of social phobia among children and adolescents. *Journal of Abnormal Child Psychology*, 34(2), 189–201.

Alkin, M. C., & Christie, C. A. (2002). The use of role-play in teaching evaluation. *American Journal of Evaluation*, 23(2), 209–18.

Anderson, C. M., English, C. L., & Hedrick, T. M. (2006). Use of the structured descriptive assessment with typically developing children. *Behavior Modification*, 30(3), 352–78.

Armstrong, J. (2001). Role playing: A method to forecast decisions. In J. S. Armstrong (Ed.), *Principles of forecasting: A handbook for researchers and practitioners* (15–30). New York: Springer.

Bailey, S., & Watson, R. (1998). Understanding in younger pupils: A pilot evaluation of a strategy based on drama/role play. *International Journal of Science Education, 20*(2), 139–52.

Beebe, D. W., & Risi, S. (1993). Treatment of adolescents and young adults with high-functioning autism or Asperger syndrome. In M. A. Reinecke, F. M. Dattilio, & A. Freeman (Eds.), *Cognitive therapy with children and adolescents* (369–401). New York: Guilford.

Beidel, D. C., Turner, S. M., & Morris, T. L. (1999). Psychopathology of childhood social phobia. *Journal of the American Academy of Child and Adolescent Psychiatry, 38*(6), 643–50.

Bergin, J., Eckstein, J., Manns, M. L., & Wallingford, E. (2001). Patterns for gaining different perspectives: A part of a pedagogical patterns project pattern language. *Proceedings ofEuroPLoP'01*, Universitaetsverlag Konstanz. Retrieved May 24, 2007, from http://www.jeckstein.de/pedagogical/PedagogicalPatterns/gain diffperspective.pdf.

Brandt, J. C., & Bateman, S. W. (2006). Senior veterinary students' perceptions of using role-play to learn communication skills. *Journal of Veterinary Medical Education, 33*(1), 76–80.

Brown, L. K., Kessel, S. M., Lourie, K. J., & Ford, H. H. (1997). Influence of sexual abuse on HIV-related attitudes and behaviors in adolescent psychiatric inpatients. *Journal of the American Academy of Child & Adolescent Psychiatry, 6*(3), 316–22.

Ceballo, R., Ramirez, C., Maltese, K. L., & Bautista, E. M. (2006). A bilingual "neighborhood club": Intervening with children exposed to urban violence. *American Journal of Community Psychology, 37*(3–4), 167–74.

Chen, K. (2006). Social skills intervention for students with emotional/behavioral disorders: A literature review from the American perspective. *Educational Research and Reviews, 1*(3), 143–49.

Cook, M. (2000). Writing and role play: A case for inclusion. *Reading, 34*(2), 74–78.

Curwin, R. L., & Mendler, A. N. (2000). Preventing violence with values-based schools. *Reclaiming Children and Youth: Journal of Emotional and Behavioral Problems, 9*(1), 41–44.

Cutler, C., & Hay, I. (2000). 'Club Dread': Applying and refining an issues-based role play on environment, economy, and culture. *Journal of Geography in Higher Education, 24*(5), 179–97.

Elksnin, L. K., & Elksnin, N. (1998). Teaching social skills to students with learning and behavior problems. *Intervention in School and Clinic, 33*(3), 131–40.

FitzGerald, M., Crowley, T., Greenhouse, P., Robert, C., et al. (2003). Teaching sexual history taking to medical students and examining it: Experience in one medical school and a national survey. *Medical Education 37*(2), 94–98.

Forgatch, M. S., Bullock, B. M., & Patterson, G. R. (2004). From theory to practice: Increasing effective parenting through role-play. In H. Steiner (Ed.), *Handbook of mental health interventions in children and adolescents: An integrated developmental approach* (782–814). San Francisco: Jossey-Bass.

Fox, L., Dunlap, G., & Powell, D. (2002). Young children with challenging behavior: Issues and considerations for behavior support. *Journal of Positive Behavior Interventions, 4*(4): 208–17.

Frey, K. S., Hirschstein, M. K., & Guzzo, B. A. (2000). Second step: Preventing aggression by promoting social competence. *Journal of Emotional and Behavioral Disorders, 6*(2), 66–80.

Frick-Helms, S. B. (2002a). Play therapy question 1: In client-centered play therapy, what is the ideal frequency of empathic responses? *SCAPT NewsLetter, 4*(1), 3–4. (Also published in British *Play Therapy* magazine (March 2007); CalAPT, GAPT newsletters.)

———. (2002b). Play therapy question 2: How should a client-centered play therapist respond to a child's profanity? *SCAPT NewsLetter, 4*(3), 3–6. (Also published in British *Play Therapy* magazine, June 2007; CalAPT, GAPT newsletters.)

Glaser, R. (2000). *Advances in instructional psychology (Vol. 5): Educational design and cognitive science.* London: Laurence Erlbaum Associates.

Good, J., & Robertson, J. (2003). Using a collaborative virtual role-play environment to foster characterization in stories. *Journal of Interactive Learning Research, 14*, 5–29.

Gray, R., Wykes, T., & Gournay, K. (2003). The effect of medication management training on community mental health nurse's clinical skills. *International Journal of Nursing Studies, 40*(2), 163–69.

Green, K. C. (2002). Forecasting decisions in conflict situations: A comparison of game theory, role-playing, and unaided judgment. *International Journal of Forecasting, 18*, 321–44.

Hardoff, D., & Schonmann, S. (2001). Training physicians in communication skills with adolescents using teenage actors as simulated patients. *Medical Education, 35*(3), 206–10.

Harper, D. C., & Wadsworth, J. S. (1992). Improving health care communication for persons with mental retardation. *Public Health Reports, 107*(3), 297–302.

Hillcox, S. (2006). The survival game: Teaching ecology through role-play. *School Science Review, 87*(320), 75–81.

Himle, M. B., Miltenberger, R. G., Gatheridge, B. J., & Flessner, C. A. (2004). An evaluation of two procedures for training skills to prevent gunplay in children. *Pediatrics, 113*(1), 70–77.

Hodson, D., & Reid, D. J. (1988). Science for all: Motives, meanings and implications. *School Science Review, 69*(249), 653–61.

Hurd, T., Muti, P., Erwin, D., & Womack, S. (2003). An evaluation of the integration of non-traditional learning tools into a community based breast and cervical cancer education program: The witness project of Buffalo *BMC Cancer 3,* 18, 1471–2407. Retrieved July 20, 2007, from http://www.biomedcentral.com/1471-2407/3/18.

Ihnen, G. H., Penn, D. L., Corrigan, P. W., & Martin, J. (1998). Social perception and social skill in schizophrenia. *Psychiatry Research, 80*(3), 275–86.

Ip, A. & Linser, R. (2001). Evaluation of a role-play simulation in political science. *The Technology Source* (http://ts.mivu.org/) (Feb.). Available online at http://ts.mivu.org/default.asp?show=article&id=1034.

Johnson, D. D. P., McDermott, R., Barrett, E. S., & Cowden, J. (2006). Overconfidence in war games: Experimental evidence on expectations, aggression, gender and testosterone. *Proceedings of the Royal Society: Biological Sciences, 273*(1600), 2513–20.

Kelly, G. A. (1955). *The psychology of personal constructs, Vol. II.* New York: Norton.

Knowles, C., Kinchington, F., Erwin, J., & Peters, B. (2001) A randomized controlled trial of the effectiveness of combining video role play with traditional methods of delivering undergraduate medical education. *Sexually Transmitted Infections, 77,* 376–80.

Kofoed, M. H. (2006). The Hiroshima and Nagasaki bombs: Role-play and students' interest in physics. *Physics Education, 41*(6), 502–7.

Kolb, D. A. (1984). Experiential learning: Experience the source of learning and development. Englewood Cliffs, NJ: Prentice Hall.

Korabik, K., Baril, G. L., & Watson, C. (1993). Managers' conflict management style and leadership effectiveness: The moderating effects of gender. *Sex Roles, 29*(5–6), 405–20.

Lam, D. H., Kuipers, L., & Leff, J. P. (1993). Family work with patients suffering from schizophrenia: The impact of training on psychiatric nurses. *Journal of Advanced Nursing, 18*(2), 233–37.

Larson, L. M., Clark, M. P., Wesely, L. A., Koraleski, S. F., et al. (1999). Videos versus role plays to increase counseling self-efficacy in prepractica trainees. *Counselor Education and Supervision, 38*(4), 237–48.

Loudon, R. F., Anderson, P. M., Gill, P. S., & Greenfield, S. M. (1999). Educating medical students for work in culturally diverse societies. *JAMA, 282*(9), 875–80.

Lutzker, J. R., Bigelow, K. M., Doctor, R. M., & Kessler, M. L. (1998). Safety, health care, and bonding within an ecobehavioral approach to beating and preventing child abuse and neglect. *Journal of Family Violence, 13*(2), 163–85.

Marcotte, D. (1997). Treating depression in adolescence: A review of the effectiveness of cognitive-behavioral treatments. *Journal of Youth and Adolescence, 26*(3), 273–83.

McSharry, G., & Jones, S. (2000). Role-play in science teaching and learning. *School Science Review, 82*(298), 73–81.

Mercado, S. A. (2000). Pre-managerial business education: A role for role-plays? *Journal of Further and Higher Education, 24*(1), 117–26.

Minghella, E., & Benson, A. (1995). Developing reflective practice in mental health nursing through critical incident analysis. *Journal of Advanced Nursing, 21*(2), 205–13.

Monti, P. M., Rohsenow, D. J., & Hutchison, K. E. (2000). Toward bridging the gap between biological, psychobiological and psychosocial models of alcohol craving. *Addiction, 95*(Supplement 2), S229–36.

O'Donnell, N., & Shaver, L. (1990). The use of role-play to teach communication skills. Paper presented at Conference on Successful College Teaching (14th, Orlando, FL, March 1–3, 1990).

Out, J. W., & Lafreniere, K. D. (2001). Baby think it over: Using role-play to prevent teen pregnancy. *Adolescence, 36*(143), 571–82.

Penn, D. L., Kohlmaier, J. R., & Corrigan, P. W. (2000). Interpersonal factors contributing to the stigma of schizophrenia: Social skills, perceived attractiveness, and symptoms. *Schizophrenia Research, 45*(1–2), 37–45.

Pillemer, K., & Hudson, B. (1993). A model abuse prevention program for nursing assistants. *The Gerontologist, 33*(1), 128–31.

Reisman, J. M., & Reibordy, S. (1993). *Principles of psychotherapy with children.* Lexington, KY: Lexington Books.

Rollnick, S., Kinnersley, P., & Butler, C. (2002). Context-bound communication skills training: Development of a new method. *Medical Education, 36*(4), 377–83.

Sadler-Smith, E., & Riding, R. (1999). Cognitive style and instructional preferences. *Instructional Science, 27*(5), 355–71.

Sander, P., Stevenson, K., King, M., & Coates, D. (2000). University students' expectations of teaching. *Studies in Higher Education, 25*(3), 309–23.

Shanks, D. R. (1995). *The psychology of associative learning.* Cambridge, England: Cambridge University Press.

Shearer, D. (2003). Using role play to develop cultural competence. *Journal of Nursing Education, 42*(6), 273–76.

Shuell, T. J. (1986). Cognitive conceptions of learning. *Review of Educational Research, 56*(4), 1–36.

Smith, S. N. (2004). Teaching for civic participation with negotiation role plays. *Social Education, 68*(3), 194.

Tsang, H. W. H. (2001). Applying social skills training in the context of vocational rehabilitation for people with schizophrenia. *The Journal of Nervous and Mental Disease, 189*(2), 90–98.

Vincent, A., & Shepherd, J. (1998). Experiences in teaching Middle East politics via internet-based role-play simulations. *Journal of Interactive Media in Education, 98*(11), www-jime.open.ac.uk/98/11.

Part III

FACILITATING
SELF-AWARENESS

12

⌘

The Play Space of Supervision

Arthur Robbins

A new supervisee enters my office, and I am immediately pulled into an atmosphere of glum dysphoria. Her voice sounds flat; her body appears heavy. There is a faraway look in her eyes. I rarely make direct eye contact. We speak briefly about her reasons for entering supervision. She pleads that she does not know what she is doing and needs help with her clients. I inquire as to her background, but it is of little help in developing any real rapport. I reflect to myself: this will not be an easy relationship. She reviews her cases with pain and incomprehension. She is brief and gives few details. I learn that her client load consists of both children and adults. The supervision session becomes oppressive. I am feeling heavy, as though I were carrying a large stone on my back.

TRANSITIONAL PHENOMENA IN THE
SUPERVISORY RELATIONSHIP

I suspect that she is both depressed and traumatized. After many dead spots in our supervisory dialogue, out of desperation, I ask her what she is going to eat when she leaves the office. Her face starts to brighten up, and a long mutual education begins on the pros and cons connected to different restaurants located in the area. We are both interested in this topic and share our particular preferences regarding styles of cooking as well as prices. In this mix we also stumble into another mutual area of interest: movies. Both of us subscribe to Netflix, and we learn that we have similar tastes regarding old and new movies. Excitement develops in our interchange of information. We smile together and occasionally laugh at our mutual discoveries. A space develops between us. D. W. Winnicott (2005) refers to this space as "play space." This space is neither inside the supervisee or myself but is at an intermediate joining point where our fantasies and affects meet and commingle. From another perspective, a certain chemistry and resonance develops between us. The introduction of the topic reads easily and has a "that makes sense" quality to it.

Using a Winnicott framework, we share a piece of mutual reality that touches both our inside and outside life. Food and movies have become akin to a transitional object: here our mutual "blankie"—food and movies—creates a deep connection that fosters the continuity of our most primary identifications. This notion of space and time has been elaborated by Winnicott and provides a way to organize this chapter.

PLAY SPACE IN SUPERVISION

Winnicott describes play as a meeting ground between our inner world and the outside reality. Metaphors, symbols, and imaginative interactions provide a creative synthesis between the inner and outer life of the child. Bridging these inner and outer worlds are sensations of singing, dancing, touching, and listening, to name a few—the byways of affect states that ultimately become part of our cognitive world.

Why then do we use the metaphor of play? For one, our interactions with the infant/child become an imaginative and generative meeting ground for the development of symbols. This ultimately becomes the fertile ground for the development of a creative spirit. Indeed the very harnessing of these symbolic expressions that connect the inside and outside become an important means of nurturing the very soul of the individual. The world of play for the child serves an important developmental function in contributing to the integration of self and other.

The therapist, according to Winnicott, facilitates the sharing of a play space. Thus, when client and therapist, or supervisor and supervisee, are unable to play, the object of supervision is to help regenerate the act of a playful therapeutic space. With this frame in mind, the supervisory cases I discuss in this chapter will be viewed as a form of play directed at and expanding the connections between client and therapist and supervisor and supervisee. Supervision, then, does not merely facilitate the acquisition of information or skills, but it activates development in the flow of communication in relationships. This flow moves dynamically in a rhythm from inside to outside, back and forth. However, this rhythm of energy can be chaotic, still, or an ongoing dance. Most importantly, play should not be confused with "having fun." The play space is a deep meeting of the minds through a range of different nonverbal and verbal interactions. Particular attention is paid to body cues, for they become the contact points for the development of an affective connection. In this triad of client, supervisee, and supervisor, we attune ourselves to the nonlinear primary process communications that are buried in our bodies. These communications make impressive inroads to our therapeutic experiences and become very important data to which we devote our therapeutic attention. Ultimately, the path from sensory, affective, and cognitive experiences organizes the therapeutic relationship.

PLAY PROVIDES A SAFE DISTANCE FOR SUPERVISOR AND SUPERVISEE INTERACTION

Let us return to the opening paragraph. I learn that this supervisee internally carries a powerful and critical father who demands perfection; he is described as emotionally bombastic and demands obedience as well as perfectionism. The inner child of the supervisee is frozen in terror. The symptom of this frozen state is expressed in a constant complaint: "I don't know what I'm doing, and I make too many mistakes; I am not perfect." However, her protective haze lifts as we start to develop a play space of communication and excitement with the shared metaphors of food and DVDs. I do not merge or become identified with the critical father or frozen child. This new space unlocks a therapist who previously was hidden behind all this terror. I discover the competent therapist who is both grounded and centered in her interactions with clients. With the diminishment of defenses that are associated with supervision, her authenticity emerges and I receive a far clearer understanding of her work as a therapist. Apparently, this structure of therapy permits the supervisee to relax and engage her clients within our complex triadic intermingling in the play space.

At the same time, the toll of her early background interferes with her going more deeply into the material with her clients. There is a whole area of interaction that requires work. Yet, I do not wish to fall into the role of her demanding father. I observe that her body holds the affects of rage, helplessness, and confusion. The tightness in her musculature, the lack of joy in her face tells their own story. However, our "nonsupervisory" interchange of movies and food humanizes our encounter and places us on more equal footing. This valuable concept perhaps could be developed further. Our actions and reactions around food and movies enlarge our play space. Her defenses loosen up, and over a period of time, her subtle sense of humor and playfulness come through. I stay away from any character analysis of her defenses and minimize any comments regarding countertransference issues. I am a supportive supervisor, and we both learn how to enjoy our contact with one another.

The evolution of a play space through a transitional object was discovered very early in my work with clients. I recall one woman who was virtually frozen in her initial therapeutic contact. Pizza shops became our transitional phenomenon, and slowly we started to trust one another over an imaginary piece of pizza. The latest discovery of a new shop was met with mutual excitement. Energy and affects became permissible and safe. The pizza metaphor offered sufficient safe distance within our dialogue. Holding and containment, then, are important dimensions of supervisory play.

EXPLORING THE DIMENSIONS OF SYMBOLIC PLAY

In order to familiarize beginners with the act of symbolic play, I often inquire how their mothers held them. Some hold little memory of this experience. Others report the holding as sensuous and pleasurable. In my teaching of art therapy students, I request that they imagine their mothers holding them. I present the following questions: When your mother holds you, what do you imagine the experience to be; do you feel safe, suffocated, or floating in the air? What kind of hands does she have? Can you draw a picture of you and your mother? I then proceed to inquire how they held their clients. At times I request they move and talk like their client and call upon the mother inside of them that resonates and contains their nonverbal sensory communications. Some report how difficult it is to go past the limitations of their own internal mother. I encourage them to develop new internalizations that will act as a substitute and are able to contain them. I suggest that they think of a positive experience with a therapist, teacher, or mentor who plays this role of a positive force for holding to develop a new internal repertoire of holding.

Occasionally, I ask students to draw a container and place something in it. Often it is a vase with a flower. I then inquire: Does the flower really fit the vase, or does it look like separate entities that do not belong together? Here, I develop a kinesthetic sense of nonverbal communication that is inherent in acquiring the feeling of play space.

Holding is a very complex act. We are constantly responding to a closeness/distance continuum of contact. I ask supervisees where they would like to place their chairs. Is it close enough or too far away? How tightly or loosely do they require this holding? Do they feel controlled or secure? Can they experience the flow of energy? Rhythm becomes a dynamic of this holding space. Can they imagine the flow of energy moving from inside to outside and back? First, being preoccupied with the self, and then with the other?

Stimulation also becomes another dimension of a playful interchange. Some materials simply overwhelm the client or supervisee who opposes the state of formless regression. Other clients require clear pencil lines, while many are best suited for a craypa interaction. There are differences in the inherent qualities of the modalities of art, movement, and music. Do we want a very primitive contact? I might think of drums along with dance. Art usually has more cognitive structure, which creates reflection. I play out these various modalities with the supervisee so that they can experience the power of each modality.

TRANSFERENCE/COUNTERTRANSFERENCE IN THE SUPERVISORY PLAY SPACE

A major area of supervisory preoccupation concerns the reaction and interaction of transference and countertransference communications. Countertransference problems take the form of projections that throw supervisees off their center and sense of being grounded. If they are not familiar with these two energetic notions of space, I offer the example of a tree that is rooted in the ground. Can they picture themselves as a tree and discover how deep their roots go, and whether they can feel their personal energy flowing into the earth? The metaphor becomes an imaginative exploration of how we encounter the safety of being grounded. Can they speak from the center of their being and discern when others are either "too much in their heads" or discharging impulses? The work, then, of transference and countertransference becomes an interchange as well as an articulation of projected affects and images. These projected affects engage very personal conflicts of the supervisee, creating a loss of center and being grounded. By implication, affects and sensations that do not create a loss of center and being grounded are not considered countertransference material. However, how we work through the personal issues of countertransference depends upon the sophistication and depth of the supervisee's past therapeutic experience.

The experience of being centered and grounded becomes likened to an ego state. There is a sense of wholeness and openness to a multitude of stimuli. On the other hand, I investigate with supervisees their ability to detect when they are scattered or intellectualized. I determine the nature of this engagement from my own particular inner state in listening to cases. I might well be working on my own countertransference to a particular supervisee.

On the other hand, I might also be picking up the supervisee's counter-transference problem. This often happens when I listen to trauma cases. Here, the supervisee becomes either dissociated or scattered, and when listening to their reporting, I am completely overwhelmed or disconnected. I then know that there is a good chance that we live in the land of trauma. As therapists, we do not ask ourselves the question, what are we feeling in a moment of time? Yet the awareness of our inner experience, while still remaining in the therapeutic dialogue, becomes an important part of the art of therapeutic play.

Quite often supervisees present a very ambivalent relationship to their inner child that undermines the therapeutic dialogue. Is the child sorrowful, or for that matter, frightened? Does this child know the sensation of joy and glee? At times, the very existence of an inside image of a child can be covered by many complex defenses.

A supervisee, Mary, comes to mind. She has undergone eight years of intensive therapy but believes it has had little impact on her life. She left an institute training program because she felt uninvolved with the material. Most of her relationships have gone nowhere. She is in her mid-forties and desperately wants something meaningful to happen. She communicates all this to me in the most bland and cutoff manner. I feel little energy in our relationship and realize that a drastic shift in the affect state must occur if we are both to survive this relationship. She complains that her clients bore her, because all they want to do is to play games. She sees very little therapeutic value in this but does not know what else to do. She is unable to transform the linear structure of a game into a playful symbolic interchange. Her background consists of an overwhelming but caring mother and a father who is critical and contemptuous. She suspects that behind his contempt lies a scary sexual attraction, although she does not have enough evidence to back up her assertion. By objective standards, I am aware of the supervisee's beauty, although there is a flat, cutoff quality to her presence. She works with children, as this is the area where she receives most of her referrals. She readily confesses to a complete unawareness of body cues.

PLAYING WITH PROJECTIVE IDENTIFICATIONS

As a supervisor, I am faced with a dilemma. If I start becoming playful, will she interpret my behavior as being seductive? Yet I feel that I have no recourse but to start opening up the "play space" that is largely absent between us. I tell her of my plans to change the direction of our supervisee/supervisor dialogue. We need much more play and an attention to body cues. I note that she makes eye contact and walks with a sense of assurance. Yet it feels like a veneer or a practiced stance rather than something that is felt inside. Mary reports that she has been a performer, although not a very successful one. However, she has mastered the trick of looking self-assured. I comment that her neck and shoulders seem full of tension; she agrees. She then adds that she is not a person who spends a good deal of time in being connected to these cues, for her orientation to life is one of seeking outside stimulation and pleasure. She also admits that she is easily distracted and has an underlying sense of anxiety.

In the next session, Mary comes in late and admits that this is her usual pattern. She keeps people waiting in spite of all her efforts to come on time. I decide to be playful and respond that I was beginning to feel she didn't want to see me. "Oh no," she protests, "That is not the case." "Well," I say, "I shall be waiting for you and thinking about you even when you are not here." She does not know whether I am being serious or not and inquires as to what I mean by that statement. "I mean exactly what I said. Your time is our time and when you are not here, the session still begins even though you are absent." She smiles vaguely and drops the subject. It is the beginning of my attempt to engage her with metaphors and symbols. I wonder to myself if this direction change is too much for her, but I do observe her body begin to relax.

Mary once again comes late for her next session. "You must be exasperated and hate me," she confesses. I retort, "I am more curious than exasperated." She replies, "I do this with everyone, and it's nothing personal." She then describes her family: "There is nothing constant about it. My parents were both performers and would keep crazy hours. They would constantly fight with one another, and I often tried to distract them with my provocativeness. Both of them yelled a good deal and I wanted attention, even if it was negative." She returns to talking about our relationship: "I firmly believe that I am certainly not your favorite; I think there are a few others you like better in the supervisory group. I truly believe you don't think much of my ability." I retort, "You certainly give me a good deal of power to decide how smart or valuable you are. What do you think of yourself? Do you value what's inside?" We leave this as a question.

She then goes on to discuss her client, whom she confesses is fat and ugly. She simply does not look forward to being with this girl. The mother is cruel, and the father yells a lot. "I wonder," I said, "if this little girl wants desperately to be seen, and at the same time doesn't feel she deserves it. Are you picking up something negative about her and a hunger that resonates with your own?" She reflects upon this and proceeds to tell me about ways she was trying to engage the child. She struggles not only with the client but also with a part of herself she simply didn't like. We both reflect, "Well let's see how all this develops," and our supervisory session ends.

In the following group training session, Mary becomes enmeshed in my countertransference response. A discussion ensues by another member who affirms her power and growth. She wants this recognized by me. When I try to divert her comments in a presentation, she feels squashed and misunderstood. A very lively discussion of power and specialness follows. Mary, the trainee under discussion, keeps very quiet. I confront her and wonder why she is not expressing her feelings regarding competition. My comment breaks the group right open: "I did not know we could see you individually," "You never told us . . . ," "Aren't you breaking confidentiality?" "You're putting Mary on the spot, what's going on with you?" Mary shares with me in an individual session her blowing up at her therapist. She felt murderous, and they both figured out that it was really directed at me. Mary is not one to readily feel anger. She feels excited and released, although she also adds, "I am not sure I feel safe anymore." I reiterate my policy that supervision is not a confidential relationship. If she is in both individual and group supervision, then I feel no compunction to separate one experience from the other. "Yes," she protests, "but you didn't tell me ahead of time." I say to her, "I just can't give a list of rules ahead of time regarding my policy; nevertheless, I certainly can understand that you are both shocked and upset with me." The supervisee does not look threatened by this new development. She is reassured by the group support and admits that anger is a most difficult feeling to own. She is hungry for approval and buries any glimmer of anger that she may feel. We certainly are making contact, and our relationship takes on a new level of intimacy. By contrast, I would not take this form of intervention with my first supervisee. The former I suspect could be easily retraumatized and not find such an interaction productive or safe. With the second supervisee, the characterological issues are prominent in contributing to a restriction of the play space. The group, after this incident, sets out on a very lively course. I seem to have lost my lofty perch, and the members seem to feel liberated by their perception that I am both human and make mistakes. Mary's newfound comfort with anger may well open up a channel to unconscious imagery and symbols. There is far less control and more energy in our relationship.

STRUCTURE IN PROVIDING A SAFE SPACE FOR
THE EXPLORATION OF TRANSFERENCE
AND COUNTERTRANSFERENCE

Directed questions, restrictive limit setting, and clear and defined directives create a safe structure for beginning students. On the other hand, more advanced practitioners and students can tolerate a certain amount of ambiguity and openness to explore personal areas. Any form of personal investigation threatens some students. Others may plunge in and reveal personal material that may precipitate a good deal of anxiety. Nevertheless, the imparting of various levels of structure makes the exploration of transference and countertransference a very real possibility.

As a professor of art therapy, I teach both introductory and advanced courses in symbolic play, formally titled Introduction to Art Therapy or Advanced Seminar in Art Therapy. But, basically, I introduce the students to the whole range of symbolic connections. In the following sections, I will offer different examples of working with both introductory and advanced students' classes. I will also contrast these experiences with working with a supervisee who functions on an advanced level.

An Example of Tight Structure

In the introductory classes, the students are often overwhelmed. Internships, assigned readings, and reports flood their very beings. Clients who function on a primitive level of communication tell their stories through nonverbal gestures and intonations. Invariably, these communications filter through and create enormous amounts of anxiety and unrest. Many of the students are strangers to the city and have given up past lifestyles to enter the program. On one hand, they are emotionally wide open and need clear and straightforward holding. They also require structure and organization to make some sense out of a chaotic introductory experience. Consequently, a good deal of my class is fairly structured and yet open to experiences regarding symbolic language. We work around the concept of boundaries and holding. Information is supplied, and we talk about the value of different modalities. However, disturbing issues become apparent. Many of their clients sneak under their skin, touching very deep conflicts within their families of origin. Many of the students enter the program with extensive therapy; others are not even sure why they need therapy. They are familiar with images from an aesthetic point of view; however, the translation of images into therapeutic meaning opens up a vast area of learning.

In the introductory class, I introduce students to the theory and framework of play. There are generous quotes from Winnicott, and I offer examples of what play is all about. I emphasize the mind-body connection. They listen, but that is nothing like the hands-on experience that comes in their internship or the exercises that are conducted in class. The following class exercise opens up the entire issue regarding the role of family and its relationship to transference and countertransference.

In a particular class, I request that students draw a picture of their family. After they have completed the task, I give them the following questions

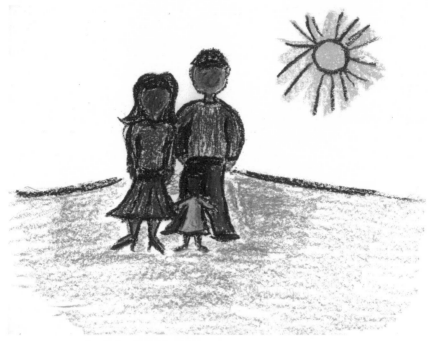

Figure 12.1.   A Student's Family Picture.

and offer time to formulate their answers in writing. The following are both the questions and the answers from a student regarding the picture of her family. Please refer to figure 12.1.

(1) *When I look at my child I feel:*
   • *Sad that she is almost invisible except her dress, she is disconnected, almost missing; she is waving her arms to be noticed.*
(2) *When I look at my mother I feel:*
   • *Constricted, uptight; looks like she has a flowery dress but it isn't so flowery. She is disconnected and untouched/not touching.*
(3) *When I look at my father I feel:*
   • *Aloof, disconnected, void, alone.*
(4) *When I look at my family I feel:*
   • *Empty, disconnected, unloving, unsure of what is going on, mysterious.*
(5) *When I look at my family, holding becomes:*
   • *An important element for support; love connections, that's what's missing.*
(6) *Authority in my family is:*
   • *The mother, father, and child, uncertain from the picture.*

(7) Connections in my family are:
- *Individual, weak, limited, unsure.*

(8) The child plays with:
- *Other children, siblings.*

I then divide the class into dyads. A student volunteers to present a case. The client is a fourteen-year-old girl who has been diagnosed as psychotic. She has been hospitalized on three different occasions. Her father, who died when she was nine, was imprisoned three times for sexual assault. He also had a history of assaulting one of her girlfriends. Her mother abandoned her, and she was farmed out to her father's family; the grandmother and aunt became the main caretakers. Her symptoms of hyperactivity and bizarre behavior warranted hospitalization; she has choked and taken off the head of a cat and stuck instruments up a dog's anus.

The presenter acts out the role of the client, moving and talking like her. After a suitable period of time, the presenter of this case becomes the therapeutic consultant for each pair of students. Each member of the dyad plays the role of either client or therapist and takes on the part of this relationship with which they are most comfortable. The presenting student moves from pair to pair, offers information, and comments as to whether the student has captured the image of the client. Roleplaying continues for thirty minutes. I instruct the group to come back into the circle and ask the following questions. Once again, I request that the group write down both the questions and their answers. The student who initially volunteered to offer her answers to the family picture now continues to give her answers:

(1) What was the client expressing in play, and how does it relate to you?
- *The client was hyperactive, had a lot of high energy, and I in return related with a sense of calmness and curiosity.*

(2) What could I offer the child in light of what was happening?
- *I tried to offer the child an outlet for her energy and to meet her resistance where it was. Looking at the child in my family picture, standing separate and disconnected from my parents, helped me to connect to this child who felt alone. This sense of isolation helped me to connect with my client.*

(3) How did the play space develop?
- *Space developed at the end when she became interested in wrapping a string around clay. I noticed it looked like an animal and wanted to walk around with it.*

We then proceed to discuss the symbolic expression of string wrapped around the clay. We hypothesized that perhaps it was an expression of a wish to be tightly held and supported.

As we view the student's picture of her family, there is an illusion of closeness that quickly falls to the wayside, as father and mother seem preoccupied and involved with themselves (figure 12.1). The child fades into the picture and is not clearly demarcated. She reaches out with her hands but does not really make contact. None of the figures express any real definition or expression in their faces. Their smiles are stereotypical and offer an illusion of friendliness. Paradoxically, the figures do seem grounded. From the student's answers to the questions, she exhibits a degree of self-awareness regarding her aloneness. She is able to take sufficient distance from the alone child, and yet is able to employ this image as a bridge to connection. She seems less aware of what the family does offer her. In this very insecure setting, all members seem grounded. What is most interesting to note, her partner reports, is that the therapist ultimately was able to calm her down through a very steady and grounded approach to her hyperactivity. What about that is so surprising?

Another student, Mirako, offers a very different set of responses to the structured questions regarding her family picture. Her answers are terse and often unrevealing:

(1) *When I look at my child I feel:*
     • *Happy, protected, and strong.*
(2) *When I look at my mother I feel:*
     • *Warm and supported.*
(3) *When I look at my father I feel:*
     • *Depressed and sad.*
(4) *When I look at my family I feel:*
     • *Good and safe.*
(5) *When I look at my family holding becomes:*
     • *Complete.*
(6) *Authority in my family is:*
     • *Equal.*
(7) *Connections in my family are:*
     • *There and still building.*
(8) *Child plays with:*
     • *Herself.*

As we review the family picture (figure 12.2) the figures exhibit minimal differentiation. The picture of the family contains different energetic qualities and appears to be more connected to the air than the earth. They are all part of a self-contained unit that is designated by a soft pastel quality. In her role play as therapist, I observe the student wandering around looking confused and lost. Her partner, who takes on the role of the child, reports minimal contact with her student therapist. The student therapist,

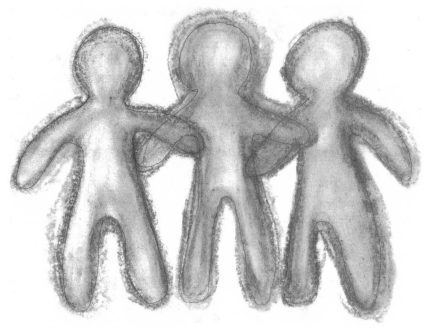

Figure 12.2. Mirako's Family Picture.

who was born and raised in Japan, retorts that she needs more time to make contact. I then ask the student therapist to move her chair and place it in the room where she feels most comfortable in being with my presence. She moves her chair approximately three to four feet away from me. I ask her partner to also move her chair where she feels most comfortable; she moves her chair approximately eight feet away from me. The class then receives a concrete example of the aesthetics of play space. The student therapist sits rather comfortably close to me. I become immediately aware of the subtleties of communication that are expressed in the student's face. I request that her partner offer a movement expression of her experience playing the client. She proceeds to move and states, "I feel like a closed door." The student therapist reports, "People often say that about me." Yet, when the student sits close to me, I perceive subtle expressions of confusion, curiosity, even playfulness that were not apparent when she sat as part of the circle. My reaction to this felt perception is to offer her an image of a gentle flower. In response to my image, she smiles. Her roots are in Asia, and nonverbal communication has been a basic part of her life. Her partner, on the other hand, is of the African-American culture that is full of outgoing energy. Obviously, a disjunction in resonance exists in this dyad. Given time, these two partners may meet one another.

Presently, however, they have a big gulf to cross in order to create a transitional space. I encourage the student therapist to see things that exist outside her family's world. In the meantime, I also try to be accepting of who she is and to be respectful of the internal relationship that has guided her life. Interestingly, both students for the first time go out to lunch with each other and report a most enjoyable exchange. I wonder to myself whether there is more mirroring going on in their dialogue now that they are becoming more comfortable with each other's presence. I am aware that the student therapist picture of her family, a most undifferentiated family structure, probably represents a lack of visual mirroring between all members of the family unit. I am also aware that, for the most part, feeling words in Asian cultures do not exist.

From a Western perspective, I view the student's picture as being ungrounded and undifferentiated. However, as soon as I give up this framework I see an extraordinarily sensitive and nuanced student who does not have the words to articulate her inner experiences. At the very least, I am aware that any of my impressions must be very tentative for I am not comfortably conversant with her culture and mores.

In the proceeding class I request all students to imagine that this client has now become a member of their family. I urge them to make up a story as to what they anticipate in the interaction. The first student offers a story wherein she takes complete responsibility for the parenting of this new member. Mirako, with much reluctance, goes out and plays with her new sibling. She resents the intrusion into her silence, but trusts that with acceptance the child will calm down and become one of them. We can observe, then, how one student carries within her an image of the caretaker and utilizes this image as a fulcrum for playfulness. The other creates a quiet meditative space that will be offered as her special form of healing.

Teaching within this very personal framework provides safety, for the exercises are structured. For the most part, I do not explore emotional issues that are invariably opened up by this particular structure. Many of the students have undergone minimal therapy, and as a result I move slowly, opening up possibilities and creating a beginning dialogue with their internal images. For some, this becomes an impetus to initiate personal therapy. Role playing facilitates an inner exploration of their experience, for they are action oriented by nature.

An Elastic Structure for Individual Differences in Transference and Countertransference

We now move to an advanced class: second-year students who already have experienced clinical work. They are currently at the beginning stages of a new internship. A young woman presents an adolescent case within an accompanying dialogue of liveliness and protest. "My client is all over the place; he is psychotic and is in constant power plays with me. He simply doesn't follow the rules; he goes his own way, never listens to me. He needs limits. I am at a loss of what to do, for it all seem too much. I am beside myself." She goes on with her case description. In one session they attempt to make a mask, and yet the whole aspect of working with plaster becomes too messy and regressive. We then open up the topic of limiting materials that are available in a room, but it soon becomes evident that theory and technique are not the issues; the presenter constantly returns to the control battle. She offers an example of the client throwing marbles in the garbage. He throws them all over the place. The symbolic meaning of garbage can become a metaphor to augment our understanding of the multiple meanings that are intertwined in one image. In the discussion a fellow student addresses the presenter: "I know what you're going through. When I was a teacher I tried to control the class and became a screamer. Soon I gave up and started to really listen to what they were all about and they calmed down." "I did teaching myself," said the presenter. "I taught sex education, and it was a horror. They would create all kinds of sexual messages. In the notes they wrote, 'Did I have sex?' I knew the answer, everyone does, but frankly it was all too much for me." She confides to the class that she grew up in a chaotic family where in order to survive, control became very important.

A discussion follows regarding the positive value of our defenses. I suggest to my class that if we cannot love our defenses, then we cannot love the very qualities that help us to survive. "Our defenses cannot be seen as our enemy but should be viewed as an ally." Slowly the class investigates their internal sense of shame regarding their personal problems. The student states, "I had a headache coming here; I thought I'd look foolish and act out of control." Slowly, a frame develops: our defenses help us to survive. The students investigate their issues regarding power and their ability to make choices regarding behavior. The presenter reports a good deal of impulsive acting out as a problem in the past. She now has a handle on her provocativeness. Slowly the class unwinds; there is laughter and recognition that we are all part of the "control freak club." We are making inroads and reducing our personal sense of shame regarding our history and the inherent conflicts of survival. The reduction of shame becomes an important learning tool in allowing the darker images of our unconscious to emerge.

AN OPEN STRUCTURE PROVIDING GREATER
FREEDOM FOR EXPLORATION

The following is an example from one of my training groups. All members of my training groups are licensed mental health professionals. One of the trainees, Felicia, is a fairly seasoned art therapist who works both in institutions and private practice. She has worked in art therapy for approximately six years and currently focuses her work on acting-out adolescents.

She is a perky, infectious young woman who characteristically walks with a jaunty cadence and has a quick smile. Felicia has been a member of my training group for approximately two years. She can best be described as alert and engaging, and is a pleasure to work with. She presents a fourteen-year-old girl with a promiscuous history. She socially encounters older men who she then proceeds to have sexual relations with. The girl was sexually molested by an uncle when she was twelve. This man also molested her mother many years ago. The father seems largely absent from the picture. Her mother is quite depressed. She lives out a role of minimal authority and awareness of her daughter's comings and goings. Interestingly, the mother does not believe that her daughter is ready for dates. An older sister learns of her younger sister's sexual experience and alerts the mother. Yet very little is done about this. Felicia presents the problem as an ethical question. She is aware of her responsibility to report this case to the appropriate authorities. The client is at risk, and little has been done to protect her from being exposed to AIDS or physical assault. Yet, Felicia expresses a hesitation to report this case.

Felicia continues to discuss her dilemma. She enjoys working with this young adolescent who virtually embodies a life spirit, and reports a very deep identification. Her client avidly reads books and likes her therapist. Felicia confesses that there is a great similarity to her own adolescence. Felicia, likewise, avidly reads books, but in contrast to her client, she spends most of her time retreating in her room.

Felicia reports that as an adolescent she encountered minimal parental control and supervision. Both parents are described as having been fairly permissive. On the other hand, she did not test limits and presented no challenge to the parents' authority. The mother, described as asexual, was viewed as uninteresting and not someone Felicia wished to identify herself with. By contrast, the father walked around nude, at least in the home, but Felicia thought little of this—it was considered natural and not sexually provocative. The father was described as much more responsive and involved with Felicia. In her early twenties she invited a young man home to share her bedroom. Felicia's father "went ballistic." This reaction was a complete shock, for he, as well as the mother, was rather unemotional and unresponsive. Felicia reported that she was embarrassed and confused by the father's response. But this was put aside, and she entered the world of male-female exploration. She hosted many parties and everyone "had a great time." As a young adult she developed an assertive, provocative presence and presented herself as meeting life head on. She was unconventional, but at the same time lived a socially acceptable life. She really didn't get into big trouble, but played in a gray area. She also made friends and worked her way up the professional ladder.

The group returns to her ethical question. Felicia becomes aware of all the issues regarding this case, yet something holds her back from reporting the client to the appropriate authorities. Her mind slips back into an association regarding power. She resents any man putting himself into a power role. She refers to a member of the group who enjoys exhibiting his smarts. She laughs and confesses that in her group session she wears provocative clothing so that she can get a rise out of this so-called smart aleck. Felicia comments that sex is one of the great equalizers. She reports that she enjoys sex. She suspects that the client enjoys the sexual encounters with older men. Notably, the client is very shy with boys her own age. Felicia confesses her anxiety—she will lose the client and possibly create an unsolvable crisis if she reports this case.

A member of the group told of a similar therapeutic situation. She, however, bit the bullet and reported her adolescent, Nancy, to the authorities. Nancy became furious and did not talk to the therapist. However, since this client was mandated to remain in the group, she belligerently attended, but minimally participated with the therapist. In spite of this negative response, in subsequent group interactions, a fellow adolescent exhibited similar destructive behavior, and Nancy proceeded to report this situation to the administration. The training group agreed that something positive had transpired with Nancy. In spite of all her protests and anger, the therapist's protection made a crucial impact. The group agreed that the client under discussion required protection from an authority.

Felicia leaves the group feeling angry and distraught. She is upset with the member who offers the example to the group, yet she is aware that this is the right thing to do. However, she is not one to follow the rules, and she decides to take the dangerous course of action to do nothing except continue to work. Felicia then returns to the issue of authority. She becomes aware that the issue is not ethical and expresses outrage at older men who take advantage of young girls. She understands that this is a piece of the reality of the world, but really cannot fathom the mentality of rapacious men. "Maybe," Felicia says, "it is not a matter of authority, but how unresponsive her parents' reactions were in her adolescence to her particular problems." As I listen my thoughts float in a different direction. I quietly reflect to myself that this young trainee may be an Electra winner in the family. She reports a close relationship with her father, yet on the face of it seems nonsexualized, at least according to her report. She is aware that there is one big difference between her life and that of the client's—she never crosses the gray line and places herself in jeopardy. However, as an adult, she has intimated that her life is full of sexual exploits.

I then proceed to draw an analogy. I cite the parallel of a suicidal client who applies for treatment. Does she insist on an agreement to prohibit the acting out of suicidal behavior while the client remains in treatment? She readily agrees that this is certainly the appropriate course of action. "Is there some comparison here?" Felicia protests that the administration is aware of the client's acting-out behavior. However, she refrains from taking the next step in abiding by the legal regulations; she has the ultimate responsibility of reporting this client to the appropriate authorities. Felicia confesses her difficulty in accepting the role of the authority. She leaves the session genuinely concerned but has not yet made up her mind as to the right course of action.

In the next group training session, a relatively new therapist/trainee presents a case of an adolescent boy. The therapist introduces art in the play relationship, and he reports the interplay to the group. In his report, verbalization goes nowhere. I offer a series of questions in order to gain a more accurate understanding of what goes on in the session. The group becomes restless. One man calls me a fussy old mother who is too intrusive. Another comments that I am a good teacher, but am I not interfering with the flow? I readily confess that I am doing a good deal of structuring and may be acting out a particular role for the presenting therapist. He shares with the group that a psychiatric consultant is involved in the case. He makes many assumptions about his client that are quite off the mark. He describes the consultant as pompous and arrogant; the therapist handles it well but feels rage. He says, "I'd like to crack his head open." After a long pause the presenter describes a few of the client's drawings. The first picture is that of a brain. In the second a dolphin changes into a crow. The presenter does very little with the material, but is obviously emotionally identified and communicates much empathy for his client. The child, age fourteen, lives in a family in which the father easily retreats and hides in his den. The mother invariably takes over, and presents a history of terminating therapists when she does not agree with the treatment plan.

I start to open up a discussion regarding the symbolic meaning of the images. Felicia expresses her irritation and impatience. She goes on to say, "We are the audience and onlookers." I am aware that it is the men who are very involved and are participating in this presentation. I do note that a few of the women offer helpful suggestions. I experience myself as defensive, and I blurt out that perhaps she is not a member of the men's club. She is furious at this comment, and I am aware that I am quite off the mark. I then sit back and reflect and recognize that I feel challenged and threatened in my role as the leader in the group. I take a deep breath and further reflect on my feelings in order to gain my ground and center.

After further group discussion I become aware that we are nearing the end of the session. I state that there are at least three fathers in this session. There is the arrogant father (the consultant), whom the presenter wishes to kill. There is the father (the boy's real father) who gives up and retreats into his den. And then there is the father that lives in the presenter's dialogue. He offers to assist the boy in transporting him to his office though the client is quite capable of getting there on his own. I share my thoughts with the group. With all these fathers, there may emerge a rational father who offers structure and protection. I recognize that I am not always this rational authority, but there exists a challenge to authority that is palatable and feels present in the group. I wonder out loud, "What constitutes a rational authority? Is there an authority that creates a safe structure for the expression of anger?" Felicia's combativeness to authority becomes more evident in her interactions with me. However, there is little time to go back to Felicia's case. I am still disturbed that we have not sufficiently dealt with the legal issues that place her license in jeopardy. I telephone her and inform her that even though her institution has not decided to report this case, she has the ultimate responsibility to follow through. I state, "A legal investigation may well jolt the mother and really become a gift for your client." She replies, "You were never this clear in our last consultation, and I am relieved that you place the issue so directly on the table." She agrees to take the next step and carry out her legal obligations.

CONCLUSION

The above examples illustrate a number of principles that pertain to the play space between therapist and client. They can be listed as follows:

1. Transference and countertransference reactions invariably affect the play space in supervision. These reactions create role locks, and the flow of supervisory material becomes repetitive and restrictive.
2. Transference and countertransference becomes a central part of learning therapeutic engagement. Without this understanding an important dimension of play space becomes neglected. The teaching of this material can be imparted on many levels. The structure of this investigation becomes contingent on the supervisees' personal and professional development.
3. Cultural factors invariably influence our understanding of the supervisory play space. The imparting of a Western framework upon a different cultural expression can lead to a good deal of misinformation and misperception. Verbal language and body language

organize our experiences. The cultural matrix further influences the way we see and respond to clients. Intermixed with this influence are emotional factors all of which affect the play space between supervisor and supervisee. This complicated matrix of understanding of how professionals learn and play demands a sophisticated approach to cultural influences.

4. Structure creates a boundary between the internal and external reality. This plays an important role in our ability to feel safe and comfortable with the emergent flow of material that occurs in supervision.

A play space becomes the imaginative expression of supervisory contact between client, supervisor, and supervisee. This space contracts or expands depending upon the safety and nonjudgmental parameters of the supervisory atmosphere. An appropriate supervisory structure regulates affect stimulation and creates a safe boundary for the investigation of transference and countertransference. This aspect of supervisory investigation ultimately unlocks a rigidity in roles that invariably impacts the supervisory play space.

Supervisory play space can best be nurtured by an acute awareness of such differences as cultural influences and the supervisee's ego defenses, as well as boundary formation. In this interaction the sensitive awareness of these factors furthers role modeling, an important aspect for learning. Within this context the possibilities of learning new skills and information become contingent upon the level and depth of the supervisory relationship. Without this awareness, supervisory information easily becomes lost through any number of defensive operations.

This type of supervision can be described as developmental in nature and is oriented toward an imaginative interaction with symbols and metaphors. This framework does not always work for all supervisees. However, for those professionals who are able and ready to take emotional risks, the gains of living in a supervisory play space are invaluable.

REFERENCE

Winnicott, D. W. (2005). *Playing and reality*. New York: Routledge.

All therapists need self-understanding and insight into their own motivations, needs, blind spots, biases, personal conflicts, and areas of emotional
difficulty as well as personal strengths. . . . The therapist is a real person, not
a robot. Therefore, personal needs and values are part of the person and thus
become a part of the relationship. The question, then, is not whether or not
the therapist's personality will enter into the relationship but, rather, to what
extent it will do so. (p. 102)

Moustakas (1959) suggested a humanistic approach to play therapy supervision that focused on the growth of supervisees' self-awareness, arguing that when supervisees integrate newly gained awareness into
their practice they can improve their relationship with their clients.
Kranz and Lund (1994) also promoted a humanistic approach to supervising play therapists in efforts to encourage their introspection and
openness to learning and to enhance the supervisor-supervisee relationship.

We further propose that therapist self-awareness may be even more important for supervision of child-centered play therapists, who must enter
into and experience the child's graphically displayed world—a world that
is often marked by difficult and painful experiences that are lived out in
therapy. We have found in our own supervisory experiences that issues of
countertransference are more frequently expressed when supervising
play therapists than when supervising counselors who rely solely on verbalization in their work with clients. For example, a supervisee's unad-
dressed issues around aggression may result in her responding to her
child client's overt expression of anger and aggression in subtle ways that
discourage expression of these feelings and related experiences in the
playroom.

RATIONALE FOR EXPRESSIVE ARTS IN SUPERVISION

Several authors have advocated for the therapeutic benefits of expressive
arts for clients of all ages (Bratton & Ferebee, 1999; Gladding, 1998; Oaklander, 1988; Oaklander, 2006; Rogers, 1993), while a few authors have
specifically encouraged the use of expressive arts as a means to facilitate
growth during supervision (Lahad, 2000; Lett, 1995; Newsome, Henderson, & Veach, 2005). Gladding (2005) emphasized the value of the creative
process for counselors as well as clients. He further explained that creative arts can enhance the lives of all individuals, creating within them "a
greater awareness of possibility" (p. 2). Bratton and Ferebee (1999) proposed that the use of expressive arts facilitates a process of creative self-
development—a process in which the individual uses realized inner resources to continue to grow in self-awareness long after the experience
has ended, thus continually creating self anew. Gladding (1998) described

a six-step experiential process involved in using creative arts with clients, culminating in the person being changed as the experience is integrated into the persona.

According to Lahad (2000) one of the main advantages of using creative arts in supervision is that it engages the right hemisphere of the brain that enables supervisees to access their experiences, feelings, and creativity. The author emphasized that most supervisees rely heavily on the left side of the brain, which activates thoughts and logic. Thus, it is difficult for supervisees to engage fully in the process of self-awareness that requires the accessing of one's experiences and feelings. Lahad further explained that the use of creative arts does not substitute for one's supervision method or theory; rather, it is used as a tool to gain different perspectives during supervision to facilitate self-awareness.

Wilkins (1995) supported the use of expressive/creative arts as a tool in supervision to enhance supervisees' intuition and ability to reflect on experiences. The author emphasized that the use of creative arts in supervision opens a channel for self-awareness that other supervision methods do not permit. Lett (1995) supported the notion that by reexperiencing the client-therapist interactions supervisees can gain insight that promotes self-awareness and professional growth. Newsome, Henderson, and Veach (2005) advocated for the use of expressive arts in group supervision to access supervisees' perceptions and emotions in relation to their clients.

Supervisors can use expressive arts to help supervisees conceptualize cases, reflect on the client-therapist relationship, increase self-awareness, gain perspective of the clients' experience, and understand the counseling process (Lahad, 2000). Play therapists in training can also benefit from exposure to the use of a variety of experiential activities during supervision. Because play in itself is a form of self-expression that relies on reliving past experiences in the immediacy of the play, play therapists are provided an enhanced means for self-understanding that parallels their clients' experiences. Additional benefits of using expressive art activities in supervision are first, enhancing the play therapist's ability to engage in the creative process and, second, increasing their appreciation of the process and power of play.

Although expressive art activities have been utilized within various theoretical frameworks, our approach is grounded in humanistic principles and procedures and thus can be described as process oriented rather than problem focused. A basic tenet of this approach is a belief in the individual's capacity for self-directed, creative growth, including a desire for understanding of self and others. The environment for growth is one of safety, empathy, care, authenticity, and immediacy. Bratton and Ferebee (1999) stated that the value of expressive arts, within a humanistic context, lies in the individual's creative process rather than in the final product. Growth and learning occur through the process of play, activity, and expression, not through the logical analysis of the situation at hand. Creating a safe environment in which supervisees feel accepted and willing to take risks is critical. Supervisors should have prior personal experience with a variety of expressive arts activities before using them in supervision in order to develop a deeper understanding of and respect for the process.

SUPERVISION FORMAT AND STRUCTURE

Expressive arts can be used in individual and group play therapy supervision, although when appropriate, we prefer the additional process benefits of group supervision. Supervision requirements vary depending on the experience of the supervisee. For mental health professionals required to be in supervision, length of sessions and format are generally dictated by licensing bodies. For the purpose of this chapter, we suggest a structure of one and a half hours for three supervisees to allow for creating and processing activities. Allowing approximately half of the supervision time for processing is essential, because creative arts can elicit deep and sometimes unconscious emotions that need to be processed during the session. However, even the most well-meaning supervisor will find that on occasion it is impossible to attend to all supervisees in the allotted time. Arrangements can be made by the supervisor for alternative measures to ensure that supervisees' well-being is attended to. For supervisors who do not have the luxury of conducting supervision in a room fully equipped with a wide variety of expressive materials, we suggest putting together an "expressive art cart" (see appendix A) that can be wheeled easily to any location.

Selection of Activities

Expressive activities that have been suggested for use with clients to facilitate self-awareness can be easily adapted for supervision purposes (Bratton & Ferebee, 1999; Gladding, 1998; Oaklander, 1988; Oaklander, 2006). Selection of the play/expressive medium to be used in supervision is important and should rely on supervisees' preferences, needs, and readiness. Landgarten (1987) proposed a guide for understanding the relationship between art mediums and client level of control over their creations that is very useful. The chart below was adapted from Landgarten and is provided as a consideration for choosing expressive art/play activities with supervisees. The lower the expressive medium is found on the list suggests greater client/supervisee control over the experience, including over his or her emotions and thoughts.

LEAST CONTROL
Wet Clay/Wet Sand
Oil Pastels/Watercolors
Dry Sand and Miniature Figures
Miniature Figures (used without sand)
Puppets/Drama/Storytelling
Collage-type Activities
Model Magic/Modeling Clay
Crayons/Thick Felt Markers
Colored Pencils
Lead Pencils
MOST CONTROL

Supervisor's Role

When using expressive arts in supervision, the supervisor's role can be best understood by conceptualizing the process as two phases: creating and processing. During the creating phase the supervisor typically assumes the role of active observer, particularly in group supervision, with the supervisor serving as a witness to the process while supervisees are engaged in the chosen activity. The supervisor attentively observes actions, body language, comments, and the creative process of each supervisee to gain a deeper understanding of supervisees and what about their creation seems most meaningful. Once supervisees have finished the activity, the supervisor's role shifts to a more active role of facilitating verbal (tell me) and nonverbal (show me) processing of supervisees' creations in order to encourage reflection and insight. Consistent with a humanistic perspective that deeply respects the individual's capacity for self-directed growth and capacity for self-understanding, supervisors are most interested in supervisees' understanding of the meaning of their own creation. The supervisor's respect for supervisees' level of readiness to engage in processing activities reinforces that supervision is a safe place and mirrors the parallel therapist/client process. Supervisees' reluctance or refusal to participate in activities or processing of their creations is rare but respected. Processing perceived supervisee resistance can be used as a means through which supervisees gain self-awareness and experience professional and personal growth.

The following general guidelines are offered for the reader's consideration in processing expressive activities in supervision and are organized into levels with the first level considered less intrusive by providing the supervisee more control over what is shared.

- Level 1: Supervisor encourages supervisees to describe/share their creations: "Tell me about your (scene or drawing or creature)."
- Level 2: Supervisor tentatively shares her observations of the process/creation: "I noticed that Pegasus and the fairy seem very connected—and they both have wings and seem kind of sad."
- Level 3: Supervisor invites supervisees to enter into the metaphor they have created: "Pretend that you are the fairy (client) and tell Pegasus (supervisee) what you need."
- Level 4: Supervisor encourages supervisee to personalize the metaphor: "As you think about how you described Pegasus, does anything fit with how you see yourself?"

In group supervision, after supervisees have described their creation, supervisors should initially focus their comments to each supervisee based on what seemed most meaningful for each individual during the creative process. Generally, when your observations are "on target" the supervisee will naturally expand on your remarks. For example, when the supervisor shared her observations that she noticed that Pegasus and the fairy seemed very connected, the supervisee got tears in her eyes and proceeded to share how her client's experiences reminded her of her own early experiences. No question was asked, nor was a response expected. One simple observation that came from carefully attending to what seemed important to the supervisee during the creative process resulted in a profound self-realization for the supervisee.

The following examples are taken from chapter author Sue Bratton's experiences in a six-month-long supervision group with three doctoral students specializing in play therapy. A variety of expressive arts activities were used throughout the process of supervision as one means of enhancing supervisees' experience and promoting optimal personal and professional growth. For the purpose of this chapter, we chose to give brief examples of one of the supervisee's experiences—we will refer to her as Sally—with three types of expressive art activities to demonstrate how these activities promoted the supervisee's self-awareness within the group process over the course of supervision. These examples are taken from the beginning, middle, and ending phases of the supervision experience to illustrate the supervisee's movement.

BEGINNING PHASE: CREATING A CLAY ANIMAL/CREATURE TO ASSESS SUPERVISEES' NEEDS

Bratton has found that clay and similar products, such as Play-Doh and Model Magic, readily facilitate self-awareness with supervisees. The tactile nature and flexibility of the clay allow people to access feelings easily and provide for malleability (Bratton & Ferebee, 1999; Oaklander 1988). Oaklander (1988) specified that the use of clay helps clients overcome barriers to their emotions and experiences. In Bratton's experience the use of Model Magic in the following activity offers supervisees greater control over their emotions and experience than using potter's clay, which is more appropriate for the beginning phase of supervision. The use of a more structured activity, such as the "Clay Creature" described below, was selected to reduce supervisees' anxiety as they began the supervision process. The use of the metaphor of an animal/creature to represent "self" allows for psychological distance, providing a generally nonthreatening means for supervisees and supervisor to get to know each other while also permitting symbolic expression of unconscious emotions, thoughts, and needs related to supervision and professional growth.

Materials Needed

Model Magic (or similar product), paper plates, and a variety of clay tools are needed. (Note: If using potter's clay, then water, paper towels, and a wire clay cutter are necessary.) Tools may include a rubber mallet, a plastic knife, a garlic press, and any other materials that one considers helpful to shape the clay. Craft materials such as colored feathers, construction paper, cellophane paper, pipe cleaners, plastic straws, assorted beads, dried pasta shapes, markers, and scissors (see the appendix) are useful for supervisees to personalize their "creatures."

General Directions

Begin the activity by providing each supervisee with a portion of clay/ Model Magic about the size of a small orange. Relaxation exercises can be used to help supervisees focus on the immediacy of the experience. Encourage supervisees to spend a few minutes becoming familiar with the feel of the clay with their eyes open, and again with their eyes closed. Next, suggest that supervisees experiment with their clay by pinching it, squeezing it, pounding it, and rolling it. Encourage supervisees to reflect on their experiences. Ask supervisees to close their eyes and simply feel their clay as they listen to the instructions for the activity: "Imagine that you have traveled through time into the future where human life as we know it no longer exists. The world is inhabited by thousands of varieties of animals and creatures, big and small—some look like animals that we know today, and others are like no creature that you have ever seen. If you could be any animal or creature in this new world, what would you be? Think about what you look like and begin to shape your animal/creature. Now open your eyes and finish your creation, using any of these materials."

After each member has finished, the supervisor asks for each supervisee to talk about their creature. As supervisees describe their creature, the supervisor facilitates the process by asking questions such as: "What is your animal/creature good at? What is hard for your creature to do? What kinds of things does your creature like to do? What does it wish it could do? What does it wish it did not have to do? How does your creature survive in this new world? What does your creature need? What keeps your creature from getting what it needs?"

Next, the supervisor encourages supervisees to reflect on aspects of their creatures that are consistent with a need they would like to address in supervision in order to facilitate their growth as play therapists. For example, when asked what his creature needed, one doctoral student supervisee stated that his creature needed a mouth and went back and drew one on. The supervisee who was an international student for whom English was his second language was able to reflect on the meaning of his creation and revealed that he was worried that he would not be able to communicate with his clients. He further disclosed that because his spoken English was much better than his understanding of English that he had been hiding this fear from his previous supervisors.

Case Example

Figure 13.1 shows Sally's creation, a four-legged creature that she described as a bird that was having trouble getting off the ground. The creature was covered with what appeared to be a "cape" consisting of layers of blue and pink cellophane that mostly covered up the bird's colorful feathers. But when Sally described her "bird creature" she revealed that what appeared to be a cape was actually a set of large wings that the bird needed in order to fly. The wings allowed the creature to fly as high as she wanted to, but would also protect her when she needed to rest. One of the supervisees in the group asked why the bird/creature needed the large heavy wings when she had all the feathers underneath. Sally responded that the wings might weigh her down at times, but they were necessary to make sure she could always fly when she needed to. Sally also shared that her bird/creature's greatest strength was that she knew how to take care of herself.

All supervisees were asked to describe their animal/creature following the general directions provided above, and all but Sally were able to make a connection between their creature's attributes and themselves. It was clear to the supervisor that Sally was not yet feeling safe enough to personalize her metaphor. In response to the supervisor's final query, "What does your creature need and what keeps your creature from getting that need met?" Sally answered that her bird/creature needed a safe place to

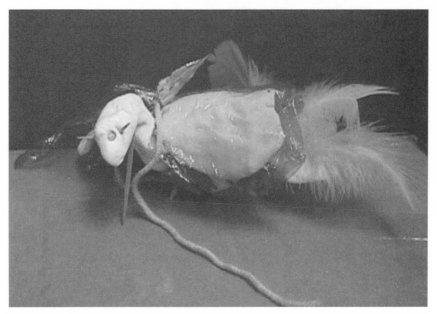

Figure 13.1. Sally's Four-Legged Creature.

rest its wings. When the supervisor encouraged supervisees to reflect on aspects of their creatures that were consistent with a need they would like to address in supervision in order to facilitate their growth as play therapists, Sally was last to respond. Although she struggled to put her needs into words, she agreed that, like her bird/creature, she needed a safe place. The supervisor added, "It must be hard for you to feel safe in here." Sally nodded, and the supervisor gently asked, "What would you need from us in order to feel safe?" To which Sally replied, "I don't know right now." Although Sally's bird/creature metaphor was ripe with additional opportunities to facilitate Sally's self-awareness, she was not ready. Instead the supervisor suggested that she take a picture of her bird creation (or take it with her) and write down anything she noticed that seemed important to her. She could bring her notes next week if she wanted to share. In later sessions and over the course of several weeks, Sally was able to use the metaphor that she had created to see how she hid herself from others, believing that she had to portray a certain image that others would find pleasing and to protect herself from rejection. Gradually, Sally was able to openly discuss that what she needed to feel safe in supervision was to not feel that she was being judged. The supervisor clarified the difference between "judging" her personhood as bad or good and the on-going assessment of a supervisee's growth that is inherent in the supervision process. Sally agreed that she would try to let the supervisor know if she was feeling judged. The group process seemed especially helpful to Sally. She seemed to particularly benefit from her peers sharing their insecurities and mistakes—something that Sally had previously not believed was allowable. As Sally was able to allow herself to be more vulnerable in supervision her ability to form relationships with her clients increased. While Sally lagged behind her peers in her development as a competent play therapist, she exhibited the most personal growth. What began as a simple activity for supervisees to get to know each other while the supervisor began to assess their supervision needs turned into a significant experience that propelled Sally on a journey of personal and professional growth.

MIDDLE PHASE: USING SAND TRAY TO FACILITATE AWARENESS OF SELF IN RELATION TO CLIENT

Sand tray has been used for many years as an expressive arts medium, and its therapeutic benefits have been widely documented (Lowenfeld, 1979; Homeyer & Sweeney, 1998; De Domenico, 1999). The kinesthetic experience sand tray provides gives the opportunity for users to access emotions that are difficult to verbalize (Homeyer & Sweeney, 1998). In supervision, sand tray can be used for a variety of purposes, including to increase self-awareness, examine relationships, conceptualize cases, and work through personal issues hindering the counseling relationship, among others. The supervisor can structure the activity around the supervisory goal. For example, the supervisor might ask a supervisee, "Can you represent the relationship you are describing between you and your client in the sand tray?" Or, "Imagine the supervision process as a movie, and depict the ending scene in the sand tray. . . . What has happened up to now; what do you think will happen?" Or, as in the example below, supervisees can be asked to represent the client's world in the sand tray.

Materials Needed

The size of the sand tray can vary depending on personal choice. Homeyer and Sweeney (1998) provided a detailed explanation of the use of sand tray with clients as well as the recommended miniatures. The "standard" size for traditional sand tray work is approximately 30 × 20 × 3 inches. For the purpose of group supervision, however, we have successfully used clay-colored plastic plant drip saucers approximately 18 inches in diameter as sand trays. These sand trays are lightweight, space efficient, stackable, and the three to four needed for group supervision will fit easily on a portable utility cart (see appendix at the end of chapter). We recommend providing as much of a variety of miniatures as space allows (Bratton & Ferebee, 1999; Homeyer & Sweeney, 1998). A variety of multicultural people/symbols is important when working with diverse populations of supervisees. Again, if supervisors do not have access to a fully equipped sand tray room, a second utility cart organized with drawer units to display the miniatures according to category can be utilized.

General Directions

Begin the activity by encouraging supervisees to use their hands to explore the sand, letting them know that they may add water if they wish. Encourage reflections on feelings that the sand evokes. The supervisor then proceeds to structure the activity in accordance with the supervision goal for that session. In the case example, the goal was to facilitate supervisees' insight into self in relation to a client they were struggling with. Supervisees were instructed to make a scene that depicted the client's world and to include themselves and any other figures that were important in the child's life.

Supervisees begin the processing phase by describing their sand tray scenes. With an awareness of supervisees' level of readiness and keeping in mind the levels of processing suggested earlier in this chapter, the supervisor facilitates the process by exploring the meaning of the selected figures and how the scene is set up. Additional questions such as, "What would you like to see happening?" or, "Could you pretend to be the child in the scene and tell your mother what you need?" can help supervisees examine the counseling relationship, gain new perspectives, and often facilitate movement. Refer to Homeyer and Sweeney (1998), Oaklander (1988), Rogers (1993), and Bratton and Ferebee (1999) for additional examples of how to process sand tray creations.

Case Example

Approximately three months into the supervision process, the supervisor asked the doctoral student supervisees to think of a play therapy case they experienced as challenging. After all supervisees had briefly described the client they wanted to focus on, they were instructed to make a sand tray scene that depicted the client's world and to include themselves and any other figures that were important in the child's life. (Note: This was not the first time that sand tray had been used with this group and, at this point in supervision, supervisees were becoming increasingly open to self-examination. This particular sand tray example was selected because it facilitated the deepest level of self-awareness in the supervisee of focus.)

Sally discussed her continued feelings of frustration with one of her play therapy clients, a six-year-old girl whose mother was bringing her for play therapy. The mother reported that the client had been "fondled" by the client's father, although there had been no legal ruling. The client's mother had primary custody, but reported that her ex-husband saw their daughter every other weekend under the supervision of his adult daughter. Sally's frustration was evident as she reported that she believed her client was in danger of being abused again and did not feel like anyone in the client's family was protecting her. Sally discussed feeling "stuck" and not knowing what else to do to help her client whom she reported becoming more anxious in her play. In previous supervision sessions, Sally had been resistant to suggestions to contact her client's father and ask him to meet with her for a parent consultation, since he had regular contact with his daughter. Sally had also not followed through on suggestions to involve the client's mother more fully in therapy.

Figure 13.2 depicts Sally's sand tray scene. She began by placing a small fairy (with one wing broken off) on top of a large rock in the middle of the sand tray and immediately identified the fairy as her six-year-old client. (She had used the figure previously in supervision to represent the same client.) Then she added a larger rock behind the fairy along with several

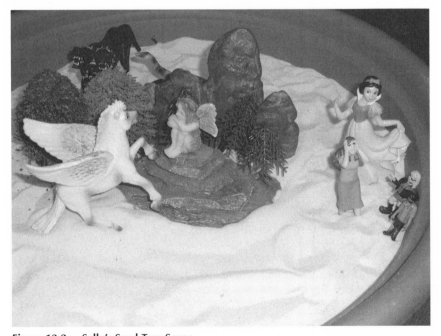

Figure 13.2. Sally's Sand Tray Scene.

trees creating a sense of protection or barrier. Next, Sally spent several minutes carefully selecting a winged horse, picking up various figures (some of which were figures she had previously chosen to represent herself) and putting them back before finally deciding on the figure that she called Pegasus. She then spent several more minutes carefully placing Pegasus close to and directly facing the fairy. She quickly took the snake (a figure she had used previously to represent her client's father) off the shelf and placed it behind the rocks and spent several more minutes deciding on a three-headed, ferocious-looking creature that she placed behind the rocks next to the snake. Almost as an afterthought, Sally added the four figures at the right of the scene and then spent several minutes arranging all the figures, making only slight modifications from where she originally placed them.

Sally asked to go first during the processing phase and began to describe her sand tray scene by telling who each figure represented, starting with the fairy (her client) and Pegasus (herself). She said the three-headed monster and the snake represented danger. The shorter female figure on the right side of the scene was described as her client's mother, and the two smallest figures represented the client's teenage half-siblings from the mother's previous marriage. Sally described the mother as overwhelmed and helpless, stating that she had her hands full with her teenage children who were often in trouble at school. Last she added that "Snow White" was her client's young first-grade teacher whom the client seemed to admire. When asked to spend a few minutes just noticing the scene she had created, she immediately began to focus on the center of her scene, commenting that she (Pegasus) was the only one that could help the fairy and that she was afraid that she would not be able to keep the danger away much longer. She noted how she had chosen the large rocks and trees to keep the danger away from her client, but then added as she stared at the scene, "and from me." She noticed that, although she had chosen the largest trees she could find to provide a thick barrier, the trees were brown and soon would lose their leaves offering little protection from the father and danger.

The supervisor remarked, "I noticed that there seems to be a strong connection between you and your client—and you both have wings and you both seem kind of sad." Sally looked intently at the figures and tears welled up. She shared that she did feel a strong connection to her client and that she felt like she could really relate to this client. Sally paused for a while as she stared at the scene and proceeded to share briefly how her client's experiences reminded her of her own early experiences. The supervisor reflected Sally's sadness and respected her unspoken decision to go no further at that moment.

After other supervisees had described their sand tray scenes, the supervisor asked that they focus on the symbol that they had chosen to represent themselves and say more about the figure. Sally noted that Pegasus had strong wings and could fly away to safety any time he wanted to. She then added, "I could easily carry the fairy away to safety with me." Another supervisee asked, "Where would you take her, and what would happen to her family?" Sally paused for a moment and was able to reflect that she was leaving the child's support system, meager as it was, out of the therapeutic process.

Another important insight for Sally developed in response to one of her peers noticing the snake seemed to be attacking the monster rather than coming toward the fairy. Sally seemed surprised by that, but then revealed, "I've felt like that," and then with strong emotion said, "I wish he were gone from her life." (This was the first time the supervisee had revealed such strong negative emotion in supervision.) The supervisor reflected, "So a part of you can identify with a snake that can attack monsters." Sally hesitated for a moment and shared more about her experiences growing up. She described the hurt from her parents' rejection of her. She never felt that she was "good enough" or lovable in her parents' eyes, although she remembered trying very hard to win their love by being a "good girl." Sally disclosed that she hated her father and had not seen him in years. As Sally shared about her early experiences and was encouraged and supported by her peers and supervisor, you could see the light bulb turn on as she began to make the connection between her early experiences and the need to protect herself from being hurt by others, and the resulting need to protect her client from pain.

As Sally was able to feel safe enough to really look at the scene she created, multiple "aha" moments began to unfold for her. This was a very complex scene that the supervisee was obviously impacted by and needed more time to process than time allowed. As is common, the supervisee was encouraged to take a picture of the scene to take with her to provide further opportunity for reflection and journaling of her thoughts. Sally gained several important insights from this sand tray experience that facilitated significant professional and personal growth (and with the supervisor's encouragement, resulted in her seeking counseling to continue to address the issues that she begun to be aware of during this session). Some of the insights were:

- She had decided the father was guilty, and she was feeling very angry toward him, which hindered her objectivity.
- She was frustrated and angry with the mother for not protecting her child from hurt, which prevented her from aligning with the mother and involving her more fully in treatment.
- She had believed that she was the only one who could help, that she must be the all-knowing expert, and that if she was not able to protect this child, she was a failure.

- The pain of parental rejection she had experienced as a child resulted in her feeling judged and inferior to others; she coped by protecting herself from further rejection by trying to be "perfect" and pleasing— not letting others see her true self. (This insight began to develop with her clay animal creation in the beginning phase of supervision, but she did not make the connection with her early experiences until this session.)
- She had been unconsciously looking for a way to escape failure and possible rejection as a play therapist. (She revealed in a later session that she had been seriously thinking about referring this client.)
- Her fear of being rejected and her lack of trust in revealing her true self, imperfections and all, were impeding her ability to develop a genuine relationship with her clients.

This activity allowed the supervisee to deepen her level of self-awareness in relation to this client, but to also begin to generalize her awareness to other clients and her personal life. The themes of safety, fear, and protection that arose early in supervision were evident in Sally's sand tray. However, this time she was able to go a step further by identifying her fear of being disliked or rejected as stemming from the hurt she had experienced as a child. Sally began to explore that she did not believe that it was okay to fully be herself; rather she believed that she must project a pleasing or perfect image to protect herself from the pain of rejection that she had experienced as a child. The major insight for Sally revolved around how her personal needs were impacting the therapeutic process. She began to explore her overidentification with her client that was resulting in Sally projecting some of her needs onto the child. She shared that she now saw how her need to protect herself and her client and to make things look okay may have resulted in her client not being able to fully express all of her feelings in play therapy. This supervision session marked a surge in Sally's professional growth that was evidenced over the next several weeks by her increased effectiveness with her clients.

ENDING PHASE: THE USE OF A MANDALA COLLAGE TO PROMOTE CLOSURE AND INTEGRATION

Even though mandalas have been used for thousands of years to invoke the spirit of healing, their use as a therapeutic medium was first acknowledged by Carl Jung (Bertoia, 1999). Mandalas provide a means for pulling together all aspects of one's life and finding one's center (Campbell, 1974), thus they are constructed in a circular fashion. Bertoia (1999) further explained that in Jungian theory, the creation of images is "the language of the unconscious" and that unconscious feelings and thoughts are projected into symbols (p. 90). According to Young (2001) the creation of a mandala allows the person to unite the different unconscious and conscious aspects within oneself, thereby fostering self-awareness. We propose that their use in play therapy supervision would be similarly beneficial for supervisees. A variety of expressive art mediums can be used in the creation of mandalas. We have found that integrating collage techniques into the construction of a mandala along with the traditionally used drawing mediums can enhance the creative process by providing supervisees with a wider range of materials for self-expression. According to Rogers (1993) a collage may be less difficult than drawing and allows for focus on the process rather than on the product.

Materials Needed

Construction paper of different sizes and colors can be used to create the circle. Similarly, paper plates provide an inexpensive, easy, and sturdy surface for creating mandalas. Provide a variety of drawing materials, including oil pastels, crayons, watercolors, markers, and chalk pastels, along with a variety of craft materials (see the appendix) and magazines for cutting out words and images.

General Directions

The mandala-collage activity was chosen as a termination/closure activity and was conducted in the next-to-last supervision session. We have found that this activity provides an opportunity for supervisees to reflect on and express how they have integrated their most meaningful supervision experiences into "self."

Begin by briefly explaining the concept of mandala to supervisees. Providing soothing music or brief guided imagery (Oaklander, 1988; Rogers, 1993) can help supervisees relax and focus on their experience in the moment. The supervisor invites supervisees to close their eyes and take a few moments to reflect on themselves, their lives, their clients, their growth as play therapists, and their supervision experiences. Next the supervisor explains, "Now, I'd like you to open your eyes and choose a circle of any size to use to create a mandala that shows how you see yourself right now in relation to your growth in supervision over the past several months. You may want to start by creating a center for your mandala to represent how you see yourself right now, what you hold most important, and what you most appreciate about yourself. Then use the rest of the circle to depict your growth this semester—your most meaningful moments and the experiences that have impacted you most. These are only suggestions; there is no right or wrong way to create your mandala."

Case Example

Sally was very intent on her creation and hummed to herself as she worked. Toward the end, she declared that this was her favorite activity of all. A photograph of Sally's mandala is not included due to the overly personal nature of her creation that would have prevented complete anonymity. Sally began her mandala by painting an entire paper plate turquoise. Next, she drew a rather large circle in the middle of her mandala and used her name to make the border for the inner circle. She spent a long time carefully selecting bits and pieces of mostly bright-colored items from the expressive art cart (see appendix) and then proceeded to use the items to make a collage inside her name. She cut a circular piece of cellophane (similar to what she had used in her first creation to hide her feathers) as the base for gluing the rest of the colorful assortment of items on, so that the edges of the cellophane stuck out around the collage—making what looked like a flower that was opening its petals. Sally spent almost twenty minutes constructing her "center" and seemed very pleased with the results. In the remaining ten minutes, Sally drew four lines radiating from the center to the outer edge of the mandala, creating four equal parts. She then proceeded to draw, write, or paint in each of the four sections. The explanation of what she included in each part is as follows:

(1) She wrote the words "safe," "happy," "sad," "fearful," "nervous," "accepted," and "courageous."
(2) She drew different sizes of figures of people without any words.
(3) She drew two people with toys surrounding with the word "connecting."
(4) She painted spots of different colors on top of the turquoise color she had initially painted the entire circle.

Sally described her mandala to the group, focusing most on her "center." She really liked how it turned out and remarked that she was "mostly no longer afraid for people to see the real Sally." She was able to talk openly about what she valued most about herself. It was clear from the amount of time and focus spent on "self" that Sally was beginning to acknowledge that she was worthy of love and acceptance for who she was, not just for her good deeds. Her peers were able to express their appreciation of being allowed to see the real Sally, especially when they knew how hard that had been and how much courage it took. Sally joked that she liked who she was in her mandala creation a lot more than her bird/creature!

Sally explained that the divisions in the outer circle were representations of what had been most meaningful in her supervision experience. The feeling words represented the myriad emotions she had experienced in the supervision process—that while it had not always been fun, she appreciated that their expression had been necessary to her growth. The drawing of two people and toys and the word "connecting" represented her clients in play therapy and how she now felt she was able to establish more genuine relationships with her clients. She added that this was one area that she would always work on now that she had experienced how important it was. The spots of colors painted on top of the turquoise background represented parts of herself that she was still in the process of understanding, accepting, and integrating—and that she would continue to do that through counseling. And finally, the four people she had drawn represented herself, her fellow supervisees, and the supervisor. While describing this part, she was sincere in her belief that it was the support and acceptance from her peers that had most allowed her to take the risk to open herself up to the feelings and experiences aroused during supervision. This activity clearly provided Sally a meaningful way to reflect on and express her personal and professional growth over the course of supervision, while providing a sense of closure. Through the use of playful and expressive activities in supervision, Sally had developed new insights and inner resources that would allow her to continue to grow in self-awareness and be open to the process of growth and self-examination—just as our clients do in play therapy.

CONCLUSION

This chapter focused on a humanistic approach to utilizing expressive arts activities with play therapist supervisees who subscribe to a similar approach in counseling clients. The use of expressive arts within clinical supervision offers many potential benefits, including the opportunity to engage in and experience the creative process. Just as play therapy and other forms of expressive therapies can enhance the therapeutic process for clients, the use of expressive arts can enhance the supervisory experience by fostering therapist self-awareness, enhancing client conceptualization, encouraging exploration and clarity of supervisees' theoretical framework, as well as facilitating development of play therapy skills. Consistent with the rationale for play therapy, the use of play, art, and other expressive materials allows supervisees a means to access and express thoughts, feelings, and experiences about themselves and their clients that they may not be able to express meaningfully through words alone.

For ease of using expressive arts activities in any space, we recommend using a three-shelf utility cart that can be easily moved. Two plastic six-drawer organizing units are placed side-by-side on the top shelf to provide an inexpensive means of organizing materials and supplies. These units are referred to as the "left drawer unit" and the "right drawer unit" in the table below.

TOP SHELF: Left Drawer Unit	**TOP SHELF: Right Drawer Unit**
Drawer 1 Crayons Markers Colored pencils Lead pencils	Drawer 1 Large color and size assortment of beads Assorted dried pasta shapes Styrofoam peanuts Foam shapes
Drawer 2 Oil pastels Watercolor paints Paint brushes Dot paints	Drawer 2 Plastic straws Toothpicks Craft sticks Pipe cleaners
Drawer 3 Scissors Stapler Hole punch Paper clips Rubber bands Tape/glue	Drawer 3 Cotton balls Yarn Assorted colors of feathers Pom poms Balloons
Drawer 4 Cutouts/cards Stickers Ink pad Ink stamps Assorted papers	Drawer 4 Ribbon Lace Felt Miscellaneous fabrics and other scrap materials
Drawer 5 Glitter glue Glitter Sequins	Drawer 5 Bubble wrap Foil Plastic colored grass Cellophane
Drawer 6 Sea shells Small stones/rocks Assortment of natural objects	Drawer 6 Assorted recycled small cardboard containers Paper/Styrofoam cups and bowls
MIDDLE SHELF: Left Plastic bin with sand art supplies	**MIDDLE SHELF: Right** Plastic bin with clay, Play-Doh, and Model Magic Clay tools
BOTTOM SHELF: Left Paper plates Construction paper Magazines	**BOTTOM SHELF: Right** Cafeteria trays (provide individual work surfaces) 3-4 round sand trays (18-in. clay-colored plant drip saucers)

REFERENCES

Bernard, J. M., & Goodyear, R. K. (2004). *Fundamentals of clinical supervision* (2nd ed.). Needham Heights, MA: Allyn & Bacon.

Bertoia, J. (1999). The invisible village: Jungian group play therapy. In D. Sweeney & L. Homeyer (Eds.), *The handbook of group play therapy* (86–104). San Francisco: Jossey-Bass.

Bratton, S., & Ferebee, K. (1999). The use of expressive art activities in group activity therapy with preadolescents. In D. Sweeney & L. Homeyer (Eds.), *The handbook of group play therapy* (192–214). San Francisco: Jossey-Bass.

Bratton, S., Landreth, G., & Homeyer, L. (1993). An intensive three-day play therapy supervision/training model. *International Journal of Play Therapy, 2*(2), 61–78.

Bratton, S., & Ray, D. (2000). What research shows about play therapy. *International Journal of Play Therapy, 1*(9), 47–88.

Bratton, S., Ray, D., Rhine, T., & Jones, L. (2005). The efficacy of play therapy with children: A meta-analytic review of treatment outcomes. *Professional Psychology: Research and Practice, 36*(4), 376–90.

Bratton, S., Ray, D., & Landreth, G. (2008). Play therapy. In M. Hersen & A. Gross (Eds.), *Handbook of clinical psychology, Volume II: Children and adolescents.* New York: Wiley & Sons.

Campbell, J. (1974). *The mythic image.* Princeton, NJ: Princeton University Press.

De Domenico, G. (1999). Group sandtray-worldplay. In D. Sweeney & L. Homeyer (Eds.), *The handbook of group play therapy* (215–33). San Francisco: Jossey-Bass.

Edwards, D. (1993). Learning about feelings: The role of supervision in art therapy training. *The Arts in Psychotherapy, 20,* 213–22.

Getz, H. G., & Protinsky, H. O. (1994). Training marriage and family counselors: A family-of-origin approach. *Counselor Education & Supervision, 33,* 183–90.

Gladding, S. T. (1998). *Family therapy: History, theory and practice.* Second edition. New York: Prentice-Hall, Inc.

———. (2005). *Counseling as an art: The creative arts in counseling* (3rd ed.). Alexandria, VA: American Counseling Association.

Homeyer, L., & Sweeney, D. (1998). *Sandtray: A practical manual.* Canyon Lake, TX: Lindan Press.

Kranz, P., & Lund, N. (1994). Recommendations for supervising play therapists. *International Journal of Play Therapy, 3*(2), 45–52.

Lahad, M. (2000). *Creative supervision: The use of expressive arts methods in supervision and self-supervision.* Philadelphia: Jessica Kingsley Publishers, Ltd.

Lambert, S. F., LeBlanc, M., Mullen, J., Ray, D., et al. (2005). Learning more about those who play in session: The national play therapy in counseling practice project (Phase I). *International Journal of Play Therapy, 14*(2), 7–23.

Landgarten, H. B. (1987). *Family art psychotherapy: A clinical guide and casebook.* New York: Brunner/Mazel.

Landreth, G. L. (2002). *Play therapy: The art of the relationship* (2nd ed.). New York: Brunner Routledge.

Lett, W. (1995). Experiential supervision through simultaneous drawing and talking. *The Arts in Psychotherapy, 22*(4), 315–28.

Lowenfeld, M. (1979). *The world technique* (2nd ed.). London: Allen & Unwin.

Moustakas, C. E. (1959). *Psychotherapy with children: The living relationship*. Greely, CO: Marron Publishers.

Newsome, D., Henderson, D., & Veach, L. (2005). Using expressive arts in group supervision to enhance awareness and foster cohesion. *Journal of Humanistic Counseling, Education & Development, 44*(2), 145–57.

Oaklander, V. (1988). *Windows to our children*. Highland, NY: Center for Gestalt Development.

Oaklander, V. (2006). *Hidden treasure: A map to the child's inner self*. London: Karnac.

Ray, D. (2004). Supervision of basic and advanced skills in play therapy. *Journal of Professional Counseling: Practice Theory and Research, 32*(2), 28–41.

Rogers, N. (1993). *The creative connection: Expressive arts in healing*. Palo Alto, CA: Science & Behavior Books.

Wilkins, P. (1995). A creative therapies model for the group supervision for counselors. *British Journal of Guidance & Counseling, 23*(2), 245–58.

Young, A. (2001). Mandalas. *Encounter, 14*(3), 25–34.

14

⌒∞⌒

Supervision in the Sand

Mary Morrison and Linda E. Homeyer

A s play therapists we work in a world of symbol, metaphor, and creativity. We offer clients of all ages the opportunity to use the modality of play for expression and communication. We provide such experiences with our child, adolescent, and adult clients to assist them in understanding self, relationships, and their world. We can use sand tray for these same experiences with supervisees. As play therapists we do not rely only on the spoken word for effective communication, yet once in the supervision relationship we typically revert to that mode. In this chapter, we hope to provide the reader with a brief overview of the sand tray therapy experience and the rationale for using sand tray as a tool within the supervisory relationship. We will also provide examples of activities for various supervisory experiences.

Homeyer and Sweeney (1998) define sand tray as, "An expressive and projective mode of psychotherapy involving the unfolding and processing of intra- and inter-personal issues through the use of specific sand tray materials as a nonverbal medium of communication, led by the client and facilitated by a trained therapist" (p. 6). Sand tray is a versatile modality that is used with children, adolescents, adults, families, and couples, individually and in groups. Advanced supervision often requires supervisees to process intra- and inter-personal difficulties and sand tray provides an opportunity for supervisees to explore these types of issues through nonverbal communication.

Play therapy is a symbolic and expressive medium for children to naturally express themselves. Play is characterized by Landreth (2002) as the natural language of children—toys are their words and play is their language. The therapist's ability to understand the symbolic expression of the child in play therapy is critical to the therapist's ability to understand the child's world. This understanding can also facilitate the therapist's own symbolic self-expression. It is reasonable for play therapists to be supervised in a manner that is consistent with the modality of therapy they use with clients. Sand tray provides a medium for therapists to experience supervision through symbol, providing them with an opportunity to view their clients and themselves through symbolic expression. Sand tray facilitates an opportunity for supervisors to access information; thoughts, feelings, and experiences, that might not be verbally disclosed by the supervisee in traditional supervision (Kwiatkowska, 1978).

Supervisors have multiple responsibilities to their supervisees, one of which is to model professional and ethical behavior (Haynes, Corey, & Moulton, 2003). Training and clinical experience in both play therapy and sand tray is critical before supervisors can ethically utilize this modality in play therapy supervision. We stress the importance of personal experience in sand tray. Sand tray is a very powerful modality and without personal experience, supervisors lack the depth of understanding to use this modality effectively. It is difficult to know how to use the content of the sand tray experience to assist the supervisee in an insightful process that is respectful and sensitive to the supervisee if one has not personally experienced its power. Indeed, whether using sand tray as a counselor or supervisor, one's own experience is the best standard of practice.

SUPERVISORY RELATIONSHIP

Supervisors have several different roles in the supervisory relationship, and an appropriate balance of these roles is challenging. It is crucial that supervisors provide a safe environment, a "free and protected space" (Kalff, 1980) for supervisees to fully engage in the supervision process. Haynes, Corey, and Moulton (2003) discussed elements of a positive supervisory relationship; the supervisor needs to display empathy, acceptance, genuineness, concreteness, confrontation, and immediacy. Supervision should be a place where supervisees feel protected in order to be vulnerable and open to the growth process of supervision. Homeyer and Sweeney (1998) discuss the necessary traits of a sand tray therapist, which include empathy, acceptance, genuineness, and immediacy. A supervisor who utilizes sand tray in the supervision process has a balanced blend of these characteristics. It is also important to note the careful balance and integration of the supervisor roles of teacher, counselor, and consultant (Bernard & Goodyear, 2004).

Clearly it is unethical for supervisors to serve as a counselor for their supervisee (American Counseling Association, 2005) and yet there are times when focus on personal strengths and weaknesses is critical for supervisee growth. Haynes, Corey, and Moulton (2003) suggest the supervisor limit such supervision issues to those related to the supervisee's clinical skills, countertransference, and coping with stress and burn-out. The supervisor in the role of counselor is brief, only as long as needed to heighten the supervisees' awareness of personal issues that are interfering with the counselor-client relationship and the supervisee's professional development. However, when a supervisor assesses that significant personal issues exist, it is a critical and an ethical responsibility that the supervisor refer supervisees to personal counseling with another therapist. In the role of counselor, the supervisor engages the supervisee sufficiently through discussions and exploration to assist the supervisee with the personal insight to understand the need for counseling to resolve those issues.

Sand tray is a dynamic addition to the supervision relationship and process. It is a powerful yet nonthreatening technique. Given the projective nature of sand tray, it is expected that the personal struggle of the supervisee will be exposed during this process. Supervisors are cautioned to stay within the roles of the supervisory relationship and process the information that is only relevant to the growth and development of the supervisee. Consequently, when used within the appropriate boundaries of the supervisory relationship, sand tray is a safe method for supervisors to quickly address personal struggles of the supervisee impacting her work. The visual image of the tray allows the supervisee to quite literally see the issue at hand, and therefore, to have insight into her own personal struggles and issues. For example, I worked with a supervisee who was a doctoral student and counseling intern at a university clinic. She was doing effective clinical work, but I could see how the stress of the doctoral program and her case load was affecting her. When I mentioned my observation of her struggle she often denied experiencing any stress or burn-out. Sensing her inability to discuss this issue openly and directly, I asked her to complete a tray, choosing miniatures that she was drawn to and arrange them in a scene. The resulting tray was three separate scenes, each in a corner of the sand tray. One scene contained several wild animals such as bears and tigers representing her feelings of school and clinic work. The second scene represented a group of close friends she rarely saw; it was an outdoor scene with a swing, a few baby animals, stones, and a few trees. The third scene was a church with a few little animals dressed as people representing her new church and friends. As she finished constructing this scene she began to cry, immediately realizing how compartmentalized her life had become and how troubling that was for her. Self-awareness occurred by simply looking at the scene in the sand of her own creation. She was then able to discuss feeling overwhelmed with her situation and how it was "wearing her down" both personally and professionally. This tray provided us a significant insight from which to discuss what a challenge her program was, and she finally gave herself permission to admit being stressed. As she released these feelings she was able to talk about how they were affecting her clinical work and to make plans to take better care of herself so that she could better attend to her clients.

ISSUES OF TRANSFERENCE AND COUNTERTRANSFERENCE

Landreth (2002) stresses that the most important resource the play therapist brings into therapy is one's own personality—one's self being the core of the therapeutic relationship. Therapists who are unaware of their biases, motivations, needs, and feelings will be ineffective with children. These characteristics of the therapist will be sensed by the child and will negatively impact the child's therapeutic process. Assuming that one can effectively compartmentalize these aspects of self is improbable (Landreth, 2002). Children are very egocentric; therefore, when therapist's feelings are revealed to or sensed by the child, the child assumes those feelings are about him or her. For example, a therapist's anger toward an abuser may be interpreted by a child as anger toward the child, damaging the therapeutic relationship and healing process (James, 1989). Landreth (2002) proposes questions therapists can ask of themselves in the play therapy relationship:

> Is your intent to change the child? Do you hope the child will play? Are you more accepting of some behaviors than others? Do you have a low tolerance for messiness? Do you have a need to rescue the child from pain or difficulty? Do you have a need to be liked by the child? Do you feel safe with the child? Do you trust the child? Do you expect the child to deal with certain issues? (p. 104)

Therapists who have not considered these questions are likely to infuse their beliefs and expectations into the play therapy relationship influencing the child's play, preventing the child from being his true self as well as impacting the therapist's ability to communicate acceptance to the child.

Children have been exposed to horrific and unimaginable experiences. The therapist who has difficulty accepting the child's reality as he plays it out in session will interfere with or halt the therapeutic process. Watching children play out their trauma is a powerful and often unnerving experience. It is critical that play therapists be prepared to experience the intensity of play with a child. Common reactions therapists experience include a desire to rescue the child, injure the responsible party, nurture the child, or be overprotective. Any of these reactions might prevent the therapist from setting limits or allowing the child to tell the full story, therefore impairing the treatment process (James, 1989). Reactions such as this to the therapeutic process must be discussed and processed in supervision. It is critical that supervisors be prepared for the variety and intensity of reactions supervisees may have to their clients.

Ray (2004) reports that therapists who have difficulty connecting with children based on their preconceived expectations of what it is like to work with children are often discouraged. Frequently therapists expect play therapy with children to be fun and rewarding, and they are surprised when they do not receive the affirmation they expect from children. Therapists also have difficulty connecting with children who reject the therapist in a vengeful and hurtful way. Exploring and understanding these feelings is critical in the supervision process in order for supervisees to grow and develop as therapists. It is also important for supervisees to be self-aware in order to anticipate and identify transference in the therapeutic relationship.

Gil (2006) defines transference as a therapist's gut reactions, feelings, behaviors, and thoughts in response to the child, or child's system, that may undermine therapeutic work. Gil and Rubin (2005) discuss the importance of exploring countertransference for child therapists. Children bring their entire system—self, parents, siblings, agencies, schools, psychiatrists, and others—to therapy, constituting many different aspects of the child to which the therapist reacts. When play therapy is used as the medium of treatment, these issues are more obvious through the physical and visual expression of play. Therefore, countertransference can occur more frequently and more pervasively when working with children in the play therapy experience. Awareness of countertransference in the therapeutic relationship is critical to understanding the child, system, and the relationship between the child and therapist that is foundational to facilitating therapeutic movement.

Because of the physical, symbolic, and externally expressive nature of play therapy, children do not hold back, tapping into the therapists' emotional difficulties more often than adult clients, evoking a more powerful countertransference experience. Gil and Rubin (2005) proposed using play-based techniques referred to as countertransference play, such as sand tray, to address countertransference issues in play therapy relationships. Countertransference play provides a way for therapists to explore countertransference in a manner more consistent with the modality of therapy used with clients. Limiting supervision regarding transference issues to talking may not be adequate given the nonverbal and symbolic nature of therapeutic work.

Play therapy is different from adult talk therapy and, therefore, supervision of play therapists should be approached differently. There are more nonverbal behaviors and symbols to which the therapist must attend in a play therapy session than in adult talk therapy. Utilizing sand tray as the modality of expression in play therapy supervision responds to this difference, providing an expressive and symbolic modality for the supervisee to explore feelings of countertransference (Gil & Rubin, 2005).

INTEGRATING SAND TRAY INTO THE
SUPERVISION PROCESS

Ray (2004) suggests that play therapy supervision frequently follows a developmental model. Stoltenberg, McNeill, and Delworth (1998) developed the Integrated Developmental Model (IDM) of supervision. As a developmental model, IDM can be applied to any supervisee regardless of the point in the supervisee's professional development. It is particularly useful with play therapy supervisees, as many play therapists initially receive training and supervision in talk therapy, returning for supervision when incorporating play therapy into their practice. The IDM provides three levels through which a supervisee grows and develops. Level 1, "Beginning the Journey," is the level of dependence on the supervisor with limited self/other awareness. Based on the supervisee's need for structure, microskills training, and level of dependency, sand tray may not be the technique of choice at this point in development. Level 2, labeled "Trial and Tribulation," contains the struggle for independence and growing awareness of the client, sometimes to the exclusion, or ambivalence, of the supervisee's own self-awareness. This is the point at which sand tray is particularly effective. Sand tray experience can assist in increased insight into the supervisee's self-awareness, transference/countertransference, and client issues. The third and final level in IDM, "Challenge and Growth," is defined by the supervisee having a stable professional identity and appropriate autonomy. The increase in supervisee acceptance of self with awareness of strengths and weaknesses provides the ability to be open to increased integration of clinical work with this deeper sense of self. The role of the supervisor is to continue to stimulate and challenge growth. Again, this is an appropriate function of the sand tray experience. Ray (2004) discusses the difference between basic and advanced play therapy skills. She states that advanced play therapy skills continue to be areas of growth throughout the play therapist's career and therefore need to be approached differently as the therapist develops as a professional and a person. Utilizing sand tray in supervision is quite conducive to these more advanced aspects of a play therapist.

SAND TRAY AS A SUPERVISORY INTERVENTION

Supervision of play therapy can be a challenging and exciting adventure. Supervisors challenge supervisees to look at the world through the child's eyes, experience what the child experiences, and understand the child's perspective. So why should supervisors utilize sand tray as a medium to assist in supervisees' understanding of children?

(1) Sand tray gives expression to the therapist's nonverbalized feelings and experiences of the client. As previously discussed, there are myriad issues, people, and situations therapists react to when working with children that often go unnoticed when supervisees verbally report on cases. Sand tray allows the unspoken and "unaware" to be expressed. For example, supervisees often have difficulty managing their feelings about a child who plays aggressively. However, rarely would a supervisee confess they do not like the child. Sand tray may facilitate a discussion that is critical to the supervisee's growth as well as the treatment of the client.

(2) Sand tray makes visual and concrete what is abstract. Supervision is often a cognitive and abstract experience as supervisees spend significant time "talking about" the case, often directing their focus away from other dynamics occurring in session. Building a sand tray creates a picture and allows the supervisee to see the dynamics and feelings of the session, moving concepts and dynamics from abstract to visual and real, providing clarity and understanding.

(3) The kinesthetic quality of sand tray—touching the sand and arranging the figures—often ignites expression for supervisees. There is something organic and relaxing about running one's hands through the sand; it creates a sense of safety, facilitating supervisees to be open and vulnerable. This also attends to a more multimodal learning experience.

(4) Therapeutic metaphors are easily discovered when sand tray miniatures are used to capture aspects of the therapeutic process. Metaphors provide the supervisee with a safe vehicle of understanding clients and his feelings toward them. Supervisees may feel comfortable characterizing a client or parent by choosing a particular miniature. Working with the resulting metaphor assists in accessing thoughts and beliefs of which they were previously unaware.

(5) Dean (2001) refers to supervisees taking a "metaposition" regarding dynamics in the case, which decreases enmeshment in the dynamics. Inexperienced child therapists often find themselves enmeshed in the child's system, aligning with or working against one parent or caregiver over another. Taking a metaposition highlights interpersonal dynamics of which one may not have been previously aware.

(6) Sand tray can be utilized in both individual as well as small group supervision. Vicarious learning occurs as supervisees discuss and explore the contents of each other's trays. Group supervision also allows supervisees to observe how the supervisor processes trays with supervisees, thus providing a demonstration as to how to process trays with clients.

(7) Finally, sand tray supervision is an excellent modality to use with resistant supervisees. Sand tray interrupts defensive verbalization and provides an opportunity for supervisees to participate in supervision in a different way, breaking down the walls of resistance (Homeyer & Sweeney, 1998).

HOW TO USE SAND TRAY

There are many different ways supervisors can utilize sand tray as a supervisory tool. As previously mentioned it is critical that supervisors be ethical role models; therefore, training and personal experience in both sand tray and play therapy are imperative before this intervention is utilized with supervisees. Supervisors should facilitate rather than direct this process. It is important that supervisors notice the process that supervisees take in choosing and arranging miniatures. It is critical that supervisees do not feel scrutinized during the creation phase, as this will inhibit the process. Sand tray is a process in which understanding and awareness occur through a growing sense of self-control, empowerment, and safety (Homeyer & Sweeney, 1998). Supervisees who feel secure in the supervisory relationship are better able to evaluate their own therapeutic process. Supervisees who independently discover characteristics in their counseling that need to be different are more likely to be open and feel more empowered to embark in the change process if they do not feel criticized by a supervisor.

Homeyer and Sweeney (1998) provide six steps in conducting a sand tray session with a client that also apply to supervision: (1) prepare the room, (2) introduce the sand tray to the supervisee, (3) create the scene in the sand tray, (4) postcreation (processing) phase, (5) deconstruction of the sand tray and clean up, and (6) documenting the session. A detailed description of each phase of a sand tray session is beyond the scope of this chapter. However, we will discuss a variety of ways to introduce the sand tray as well as how to process the sand tray with a supervisee.

The approach you take to introduce the sand tray depends on your intent and purpose for its use with the supervisee at this point in the supervision process. For example, if your desire is for the supervisee to process a specific aspect of a case or session, then a directive prompt might be helpful. Sand tray is a very flexible medium, so there are myriad prompts one could give to supervisees. Described next are several examples of the types of prompts that might be helpful depending on the supervision goal.

Understanding the System

Choose a figure to represent the child and each member of his system (e.g., parents, teachers, agency workers, etc.). This prompt might be especially important for supervisees who are struggling with someone in the child's system, a frequent occurrence for child therapists. We find that supervisees often blame parents or teachers for the difficulties of the client, and this attitude makes it very difficult for counselors to form a strong working alliance. A sand tray prompt such as this can help the supervisee gain awareness and insight into feelings regarding the system and how they may be impacting the therapeutic process.

Understanding Their World

What is your client's world like? This prompt is general. However, it can be helpful for supervisees to look at all of the client's struggles from a global perspective. Often therapists only conceptualize a child from their experience in the playroom when the child's world is much bigger than the playroom. This prompt may also assist the supervisee in conceptualizing the client. Many beginning therapists have difficulty verbalizing the complete picture of the client, and seeing a visual representation of the client's world may facilitate this process.

Compare and Contrast

What is the client's world like today? What will the client's world be like at therapy termination? Comparing and contrasting these two trays may bring insight to what the client needs to move toward termination. This is a commonly used Adlerian technique with clients, and it can be very helpful for supervisees to create a treatment plan and gain perspective on what the client needs most. Frequently, supervisees are overwhelmed by the excessive and extreme needs of child clients. This technique can help in prioritizing what supervisees need to do for clients. Compare and contrast is a very frequent and useful category of prompts. Again, the prompt is developed by the supervisor to lead the supervisee to explore a supervisory issue. Perhaps the supervisee is becoming too enmeshed with a child's issues. A prompt like, "Make a scene in one half of the tray of how you feel before seeing your client, and in the other half, what you feel like after the session," might reveal issues.

Understanding Parents

Create a scene showing the parent's world. This prompt is to help supervisees gain perspective and understanding of parents. As previously mentioned, supervisees often struggle with forming a cohesive bond with parents and are therefore frequently critical of parents. Supervisees who look at things from the parents' perspective may gain more appreciation and empathy for parents.

Understanding the Session

A prompt like, "Create a scene showing your experience of your session last week," will be helpful for supervisees to process very specific incidents in a play therapy session. Specific play behaviors and themes are often very difficult for supervisees to understand and accept, such as sexualized or aggressive play. Trauma reenactments can also be an intense and emotional experience for supervisees processing their feelings and experiences regarding the play, but they can be healing. Supervisees may need to process their own feelings in this situation so that their perceptual experience does not interfere with the child's therapeutic process.

Understanding Countertransference

Gil and Rubin (2005) suggest processing supervisees' countertransference feelings immediately after a session, when feelings and reactions are fresh. The authors suggest the following prompt, "Allow yourself to check in and see what thoughts, feelings, and responses you have about the work you've just completed [with a specific client or over a specific period of time]. Then review the miniatures in front of you and use as few or as many as you like and place them in the sand box" (p. 96). Gil and Rubin suggest that supervisees process their feelings as they observe the scene in the tray, providing opportunity for feelings to be represented both visually and verbally.

There may also be countertransference issues between the supervisee and supervisor. Issues in the supervisory relationship must also be addressed. Sand tray can serve as a way to work through these issues as well.

Understanding Your Professional Development

Construct your world as a counselor. Mary worked with a group of elementary school counselors who were struggling in their positions. Many elementary counselors are the only counselor in their building and experience a great deal of isolation. Elementary counselors struggle with the many responsibilities in their roles of administrator, teacher, and counselor. Mary was providing support to a small group of counselors through expressive arts techniques. Each counselor had his or her own personal small sand tray—small plant saucers found at a local nursery. The prompt was to construct a tray of what their world was like at work. Once everyone completed their trays, we sat in a group and each person shared his or her tray. In group supervision it is important to connect the group members for a shared experience and vicarious learning. Linking members' similar feelings and experiences is critical in the group supervision process. This was especially important for these school counselors who were struggling in their roles and with isolation. There were consistent themes among the group of feeling stretched by so many demands, pressure from administrators, lack of time to spend counseling children, and a love of helping children. Each tray expressed these experiences differently; however, the themes were the same. One counselor chose a fairy with a magic wand to represent herself, an aggressive dinosaur representing her principal, and several nurturing animals representing the children and teachers. When she described her tray, the fairy flew around spreading magic to all the animals and protecting them from the dinosaur and his hurtful rules. As she described her tray, the other counselors were able to provide her with support and encouragement to continue to "spread magic to the children." These counselors were amazed and commented at the conclusion of our sand tray experience how helpful this was to them. The counselors reported feeling more encouraged, supported, and energized in their careers.

Play Genograms

Gil (2006) proposes utilizing play genograms with children and families in play therapy. This technique can be adapted for supervision as well. First, the supervisee constructs a genogram on a large sheet of paper including all significant caregivers in the child's system, including the play therapist/supervisee, foster parents, birth parents, social workers, teachers, daycare providers, and so forth. The first instruction is, "Choose miniatures that represent the client's feelings and thoughts about each person in the genogram, including yourself, from the client's perspective." The second direction is, "Choose miniatures that represent the client's feelings and thoughts about each person in the genogram, including yourself from your perspective." The discussion about the difference between the therapists' perspective and the client's perspective is a very interesting and noteworthy one during supervision.

This idea of using both the client's and the supervisee's perspectives occurred serendipitously as chapter author Linda Homeyer was conducting a supervision workshop. Given the prompt to think about a client with which they were not feeling particularly successful, they were then asked to make a genogram of the client's family. Several of the participants realized in the process of constructing the genogram that they were doing it from their perspective, not the client's. This demonstrates the many insights that might occur as symbolic, out-of-awareness information reveals itself.

Gil (2006) expands on this activity with clients in asking them to choose a miniature to represent their thoughts and feelings about the relationship the client has with each person in the genogram. Supervisees can construct this genogram from both the client's perspective and their own perspectives. Another interesting twist to this activity would be for the supervisee to choose miniatures that represent his or her own thoughts and feelings regarding the relationship with each person in the client's genogram. This is a dynamic way to openly discuss the experiences the supervisee has with the other adults in the child's system.

Magnuson (2000) suggests having supervisees construct professional genograms to enhance professional identity and clarity. Professional genograms could be done in a sand tray just like play genograms, utilizing miniatures to symbolize professional influences such as theorists, supervisors, and mentors.

Nondirective prompts can also be utilized, allowing the scene in the sand to be a result of the supervisee's interaction with the sand and miniatures. Supervisees who are at a lower level of development may find a nondirective prompt difficult, in that they are preoccupied with evaluation. A nondirective approach may be a good way to challenge those beliefs and assist the supervisee in focusing on the process rather than the product. In using a nondirective approach, it is likely that the supervisee's personal struggles will be more evident. Therefore, it is important for the supervisor to not move entirely into the counselor role. This type of personal supervision may be reserved for more advanced supervisees who are no longer focused on skill building but rather on personal development within the counseling relationship.

Homeyer and Sweeney (1998) suggest this nondirective prompt:

> Here is a collection of miniatures (pointing to shelves or boxes). You may use as many or as few as you like. I would like you to take a few moments to look at them, then select a few that really "speak to you." Place them in the sand (point to the sand tray). Then add as many as you like to create a world in the sand. I will sit here quietly, until you are finished. Take your time and let me know when you are done. (p. 62)

This prompt will provide supervisors with a picture of the supervisee's experience in the moment, providing insight as to the various factors that are contributing to the counseling relationship.

Processing Sand Tray

As when utilizing any expressive art modality, processing the sand tray experience with a supervisee is vital to the process. Homeyer and Sweeney (1998) give explicit instructions as to the role of the therapist during the construction and processing phases of the sand tray experience with a client, which can be adapted for supervision purposes. Creating an environment in which the supervisee feels safe and free to express is critical; Jungians refer to this concept as providing a "free and protected space." In order to provide this type of environment, supervisors must be involved in the construction of the tray through listening and observing. Involvement in this type of experience may be quite different than one might expect; supervisors are discouraged from talking much during the construction of the tray. Observations of how the supervisee approaches the tray are important to the process. A great deal of insight can be gained through observing how the supervisee approaches the construction of a sand tray, the interaction with the sand, and the choice and placement of each miniature. When processing the tray with supervisees, it is tempting to interpret the symbolism of the tray utilizing your knowledge of the supervisee and his client cases. However, it is the supervisee's interpretation of the symbols that is most important. Allowing the supervisee to fully explore and understand his feelings in each tray enables the advanced supervisee to achieve his own sense of understanding and awareness. This self-discovery is far more valuable than a supervisor's evaluation of the tray. However, the supervisor's insights are used for the development of artfully crafted questions to assist the supervisee in fully exploring the meaning of the sand tray.

After the completion of the tray, Homeyer and Sweeney (1989) recommend several aspects of the sand tray for the supervisor to consider during the processing portion of this experience. First, visually observe the completed sand tray, look at the entire scene, and consider it as a whole unit. What emotion does the sand tray evoke? As counselors we must always be aware of the emotions within us. Self-awareness is necessary to determine which reactions are based on our own experience and which are in reference to the work before us. Evaluate the organization of the sand tray: Is it overly organized or chaotic; rigid or realistic; unpeopled? Finally, identify the theme or metaphor of the sand tray. The emotional responses that come from within are important in the processing phase of sand tray.

When processing sand tray it is important to move from global to specific to facilitate the supervisee's expressive process. Homeyer and Sweeney (1998) suggest beginning with discussing the entire scene, asking for a title, then discussing the sections or parts of the tray and finally specific miniatures. When discussing any aspect of the tray, begin with the metaphor the supervisee has already established in the tray. This allows the supervisee to stay within the safety of the metaphor. It also provides some needed emotional and psychological distancing through the discussion of the contents of the sand tray rather than the focus becoming too intensely directed at the supervisee. Enlarging the meaning of the metaphor requires the supervisor to truly understand the supervisee's world from his or her perspective. This technique allows the supervisor to make connections from the scene in the sand tray to the supervisee's experience with clients. It is important to stay within the metaphor. However, there may be times when supervisees make the connection on their own. This personal awareness and insight should be honored and processed even if it is not the interpretation the supervisor considered. It is important to note that supervisees who are not yet ready to make the connection from the metaphor to their own experience are working within their areas of comfort, which should be respected.

The sand tray can also be utilized as a springboard for discussion once the supervisor has an understanding of the supervisee's scene. Questions such as these can also facilitate insight: What will happen next? What happened just before this scene? What do the figures in the tray need most? What do you need most? It is important to remember to respect the supervisee's metaphor; if she has not stepped out of the metaphor then tailor your questions to stay within the metaphor. For example: What does this lion need most? What does this girl want to happen next? What will things be like for this figure when things are better? It is important that the questions asked are relevant, purposeful, and focused on the supervisee's development as a counselor.

CONCLUSION

Sand tray is a remarkable technique that can be utilized with existing supervision models. Sand tray provides opportunities for supervisees to grow both personally and professionally in providing an opportunity for nonverbal expression. In order to utilize sand tray in supervision, it is imperative that supervisors have their own training and supervision in the use of sand tray. It is also critical that supervisors who facilitate this growth process focus the discussion on the supervisee's professional development and resist becoming the supervisee's counselor. Sand tray is a powerful medium and many of the supervisee's personal struggles and emotional experiences may be revealed. Referrals for counseling should be ready, if needed.

Sand tray facilitates the parallel process between supervisee and client. Haynes, Corey, and Moulton (2003) describe the parallel process of the supervisee's behavior with the supervisor as a mirror of the supervisee's behavior with the client. The parallel process is a powerful aspect of supervision that when addressed appropriately can provide great insight into both the client and supervisee's growth. Sand tray can facilitate this process as scenes are created in the sand that function as springboards of discussion regarding the therapeutic and supervisory relationships.

The self-awareness developed in supervision can be greatly enhanced through the use of symbols, metaphor, and play as discovered through the use of sand tray. The play therapist who works in the world of play also benefits from the use of play in supervision, enhancing understanding of client and self simultaneously.

REFERENCES

American Counseling Association. (2005). *Code of ethics and standards of practice.* Alexandria, VA: American Counseling Association.

Bernard, J., & Goodyear, R. (2004). *Fundamentals of clinical supervision.* Boston: Allyn & Bacon.

Dean, J. E. (2001). Sand tray consultation: A method of supervision applied to couple's therapy. *The Arts in Psychotherapy, 28,* 175–80.

Gil, E. (2006). *Helping abused and traumatized children.* New York: The Guilford Press.

Gil, E., & Rubin, L. (2005).Countertransference play: Informing and enhancing therapist self-awareness through play. *International Journal of Play Therapy, 14*(2), 87–102.

Haynes, R., Corey, G., & Moulton, P. (2003). *Clinical supervision in the helping professions.* Pacific Grove, CA: Thomson Brooks/Cole.

Homeyer, L., & Sweeney, D. (1998). *Sand tray: A practical manual.* Canyon Lake, TX: Lindan Press.

James, B. (1989). *Treating traumatized children.* New York: The Free Press.

Kalff, D. (1980). *Sandplay, a psychotherapeutic approach to the psyche.* Santa Monica, CA: Sigo Press.

Kwiatkowska, H. (1978). *Family therapy and evaluation through art.* Springfield, IL: Charles C. Thomas.

Landreth, G. L. (2002). *Play therapy: The art of the relationship.* New York: Brunner-Routledge.

Magnuson, S. (2000). The professional genogram: Enhancing professional identity and clarity. *The Family Journal: Counseling and Therapy for Couples and Families, 8*(4), 399–401.

Ray, D. (2004). Supervision of basic and advanced skills in play therapy. *Journal of Professional Counseling: Practice, Theory & Research, 32*(2), 28–41.

Stoltenberg, C. D., McNeill, B. W., & Delworth, U. (1998). *IDM: An integrated developmental model for supervising counselors and therapists.* San Francisco: Jossey-Bass.

15

⹉∞⹊

Countertransference Play

Informing and Enhancing Therapist
Self-Awareness through Play

Lawrence Rubin and Eliana Gil

Since its introduction by Sigmund Freud nearly a century ago (Freud, 1910/1959), clinicians have alternately embraced the idea of countertransference either as a valuable tool for enhancing therapeutic outcome as it can "deepen therapist's awareness of relationship dynamics and provide valuable information about the course of treatment" (Hayes, et al., 1998, p. 468) or as a therapeutically limiting, defensive, and largely unconscious process. The concept of countertransference has evolved from its origins in adult psychoanalysis to a more broad applicability in the area of child and adolescent treatment. Initially and narrowly defined as the therapist's unconscious reaction to the client's transference, the concept of countertransference has expanded to include any and all of the therapist's thoughts, feelings, and behaviors that may undermine treatment, and that arise in response to the client (Fromm-Reichman, 1950), the client's family (Maddock & Larson, 1995), or even elements of the client's larger ecosystem (O'Connor, 1991).

Understanding of the therapeutic impact of countertransference has also expanded beyond both psychoanalysis and the treatment of adults to therapeutic work with children and use in nonanalytic treatment, such as family therapy. In treatment with children and adolescents, the therapist's blind spots, biases, and unrecognized emotional needs may result in inappropriate emotional and behavioral responses, intolerance, need to be liked by the client, and attempts to change the client (Landreth, 2002). Metcalf (2003) has even argued that countertransference responses in child therapists exceed those found among adult therapists.

Even in light of this expanded view of the impact of countertransference, the means of addressing and resolving it have historically been described simply as "talking about it." The literature focuses on nonspecific verbal techniques designed to help the therapist develop awareness, insight, and self-understanding through reflection, supervision, or treatment (Robbins & Jolkovski, 1987; Rosenberger & Hayes, 2002; Sarles, 1994). This emphasis on intellectual and verbal means of addressing and resolving countertransference is not necessarily a problem, particularly when the treatment is predominantly verbal or oriented to adults. However, traditional, adult-oriented, verbal therapies for addressing countertransference may not be optimal for those involved in the treatment of children and adolescents, and for those using play therapy in particular, because play therapy is not exclusively dependent on the verbal elements of traditional therapy, that is, discussion, inquiry, and interpretation. Instead, play therapy taps the child's ability to use creative imagination, pretend play, symbol language, and metaphors.

Few efforts have addressed countertransference and differential means of dealing with it, especially in the field of child and adolescent therapy. In looking at one possible reason for this neglect, Schowalter (1985) posited that child therapists may be uncomfortable with the type of self-examination required for those involved in the highly active and hands-on therapeutic work inherent in therapy for children and adolescents. Regardless of the possible reasons for this neglect, efforts must be made by child therapists to address and harness the countertransference responses that arise in play therapy with children and teenagers. To do so, an understanding of the importance of these responses is necessary.

COUNTERTRANSFERENCE WITH CHILDREN
AND ADOLESCENTS

Traditional psychoanalytically defined countertransference is conceptualized as a reciprocal relationship between the client's transference and the therapist's unconscious. This is a linear and limiting conceptualization, particularly when working with children and teenagers, with whom effective intervention often requires active involvement with family members. According to a number of writers/clinicians in the field (Bernstein & Glenn, 1988; Bettleheim, 1975; McCarthy, 1989; Wright, 1985), awareness of the countertransference that manifests itself in child therapy is the key to understanding the child's psychological issues, the child's family, and the relationship between the child and the therapist. This implies that the therapist's countertransference is not limited to his or her unconscious responses. Instead, it may be a conscious cognitive, behavioral, or affective reaction to some characteristic (or experience) of the child or the child's family. Gabel and Bemporad (1994a; 1994b) suggested that the therapist's countertransference response may be to the agency in which the treatment is taking place. Waksman (1986) warned child analysts that their persistent and unresolved childhood issues could contaminate their work with both their child clients and their clients' parents. Rogers (1995) in her book *A Shining Affliction* chronicled how countertransference can affect the therapeutic relationship as well as a clinician's professional and personal stability. Given the myriad potential sources of countertransference in working with young clients, it becomes important to ask the question, "What is it about working with young clients that is so potentially evocative of countertransference?"

WHY YOUNG CLIENTS EVOKE COUNTERTRANSFERENCE

Therapeutic work with young clients presents unique countertransference challenges. Brandell (1992) observed that unlike adults, children (1) lack conscious motivation for treatment, (2) are far more action oriented, (3) are easily frustrated, and (4) are inherently regressive. According to Brandell, for these reasons—and also because young clients readily act out, engage in primary process thinking, and tax therapists' defenses more readily than adults—they evoke powerful countertransference. In a similar vein, Gabel and Bemporad (1994b) observed that because children are behaviorally and emotionally unpredictable, have ready access to material of a sexual and aggressive nature, and may be embedded in unstable family systems, they are potential countertransference tinderboxes.

Several authors have addressed countertransference responses to clients with various pathologies and presenting problems, utilizing more expressive techniques, such as sandplay (Bradway, 1991; Bradway et al., 1990). In discussing depressed youth, Bemporad and Gabel (1992) observed that preschoolers' helplessness, teenagers' confusion, and suicidal children's anger and confusion can elicit significant countertransference reactions. Similarly, the powerlessness, anger, divided loyalty, and sadness that children experience due to losses and disruptions can be extremely emotionally taxing to their therapists (Garber, 1992; Jewett, 1994; Karr-Morse & Wiley, 1997). In addition, the plight of foster children, with their concurrent feelings of loss, frustration, and attachment difficulties, has been well documented (Boyd Webb, 2005; Fahlberg, 1994). The treatment of adolescents with borderline traits who are in constant turmoil and who regularly practice splitting and projection can push therapists beyond their ability to control their emotions and responses (Mishne, 1992). Moser, et al. (2005) drew attention to the dynamic matrix of sibling relationships and the countertransferential pull it exerts on the therapist based on their family of origin, and particularly earlier sibling ties. McElroy and McElroy (1991) warned that clinicians working with families of incest, particularly those untrained, overwhelmed, or unprepared, may be negatively affected by countertransference responses to their clients, to the obvious detriment of all involved. Finally, the evocative task of working with abused children, the most vulnerable and fragile of clients, can challenge and test therapists' skills and boundaries, push them to undermine or overfunction for parents, and create personal and professional challenges such as time management, rescue fantasies, or vicarious traumatization (Cattanach, 1994; Gil, 1991; James, 1989; Perry & Szalavitz, 2006).

TYPICAL COUNTERTRANSFERENCE RESPONSES

The specific countertransference reactions evoked by young clients and/or their families or situations are as varied and complex as the clinical problems they present. According to Sarles (1994) countertransference is "a phenomenon that exists in every encounter with a child and adolescent patient and includes the full spectrum of emotions and reactions including anger, anxiety, dreaded waiting, envy, joy, love and hate" (p. 73). For Sarles, these responses and reactions are not so much a peril, but an inherent challenge in therapy with young clients. Similarly, McCarthy (1989) suggested that countertransference may be manifest in therapists' avoidance of their own or their clients' anxiety and might take the form of avoiding certain issues in counseling that might arouse the anxiety of either therapist or client. Schowalter (1985) noted that countertransference could take many forms: (1) preemptory diagnosis or discharge planning, (2) under inclusion or over inclusion of the parents in treatment, (3) competitiveness with the parents, and (4) excessively positive or negative feelings toward the client. Gabel and Bemporad (1994b) noted that young clients may lead therapists to over identify with them, use the child in the service of their own needs, or take on a go-between role in the family.

In exploring the relationship between countertransference and childhood depression, Brandell (1992) observed that therapists experienced a range of responses, including helplessness, futility, frustration with parents, desire to protect, confusion, rescue fantasies, and boredom, as well as the need to relive their own childhood and/or adolescent experiences. Working with therapists of abused children, Marvasti (1992) found countertransference reactions that included reluctance to explore abuse-related issues, identification with the victim or the abuser, vicarious guilt and shame, and failure to report. Similarly, McElroy and McElroy (1991) found that unbridled countertransference in therapists working with incest families resulted in collusion to offer (and receive) superficial treatment, avoidance of the deep pain of incest, competition with the parents, and emotional withdrawal from the case. In an analysis of countertransference responses to children with chronic illness, Soarkes (1992) identified therapists' guilt over their own good health, inappropriate disclosure of emotions, powerlessness, and grief related to losses in their own lives. Finally, and writing specifically in the context of play therapy, O'Connor (1991) cautioned therapists to monitor their countertransference so that they could avoid frustration, savior fantasies, over identification with their clients, and burnout.

Each of the foregoing countertransference responses is extremely powerful and threatens to undermine therapeutic efficacy and outcome, and each calls for a means of resolution that creates successful opportunities for self-processing in order to overcome obstacles presented by the countertransference. We suggest that therapists can address their countertransference by using strategies that are consistent with the mode of treatment they typically use with their young clients, namely, play therapy.

ADDRESSING COUNTERTRANSFERENCE

In traditional psychoanalysis with both children and adults, countertransference is addressed and resolved through the therapist's own analysis. In a review of the general empirical literature on countertransference, Rosenberger and Hayes (2002) found that anxiety management, self-integration, and clarification were the most widely cited means of countertransference resolution. Robbins and Jolkovski (1987) noted that the most effective ways to deal with countertransference included awareness, understanding, alertness, and implementation of a theoretical framework, along with an investigative approach to self-awareness; however, they did not specify how to use these means. Hayes, et al. (1998) suggested that, "Using supervision, reflecting on sessions and meetings one's needs outside of treatment were critical countertransference management factors" (p. 469). Frawley-O'Dea and Sarnat (2001) comment that "supervisee regressive reactions can be triggered by the patient, by the supervisor, or by the learning process itself" (p. 112). Finally, Campbell (2000) suggests that supervisors may also have countertransference to their supervisees, including "the need to be needed, the need to be liked, and the need to be powerful," (p. 43) so countertransference remains a central issue for discussion in supervisory relationships.

In the arena of countertransference resolution in nonanalytic therapy for children and adolescents, McElroy and McElroy (1991) posited the importance of personal therapy for the clinician as well as a team approach that make use of outside therapists as consultants. Waksman (1986) discussed a note-taking technique, a departure from the standard traditional practices of verbal dialogues, and commented on the surprising unwillingness of clinicians to be more spontaneous and creative in addressing countertransference. Gans (1994) described an "indirect communication technique" in which the therapist soliloquizes his countertransferential thoughts and feelings in the patient's presence as a means of working it through (and deepening the therapeutic bond). In a similarly creative fashion, Rudge (1998) suggested that the therapist explore her "countertransference dreams" in order to process the intense reactions evoked in therapy earlier in the day. Processing dreams in supervision is also discussed elsewhere (Robertson and Yack, 1993).

O'Connor (1991) moved the discussion of countertransference into the realm of play therapy. He, like others before him, indicated that therapy for the therapist could be helpful. Self-awareness was also an important tool for O'Connor, who added consultation, supervision, and other techniques to the list of resources for dealing effectively with countertransference. In her review of countertransference patterns among play therapists, Metcalf (2003) noted that group supervision, consultation, and peer process groups, as well as training play therapists to recognize signs of countertransference, could be helpful. However, like others before them, neither Metcalf nor O'Connor suggested direct use of therapeutic play to address countertransference by therapists.

This chapter's co-authors strongly believe that if therapists trust and value the curative potential of play therapy, then utilizing the same tools of play therapy to inform and enhance their self-awareness is an obvious choice.

INFORMING AND ENHANCING THERAPIST
SELF-AWARENESS THROUGH PLAY

The use of play therapy to help play therapists address countertransference has been seemingly absent from the child counseling and play therapy literature; however, in the related field of art therapy, art media in supervision has been documented by Malchiodi and Riley (1996). Rubin (1984, p. 58) asserts that, "The therapist can use his/her artwork as an aid to self-understanding in addition to helping the patient." Rubin suggested that therapists could verbally interact with their clients in session by sharing their thoughts through artwork and could also draw portraits of their clients outside the session in order to resolve countertransference. Similarly, Wadeson (1995) encouraged art therapists to draw pictures of themselves with their clients; of the therapy hour; of themselves with their clients' illnesses; and of the beginning, middle, and end of treatment.

Countertransference Play

The chapter authors suggest exploring and then incorporating play therapy strategies as a way to expand and/or strengthen those techniques already used to address countertransference—we do not propose an either/or dichotomy. We also think that it's possible that nonplay therapists might explore or experiment with these ideas to further enhance their self-understanding. At the same time, it is likely that personal familiarity with the curative properties of generic and therapeutic play will facilitate clinical experimentation. We have also found that therapeutic play may prove beneficial in the context of clinical supervision to help supervisees address their countertransferential responses.

The practice of therapists or clinical supervisors "checking in" with themselves and/or their supervisees is not unusual. This checking-in process may or may not result in substantive insights or discussions, but post-session processing can also be fascinating and can lead to deeper introspection, understanding, or therapist behavioral changes. The use of therapeutic play can augment perceptions, narrow or expand focal points, provide metaphors for exploration, and access and use affect and energy in the therapy or supervisory relationship.

In the following sections we demonstrate how various forms of play and play therapy can amplify self-awareness of countertransference and its impact through both nondirective and directive means. As will be apparent, either or both of these approaches can be readily applied to therapists' self-work and in supervision and can serve as a springboard for other creative methodologies.

Countertransference Art

As mentioned above, art therapists and other clinicians have been encouraged to use art to understand themselves and their clients. Many adults resist or withdraw from art experiences because of feelings of performance anxiety. The art task must therefore be user-friendly, inviting, and nonthreatening.

Most clinicians will not have the time or the energy to process their countertransference responses after every session. However, a structured art activity to process countertransference responses may be most relevant after frustrating, disturbing, or exhilarating sessions or when clinicians begin to experience unexplained feelings of fatigue, irritability, emotionality, hyper vigilance, or hyper arousal. Integrating any new or unfamiliar clinical habit requires time management skills, recognition of its value, and the willingness to promote personal and professional self-growth.

The training process to become a registered art therapist (ATR) includes an emphasis on self-introspection through art. During my (chapter author Eliana Gil's) own art therapy training process at George Washington University's art therapy program, I was taught to use an art activity called "countertransference art." I have found this activity immensely valuable and have come to appreciate its profound value in my therapeutic work as well as in my clinical supervision of others.

Making countertransference art requires a few tools: a box of Nupastels (colored chalks) available at any art or crafts store, white paper (standard 8½-inch × 11-inch paper suffices), slightly wet paper towels, and felt-tip black ink pens. The directive is: "Use these chalks and pens to make lines, shapes, images, symbols, and/or words, filling in as much or as little of the page with whatever comes to mind." This is obviously a request for abstract art (versus representational art) and as such, can decrease the performance anxiety and/or self-consciousness associated with drawing or painting. After making the countertransference art, clinicians allow themselves some time to evaluate their responses. Specifically, clinicians can reflect on the art-making process (physical energy, affective state, movement, intensity of line pressure, or physiological changes), content (images, symbols, words, or shapes), and associations (what does the artwork suggest to you about your thoughts and feelings regarding your client or session?). A useful approach is to view the page from all directions, hold it close or near, leave it and return to it, and document initial as well as subsequent responses. When using the countertransference art in supervision (that is, you as supervisor have instructed your supervisee to use this art activity in reference to his or her clients and countertransferential responses), you guide the supervisee toward self-introspection and maintain a structured discussion of the art product, the art-making process, and the emotional and physical responses to viewing the art.

In addition to this particular countertransference art activity for processing clinical countertransference in therapists and/or their supervisees, a more directive approach can be taken. Chapter author Lawrence Rubin has used this strategy successfully in his supervision with students. Using a more directive stance, the instruction to the supervisee is, "Draw a picture of a particularly troubling or challenging therapy session . . . one that left you with a lingering, and perhaps bothersome, feeling." The therapist may, of course, do this for a supervision session that left him or her feeling similarly. The supervisor may expand this directive art technique by asking himself or another to "depict a troubling session, placing yourself, or your feelings, or even the client's issue(s) directly into the artwork."

We will illustrate these two different techniques with clinical case examples. Gil discusses how she processed her own countertransference through her use of art, and Rubin gives an example of the use of art in supervision.

Case Example of Therapeutic Use of Countertransference Art with a Client (Gil)

Fifteen-year-old Jason came willingly to therapy with his parents who were concerned about his moodiness, isolation, and unwillingness to spend time with his family. Jason's parents seemed angry and resentful of each other. They were unable to articulate why they thought their family seemed so unhappy and disconnected, but something unspoken seemed to be underlying this family's pain. I met with Jason's parents to take a developmental history and to see if I could gain some insight about what was going on. Jason's father, Tom, made many obscure references to how different he was from his son Jason, how Jason could have been someone else's son and he wouldn't be shocked, and how Jason had never acted "in ways that fathers expect." His disappointment was palpable, much to the chagrin of Tom's wife, Kathy. Kathy cried quietly and dabbed her tears with a crumpled tissue. She looked at me at one point and said "it might have been better if Jason hadn't been born to this cruel world." When this family left the session, I felt mystified, unsettled, and uncertain—countertransferential responses that informed me about the family's problem: They were uncertain about their family functioning, lacking direction, and emotionally disconnected from each other. I felt a heaviness as the family left, and decided to pull out my chalks and paper and produce a countertransference drawing.

When I reviewed this drawing, I had the following responses: "This looks like a dragon emerging from water. The dragon has a male presence with female features—it looks both mature and childlike." I pondered my process (quiet, careful, with sudden spurts of color) as well as the content (a dragon emerging from the sea). My associations were "coming out," gender ambivalence, and the context of water. Something about a birth occurred to me. I also noted that the dragon seemed to rise to the sun and the warm and bright yellow color, while on the left side of the page, there appeared to be a presence in the darker color, black (perhaps a face, perhaps two figures with a small figure). My reactions were either the dragon being watched or the dragon being separate from a family. As I drove home I let my mind wonder, an important part of self-reflection, and I thought about the art that I had created and the feelings I experienced during and after the session. I revisited Tom's words, and new insights emerged about his harsh descriptions of his son. I wondered if Tom had somehow conveyed his dissatisfaction directly to his son and whether Jason withdrew from his parents in an effort to avoid his father's apparent rejection of him. I decided to meet with Jason alone (as opposed to meeting in family therapy, as we had arranged). I wanted to see if Jason would be more communicative in an individual session since he had been so reticent in the family therapy session. I wanted to ask Jason his view of his family, how close or distant he felt, if he would turn to his mother or father if he had a problem or worry, and I wanted to hear his perceptions of what was going on in his family. Before I knew it, Jason "came out" to me, stating his relief at being able to tell me what was really going on with him. Jason noted that he was convinced that his parents already knew that he was gay and that his father would never accept him. As I listened to Jason, my countertransference art made more sense, and I was interested to see how Jason's parents had somehow transmitted what they knew and had not yet articulated. Although this example may be dramatic, it is a memorable example of how useful countertransference art can be in allowing us to both identify and then process our countertransference responses. Once we make countertransference art, it stands as a separate art production that can be pondered, felt, and possibly understood on many conscious and unconscious levels.

Example of the Use of Directive Countertransference Art in Supervision (Rubin)

Jennifer, my supervisee and a recently divorced mother of two, struggled with intense feelings of resentment and rage toward her ex-husband, whose irresponsible financial decisions had bankrupted the family and whose emotional unavailability had similarly undermined their marriage. Jennifer had difficulty suppressing these feelings at home and was often short-tempered with her children, who had reacted with fear and insecurity that originated in their parents' divorce. During supervision, Jennifer was describing her anger toward her young client's mother for not protecting him. I noticed that she became progressively unable to process her feelings about this case. Frustrated with my own difficulty moving Jennifer into a more productive processing of the case, I directed her to draw a picture of the relationship between herself, her young female client, and the client's mother.

She drew a picture of herself and her client protected under a table from the raging mother, who was perched threateningly atop the table (see figure 15.1). Previously unaware of how she tended to protect, and thus isolate, clients from angry and abusive parents, the therapist drew connections to similar patterns both in her own marriage and in her family of origin, in which her own father had acted similarly to her ex-husband.

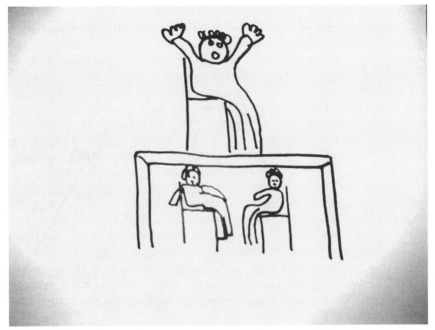

Figure 15.1. Jennifer's Drawing of Herself and Her Client (Under the Table) and the Client's Mother (on Top of the Table).

Countertransference Sand World

Even though sand therapy has been used for a number of years, it has gained steady popularity in the last two decades (Amman, 1996; Boik & Goodwin, 2000; Kalff, 1980; Lowenfeld, 1935/1967; Mitchell & Friedman, 1994; Ryce-Menuhin, 1992). As mentioned at the outset of this chapter, if clinicians value the therapeutic approaches they offer their clients, these same approaches can form the basis for exploring countertransference responses during clinical work. In countertransference sand therapy, therapists build miniature scenarios in the sandbox immediately after stressful or mystifying sessions, or undertake the sand therapy task while keeping a specific client or session in the forefront of their minds. The instruction is, "Use as few or as many miniatures and make whatever comes to mind in the sand tray, allowing yourself to be guided by your thoughts, feelings, and reactions to your client, your client's family, your client's problem, or a single session." This countertransference technique will be more accessible to those already practicing sand therapy because it requires traditional sand therapy equipment, such as a sandbox, fine white sand, a collection of miniatures, and water. Contemporary sand therapy includes the use of sandboxes of many sizes and shapes as well as the use of containers, such as Tupperware boxes, kitty litter boxes, and shoe boxes. The formality and structure of the technique will vary, as will the size and scope of the miniatures that have been collected (Bradway et al., 1990; Homeyer & Sweeney, 1988).

Clinicians should prepare themselves to make their countertransference tray by making sure they will be free of interruptions, by giving themselves permission to take time without internal pressure to rush, and by making the environment as quiet and comfortable as possible. Once the sand therapy process feels complete, clinicians can explore their reactions to the miniature scenario they have created in the sandbox.

In addition to this more nondirective approach, supervisors may guide their supervisees to create a miniature scenario that "depicts a particularly troubling session you had with a client or the relationship between you and a client that seems to elicit unusual or troubling feelings in you." As an example, a therapist struggling with her own impending divorce and feeling overwhelmed, angry, and depressed conducted a session with a child who was neglected and who was extremely needy and dependent. At Rubin's suggestion, she made two sand tray scenes in a supervisory session.

The first tray, which represents the therapist's sand depiction of the first half of a session in which she was unable to nurture the child, shows how she equated herself with the client by using the same animal to represent both of them (see figure 15.2). The only difference was that the therapist gave herself a boat to float in and used a traffic light in an attempt to control her anger. In the second sand scene (figure 15.3), which represented the second half of the same session, the therapist regained control, using a turtle to slow herself down and trees to soften the scene, and thus her emotions. While both characters were spotted dogs, suggesting not equality but equivalence, the therapist's character was larger, and therefore in a better position to nurture. Through this sand work, the therapist/supervisee developed considerable understanding into how her countertransference had played itself out in the session.

Gil routinely utilizes a group supervision technique that appears to promote self-introspection and exploration of countertransference. In small supervision groups (no more than six supervisees), one group member presents a clinical case imbedded with a specific clinical question. Other group members are then asked to take small sandboxes in their hands and find miniatures that best show their thoughts and feelings about the case that they have just heard. They are then asked to place these miniatures in the boxes and bring them back for further group discussion.

A supervisee presented a complex child abuse case in which three children had been severely injured. The supervisee was struggling with

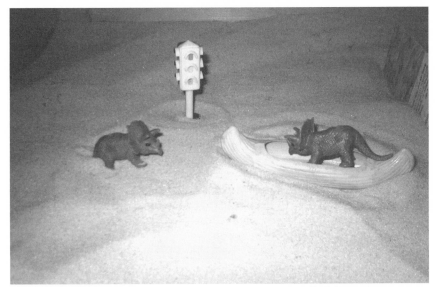

Figure 15.2. Therapist's Sand Tray Representing the First Half of the Session.

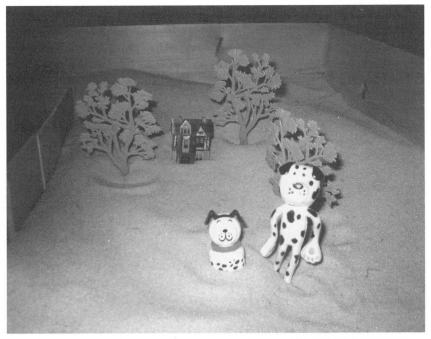

Figure 15.3. Therapist's Sand Scene Representing the Second Half of the Session.

overwhelming countertransference responses including fear, overprotection, a desire to overfunction, and anger. Her clinical question was how to proceed. Overwhelmed with strong emotions, she was unable to think through how to prioritize her interventions with the family. Group members filled their sandboxes, brought them back for group discussion, and spoke some about what they had created in the box.

When this supervisee saw each group member's sandbox, she felt suddenly energized and noted, "I can't believe how each of you has some of my feelings in your sand trays. I was thinking there was something wrong with me to have so many emotions in my work . . . now I see that it's okay, it's normal." Somehow "seeing" other supervisees' responses to this family normalized her responses. When the group discussed their responses, it was clear that everyone had utilized symbols of boundaries (fences, gates, enclosures) and that the first priority was to ensure that these child clients were now in a safe and nurturing environment. Note that creating images using art or sand can be an evocative and powerful experience. As informative and useful as these tools might be, they may also be disquieting in the type or level of affect that they generate. Clinicians may find processing their work with colleagues or consultants to be helpful, and may use other methods such as collage, dollhouse play, and metaphoric storytelling to enhance self-awareness and address countertransference.

Countertransference Symbol Work

Symbol work requires an investment in creative imagination and a basic trust in the richness and reliability of symbol language. Mental health professionals are more or less comfortable with leaving the realm of verbal communication; however, this countertransference technique has vast possibilities for mobilizing clinical energy and promoting understanding. With symbols we can see our underlying concerns, "shrink" the problem, move miniatures, and express our thoughts and emotions. Art and sand tray activities also use symbols, but the symbols are in a more confined context that utilizes boundaries (edges of a page, confines of the sandbox). Art includes interaction with the art medium (chalks, paints, pencils, watercolors, etc.), and sand therapy includes the use of fine, white sand, which is evocative in its own right.

Symbol work can be done by simple selection and manipulation of symbols out of a designated context. This can happen any time and anywhere, and it can yield remarkable insights or opportunities for processing a particular issue in a quiet way. The directive is simple: find a symbol that shows your thoughts and feelings about your work with a specific person or over a particular period of time. This activity is then

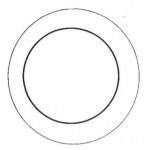

Figure 15.4   Circle Exercise

processed (for example, as it has been described in the art and sand countertransference exercises).

To make use of symbol work with adolescents or children, I (Gil) have created a technique in which two circles are placed on a page, creating a donut effect (see figure 15.4).

In the center circle, clients are instructed to place miniatures that suggest worries, problems, or concerns. In the outside circle, clients place miniatures that represent steps toward resolving or addressing their expressed problem. Of course this exercise is useful for both therapist and client. After a difficult session with an adolescent girl who seemed unable to make good decisions and ended up putting herself in harm's way, I took some time to process my countertransference by using this circle exercise. In the center, I placed symbols of my perception of my work with this youngster. I was struck by the images of being bound up (the mummy), covering her ears, a person shooting a gun, and a stop sign. This summed up my feelings of helplessness in working with this challenging teen. I immediately placed different miniatures in the outer circle, and I noticed that several of them seemed to gap the inner and outer circle. I placed a magic lamp, a bridge with a wise man sitting at the top, and grasping hands. In addition, I placed Pocahontas with daisies, a laughing Buddha, an Alaskan child holding a mask in her lap, a police officer reaching out, a woman doing yoga, and a small figure of an African American mother and child.

As I utilized this technique, it became very clear to me that my frustration and despair were reflective of this youngster's experience of isolation and helplessness. At the same time, this exercise clarified my own hopefulness and directed me in a couple of areas that I had neglected—especially, my need to provide unconditional acceptance, to continue to reach out and make contact, to anchor myself, and to use a sense of humor. As I did this exercise, I was led to offering my teenage client the opportunity to work with the circles herself. Amazingly, she was immediately engaged with the miniatures, and this work allowed her to both acknowledge her isolation and find signs of resiliency and optimism. It was interesting to note that the laughing Buddha also appeared in her outer circle.

CONCLUSION

The study of countertransference dates back nearly a century, with roots that are deeply embedded within the psychoanalytic tradition. With countertransference historically defined within that tradition as the therapist's unconscious response to that of the client, early countertransference literature focused on traditional verbal therapies with adults. While clinical attention was later broadened to encompass therapy with children, even after it became quite evident that children could evoke powerful countertransference, little research or clinical discussion was directed at dealing with countertransference that arises in child therapy. Only recently has the clinical study of countertransference been untethered from the unconscious and expanded beyond the therapy room to include the client's entire ecosystem. While this represents a considerable advance in understanding of the phenomenon, the means of addressing and resolving it has been exclusively verbal. This chapter has taken a step toward remedying this deficiency by suggesting how the modality of play, the same modality used in therapy with children and teenagers, can be applied to countertransference awareness and resolution in self-work and supervision.

Countertransference play is a logical outward extension of play therapy, whereby therapists experienced with play can explore their responses to a client, as well as to members of the client's system, or even to agencies involved in the client's care. Therapists can use countertransference play before a session with a particularly troubling client or after a session that leaves them with strong, inexplicable, and/or uncomfortable feelings or thoughts. This technique may also lend itself to both individual and group supervision that is either directive or nondirective and that incorporates a wide range of expressive media including art, sand, and symbol work. Other possibilities may include collage work, role playing, and storytelling.

While the development of countertransference play was both logically derived from our clinical work and based on our collective intuitive approach to play therapy and play therapy supervision, we are not suggesting that it is a simple technique that can be readily applied by anyone with a modicum of play therapy experience. This would be the equivalent of saying that play therapy itself is nothing more than a simple technique to be applied expediently. Instead, countertransference play, like play therapy, is a potentially rich and complex resource for clinicians who have dedicated significant efforts to acquiring a firm foundation in the theories and practice of counseling children and teenagers in general, and of play therapy in particular. Just as the discipline of play therapy has increased its empirical foundation through experimental outcome study, we recommend that similar efforts be directed at countertransference play; readers are encouraged to use the examples provided in this brief chapter as a springboard for creative applications of their own.

REFERENCES

Ammann, R. (1996). *Healing and transformation in sandplay: Creative processes become visible*. Peru, IL: Carus Publishing.

Bemporad, J. R., & Gabel, S. (1992). Depression and suicidal children and adolescents. In J. R. Brandell (Ed.), *Countertransference in psychotherapy with children and adolescents*. Northvale, NJ: Jason Aronson.

Bernstein, I., & Glenn, J. (1988). The child and adolescent analyst's emotional reactions to his patients and their parents. *International Review of Psycho-Analysis, 15,* 225–41.

Bettleheim, B. (1975). The love that is enough: Countertransference and ego processes of staff members in the therapeutic milieu. In P. Giovacchini (Ed.), *Tactics and techniques in psychoanalytic therapy*. Northvale, NJ: Jason Aronson.

Boik, B. L., & Goodwin, E. A. (2000). *Sandplay therapy: A step-by-step manual for psychotherapists of diverse orientations*. New York: W. W. Norton.

Boyd Webb, N. (Ed.). (2005). *Working with traumatized children in child welfare: Social work practice with children and families*. New York: Guilford Press.

Bradway, K. (1991). Transference and countertransference in sandplay therapy. *Journal of Sandplay Therapy, 1*(1), 25–43.

Bradway, K., Signell, K., Spare, G., Stewart, C. T., et al. (1990). *Sandplay studies: Origins, theory, and practice*. Boston: Sigo Press.

Brandell, J. R. (Ed.). (1992). *Countertransference in psychotherapy with children and adolescents*. Northvale, NJ: Jason Aronson.

Campbell, J. M. (2000). *Becoming an effective supervisor: A workbook for counselors and psychotherapists*. Philadelphia, PA: Accelerated Development.

Cattanach, A. (1994). *Play therapy: Where the sky meets the underworld*. Bristol, PA: Jessica Kingsley Publishers.

Fahlberg, V. I. (1994). *A child's journey through placement*. Indianapolis, IN: Perspectives Press.

Frawley-O'Dea, M. G., & Sarnat, J. E. (2001). *The supervisory relationship: A contemporary psychodynamic approach*. New York: Guilford Press.

Freud, S. (1910/1959). Future prospects of psychoanalytic psychotherapy. In J. Strachey (Ed. and Trans.), *The standard edition of the complete works of Sigmund Freud* (Vol. 20, 87–172). London: Hogarth Press.

Fromm-Reichman, F. (1950). *Principles of intensive psychotherapy*. Chicago: University of Chicago Press.

Gabel, S., & Bemporad, J. (1994a). An expanded concept of countertransference. *Journal of the American Academy of Child and Adolescent Psychiatry, 33*(2), 140–44.

Gabel, S., & Bemporad, J. (1994b). Variations in countertransference reactions in psychotherapy with children. *American Journal of Psychiatry, 48*(1), 111–20.

Gans, J. (1994). Indirect communication as a therapeutic technique: A novel use of countertransference. *American Journal of Psychotherapy, 48*(1), 120–29.

Garber, B. (1992). Children who have experienced parental loss and divorce. In J. Brandel (Ed.), *Countertransference in psychotherapy with children and adolescents.* Northvale, NJ: Jason Aronson.

Gil, E. (1991). *The healing power of play.* New York: Guilford Press.

Hayes, J., McCracken, J., McClanahan, M., & Hill, C. (1998). Therapists' perspectives on countertransference: Qualitative data in search of a theory. *Journal of Counseling Psychology, 45*(4), 468–82.

Homeyer, L., & Sweeney, D. (1988). *Sandtray: A practical manual.* Canyon Lake, TX: Lindan Press.

James, B. (1989). *Treating traumatized children.* Lexington, KY: Lexington Books.

Jewett, C. (1994). *Helping children cope with separation and loss* (Rev. ed.). Boston, MA: Harvard Common Press.

Kalff, D. (1980). *Sandplay.* Santa Monica, CA: Sigo Press.

Karr-Morse, R., & Wiley, M. S. (1997). *Ghosts in the nursery: Tracing the roots of violence.* New York: Atlantic Monthly Press.

Landreth, G. (2002). *Play therapy: The art of the relationship.* New York: Brunner Mazel.

Lowenfeld, M. (1935/1967). *Play in childhood.* New York: Wiley.

Maddock, J. W., & Larson, N. R. (1995). The social ecology of incest treatment. In J. W. Maddock & N. R. Larson, *Incestuous families: An ecological approach to understanding and treatment* (345–82). New York: Norton.

Malchiodi, C., & Riley, S. (1996). *Supervision and related issues: A handbook for professionals.* Chicago, IL: Magnolia Street Publishers.

Marvasti, J. (1992). Psychotherapy with abused children and adolescents. In J. Brandel (Ed.), *Countertransference in psychotherapy with children and adolescents.* Northvale, NJ: Jason Aronson.

McCarthy, J. M. (1989). Resistance and countertransference in child and adolescent psychotherapy. *American Journal of Psychoanalysis, 49*(1), 67–76.

McElroy, L., & McElroy, R. (1991). Countertransference issues in the treatment of incest families. *Psychotherapy, 28*(Spring), 48–54.

Metcalf, L. M. (2003). Countertransference among play therapists: Implications for therapist development and supervision. *International Journal of Play Therapy, 12*(2), 32–48.

Mishne, J. (1992). Treatment of borderline children and adolescents. In J. R. Brandell (Ed.), *Countertransference in psychotherapy with children and adolescents.* Northvale, NJ: Jason Aronson.

Mitchell, R. R., & Friedman, H. S. (1994). *Sandplay: Past, present, and future.* New York: Routledge.

Moser, C., Luchner, A., Jones, R., Zaroski, D., et al. (2005). The impact of the sibling in clinical practice: Transference and countertransference dynamics. *Psychotherapy: Research and Practice, 42*(3), 262–78.

O'Connor, K. (1991). *The play therapy primer.* New York: John Wiley.

Perry, B. D. & Szalavitz, M. (2006). *The boy who was raised as a dog: And other stories from a child psychiatrist's notebook.* New York: Guilford Press.

Robbins, S., & Jolkovski, M. (1987). Managing countertransference feelings: An interactional model using awareness of feelings and theoretical framework. *Journal of Counseling Psychology, 34*(3), 276–82.

Robertson, B., & Yack, M. (1993). A candidate dreams of her patient: A report and some observations on the supervisory process. *International Journal of Psycho-Analysis, 74*(5), 993–1003.

Rogers, A. (1995). *A shining affliction: A story of harm and healing in psychotherapy.* New York: Penguin Books.

Rosenberger, E., & Hayes, J. (2002). A review of the empirical countertransference literature. *Journal of Counseling and Development, 80*(3), 264–70.

Rubin, J. A. (1984). *The Art of Art Therapy.* New York: Brunner Mazel.

Rudge, A. (1998). A countertransference dream: An instrument to deal with a difficult transference situation. *International Forum of Psychoanalysis, 7,* 105–11.

Ryce-Menuhin, J. (1992). *Jungian sandplay: The wonderful therapy.* New York: Routledge.

Sarles, R. (1994). Transforming countertransference issues with adolescents: A personal reflection. *American Journal of Psychotherapy, 48*(1), 64–74.

Schowalter, J. E. (1985). Countertransference in work with children: Review of a neglected concept. *Journal of the American Academy of Child Psychiatry, 25*(1), 40–45.

Soarkes, B. (1992). Treating children with a life-threatening illness. In J. R. Brandell (Ed.), *Countertransference in psychotherapy with children and adolescents.* Northvale, NJ: Jason Aronson.

Wadeson, H. (1995). *The dynamics of art psychotherapy.* New York: John Wiley.

Waksman, J. (1986). The countertransference of the child analyst. *International Review of Psychoanalysis, 13,* 405–15.

Wright, B. (1985). An approach to infant-parent psychotherapy. *Infant Mental Health Journal, 4,* 247–63.

Part IV

POTPOURRI OF
PLAYFUL TECHNIQUES

16

⟡

Playful Activities for Supervisors and Trainers

Evangeline Munns

Na matter what therapeutic treatment method we may use, it is imperative that we have insight into our own intrapsychic responses (Jernberg, 1983). Healer, know thyself first! With ever-increasing caseloads and shorter time frames for treatment, it is easy for most therapists to focus completely on the problems of their patients and spend negligible time on self-reflection. In our supervision times all of the attention too often goes into trying to solve the client's difficulties without really looking at our own responses and motivations as therapists.

The need to be in tune with our own issues is important because of the ever-present risk of countertransference—the projection of our own needs onto the client. It is important to remember that in spite of perhaps having had our own personal analysis in the past, it is highly likely that some countertransference takes place in nearly every session with our clients. Why? Because we are human. If our countertransference projections fit in with the needs of the client, then this is a less worrisome situation. However, if our own issues drive us to fulfill our own needs at the expense of the client, then we may indeed harm the client.

Countertransference issues can easily come to the fore with many treatment methods, but particularly where there are direct interactions with the client involving physical contact. There are a number of therapeutic treatment methods that involve such contact and an example of this is Theraplay, a structured form of play therapy. On a clinical level Theraplay has proven to be highly effective in enhancing parent/child relationships

271

and/or attachments (Munns, 2000). However, in Theraplay the activities are fast changing, leaving little time or space for reflections or self-examination. Therapists must be aware of their own issues and resist the temptation to re-enact their own childhood. "There is the invitation to do to the child what was done to the therapist as a child, or to do to the child what the therapist feared or wished would have been done" (Jernberg, 1983, p. 431).

REACTIONS

The therapist needs to personally ask continuing questions as to the reason for choosing a particular activity and exploring personal reactions to the child's behavior. In fairness to the therapist, there may be natural reactions, particularly to the child's misbehavior. However, "the therapist must not be so objective that he experiences neither anger nor anxiety, nor must be so vulnerable that he drowns in these experiences" (Jernberg, 1983, p. 431). There are four areas in which the therapist must be especially insightful about personal feelings (Jernberg & Booth, 1999).

Anger

Anger may be a natural reaction to a child's physical or verbal abuse such as hitting, kicking, spitting at the therapist, and so forth, but if the anger is so great that the therapist cannot overcome her feelings and move beyond them, then there is a problem. As well, if the therapist becomes angry in response to a child's behavior that normally does not evoke such feelings in others, then such feelings need to be explored (e.g., therapist feels angry while feeding the child).

Dependency

A therapist may deny her own regressive yearnings by avoiding any regressive activities with the child, such as not feeding the child or not putting powder on the hurts on a child's hands even with children who have been deprived or neglected and clearly need it. On the other hand, the therapist may prolong such activities in order to satisfy her own passive, dependent longings.

Sexuality

When working with clients who have been sexually abused in the past and are acting out by being provocative, seductive, and so on, there may be a sexual arousal on the part of the therapist. What the therapist does with these feelings is crucial. The therapist must acknowledge such feelings, try to neutralize them, change the activity, and explore these feelings later with a supervisor or personal therapist.

Competition

We live in a competitive world and our competitive strivings are often strongly ingrained by the time we become adults. The therapist must be able to rise to challenges, but not to the point of always striving to win. The child should be winning most of the time. The therapist must also not be competitive with the parents and not put down the parents in any way. The therapist needs to form a positive alliance with parents and not be looked upon as a judge or competitor.

AVOIDING COUNTERTRANSFERENCE

There are many traditional ways to avoid or decrease countertransference feelings, such as supervisor or peer observation, viewing videotapes of one's sessions, supervision, role playing, and personal psychotherapy. Hopefully, through these methods some insight is gained by the therapist. There are other more playful ways of helping therapists gain self-knowledge that can be used during training sessions, as well as in group supervision. Some of these are described below. They are generally nonthreatening, and supervisees or trainees are not usually overwhelmed. At times there may be a few tears when someone is triggered in remembering a loss, but not to the point of being unable to recover in a group.

The following activities are presented in a sequence (which can be altered) beginning with a gentle look at some undiscovered aspects of ourselves and proceeding to a deeper level of self-knowledge. Many are derived from workshops with Dr. Viola Brody (Brody, 1997). If time permits, it is often helpful to begin with "freeing up" or "ice breaker" exercises such as keeping balloons tossed up in the air, or within a circle formation throwing balls to each other while calling out that person's name.

Getting to Know Ourselves through Voice

Close your eyes and take a deep breath and as you exhale just relax.
Repeat above but as you exhale just clear your mind of all thoughts.
Take a deep breath and as you exhale make a sound—any sound.
Take a deep breath and as you exhale make your sound louder.
Take a deep breath and as you exhale make your unique sound.

Place two fingers on your lips and feel them vibrate as you make your
sound.

Take a deep breath and as you exhale and make your sound, think of
projecting it to every corner of this room.

Take a deep breath and as you exhale, think of projecting your sound
beyond this room, beyond this building, beyond this city, and into the
universe. Hold the sound until you finish exhaling.

Take a deep breath and open your eyes as you exhale.

In one word, how was that for you? Would anyone like to share?

Note that the leader makes the first sound and the group follows, but
everyone is making their unique sound. It is amazing how often beautiful
harmony results when everyone is vocalizing their sounds together.

Getting to Know Our Bodies

Sit in a comfortable position in a space of your own that is not too near
to anyone else. Close your eyes. Take a deep breath and as you exhale
just relax. Take a deep breath and as you exhale, clear your thoughts
from your mind.

Rub the palms of your hands together for a few seconds and feel the
bumps and soft mounds and crevices of your palms as you do this.

Now place your palms facing each other about one quarter inch apart,
so they are not touching each other. Do you still feel the energy and
warmth between your hands? Do your hands like each other?

Now place both palms of your hands on top of your head and explore
the bumps and curves of your scalp and the smoothness, waves, or
curliness of your hair. Feel the roots of your hair as you run your fingers and hands through your hair.

Now feel your face with both of your hands, starting on your forehead—
the lines and furrows, the hair of your eyebrows, the furrows between your eyebrows and at the edge of your eyes, your eyelids, and
the hollows of your eye sockets.

Now press gently on your eyelids—do you see two dark pools behind
your eyes as you do this? Go in there for a minute. Pause.

Feel the ridge of your nose, your soft nostrils, your cheekbones and the
hollows of your cheeks, the dip below your nose, the softness of your
lips, the corners of your mouth, the dip below your mouth, your chin.

Now trace the hard outline of your jaw reaching to your ears. Feel the
ridges of your ears, around, behind, and in front—all the inner curves
and your soft earlobe.

Now press a fingertip into each ear for a minute and hear the powerful
throbbing of your inner body—the pulsing rhythms.

Does your head feel different now from the rest of your body?

Feel the front and back of your neck—the strong tendons and vertebrae and the hollow at the base of your neck.

With your right hand explore your left shoulder—the collarbone, the warm armpit, the muscles of your arm, the pointy elbow, the forearm, the many bones of your wrist, the knuckles of your hand, your fingers and each fingernail, the spaces between your fingers, and the palm of your hand. Now with your left hand explore your right shoulder, armpit, arm, and so on.

Now place both palms on top of your chest and moving down feel the softness of your breasts, the hardness of your ribs underneath and around, your belly button, and your tummy.

Using both hands, feel your right hip, the strong bone there, around to your back, the vertebrae there and in your tailbone, the strong muscles of your buttocks, and your thigh all around.

Now using both hands explore your left hip, and so forth. As you finish exploring your left thigh, go down to your left kneecap and feel the bumps of your kneecap and the strong tendons underneath.

Explore your calf muscles, your strong shinbone, your bony ankle, your hard heel, your feet on top and underneath, and your toes and toenails.

Now explore your right knee, calf, shinbone, ankle, heel, foot, and toes.

Now put both hands on top of your head and brush your body energy in one full sweep, from the top of your head, down the front of your body, right out past your toes and into the universe. Do this sweep once more.

Take a deep breath and open your eyes. In one word—how did that feel? Does anyone want to share?

Note that even though this exercise may seem strange to some it is very powerful. Comments are heard such as "I feel as if I have been born again," "I feel reconnected," and "I feel centered."

Body Movements

Find a partner. Decide who will be the first to move while the other observes. The person moving with his or her eyes closed moves in any way and in any direction. The partner silently observes, perhaps writing notes and verbally guiding the moving partner away from bumping into any objects, if this should be imminent. The moving partner stops after a few minutes. A discussion takes place between the two partners, with the observer personally reflecting how it felt and voicing any insights he or she may have gained about the moving partner. Next, the partners change positions and the observer now becomes the moving person, with a discussion that follows between them. A general discussion may take place at the end with everyone participating. This exercise takes approximately ten minutes.

When You Were First Seen

Everyone is seated with a note pad and pen in a space of his or her own. The leader says, "Close your eyes and take a deep breath and just relax as you exhale. Take a deep breath and as you exhale, let go of your thoughts—clear your mind. Take a deep breath and as you exhale, go back in your memories to a time when your were first truly seen by a person who saw the all of you—your positive and negative aspects—but still accepted you. Go back in your memories until you find someone. This may take some time. When you find that person that saw the whole of you, try to remember everything: how old were you, what were you doing, what were you wearing, where you were, and most importantly, how you felt. Think about this and then write down your memories and feelings. If you want, you may even try to draw yourself at that time." (Leader allows five to ten minutes to pass and when most people look as if they are finished, announces, "We will spend two more minutes on this, and then we will end.") After a short space of time the leader says: "Everyone open their eyes. Is there anyone who would like to share some of their thoughts and feelings on what they have just experienced?"

Note that the leader should have a tissue box handy as some people may cry when they think of someone that has been important to them and is now gone from their lives, or for any other reason. Signal to a group member near that person to move in closer and offer some comfort even if it is just a touch on the shoulder. (Leader should check with that person after the group is finished to see if they are okay.)

The leader should also discuss with the whole group how important it is for each of us to feel completely accepted by someone, but how difficult it may be to find someone like that. Finally, participants are asked to think about their clients and how meaningful it can be to them to have a therapist that really accepts them—that it may be the first time they have had such a feeling. This exercise takes about 10 to 15 minutes.

Baby Memories

Form an inner circle with several people standing and facing each other. Have people form an outer circle, so that everyone in the inner circle has someone standing behind them. People in the inner circle should close their eyes. People in the outer circle should now move two places to the right so they are behind a new person. Now people in the outer circle whisper into the ear of the person in front of them something they would have liked to have heard when they were a little baby. Repeat this instruction so everyone understands: "Whisper into the ear of the person in front of you whatever you wished someone had said to you when you were a little baby. You may say the same thing as you move around the circle or something new, it is up to you. When you are finished move to the right one place and whisper something into the ear of the new person in front of you. Keep doing this, moving to your right until you have whispered into everyone's ear and you are back to your original space. Reverse circles so the inner circle now becomes the outer circle." At the end everyone sits down and the leader asks, "In one word, how was that for you?"

Note that this is another powerful exercise. Some people may cry because they are not accustomed to receiving positive messages. The leader should discuss with the group how difficult it can be to receive praise. We as therapists often praise our clients in order to support them, but we must also realize how painful it can be for some people to hear positive messages when they are not used to hearing such support or it does not fit into their negative self-image. This relates to acceptance of ourselves and goes back to early acceptance by our chief caregivers. This activity can generate a lot of good insight within each therapist. The leader should open up the discussion: "Would anyone like to share how they feel?"

Strengths and Stressors and the Love Circle

This activity was obtained from a workshop given by Robert Allen in California.

Stressors and Strengths

Everyone writes down three stressors and three strengths in their lives. Divide the group into smaller groups of four to six people. Everyone finds a partner in their group and takes turns discussing their strengths and stressors with their partner. After about five minutes everyone is directed to find a new partner and to discuss their stressors and strengths with the new partner. If time allows, this is again repeated with another new partner until everyone has had discussions with everyone else.

Love Circle

Now participants go back to their circle formation, and one person volunteers to sit in the middle of the circle. This person faces each person sitting in the circle while they in turn verbalize something positive about the person sitting in the middle. When everyone has had their say (the person in the middle remains silent except maybe saying "thank you"), the next person in the circle exchanges places with the middle person and everyone says something positive about him or her. This keeps on until everyone has had a chance to be in the middle receiving compliments.

The leader opens the discussion and asks, "Would anyone like to share how they felt doing this activity?" The discussion often reveals how good it feels to receive praise, but also how difficult it can be, especially when the positive comments do not fit in with our self-image.

CONCLUSION

It is wise to start with the activities that are simply designed for participants to learn something about themselves in a new way. The activities that touch on deeper, more unconscious feelings are used when participants know each other a little better and feel safer with the leader and with each other. Although some aspects of the latter can bring painful feelings, they are generally not overwhelming. It is the author's belief that a little crying can often be beneficial, as a participant is able, at last, to release feelings that have been pent up for too long. When a participant is showing some distress it is important for the leader and others to show physical support for that person. Often, all it takes is an embracing arm or a light touch to let that person know that there is someone who cares about how they are feeling. These activities often evoke a lot of empathy from others in the group.

Overall, the exercises above have been found to enhance insight, acceptance, and nurturance. They give the feeling of being cared for, strengthened, feeling connected, and feeling good. Because the exercises are playful and generally nonthreatening the participants often let their defenses down and start experiencing thoughts and feelings that they have suppressed or repressed in the past. There is no one to judge them. They reveal only what they want to reveal in the sharing moments. If they want to remain silent, that is completely accepted. The experiences, with or without sharing, can be very moving and powerful to the individual.

REFERENCES

Brody, V. (1997). *The dialogue of touch: Developmental play therapy.* Northvale, NJ: Jason Aronson.

Jernberg, A. (1983). *Theraplay: A new treatment using structured play for problem children and their families.* San Francisco, CA: Jossey-Bass.

Jernberg, A., & Booth, P. (1999). *Theraplay: Helping parents and children build better relationships through attachment-based play.* San Francisco: Jossey-Bass.

Munns, E. (2000). *Theraplay: Innovations in attachment-enhancing play therapy.* Northvale, NJ: Jason Aronson.

17

⌒∞⌒

Playful Supervision

Sharing Exemplary Exercises in the Supervision of Play Therapists

Anne Stewart and Lennis G. Echterling

> You can discover more about a person in an hour of play than in a year of conversation.
>
> —Plato, Greek philosopher, 427–347 BCE

The word "playground" likely evokes in you a wide range of memories and emotions. We invite you to begin this chapter by taking a couple of moments to close your eyes and imagine a playground scene. In your vision, the playground might include swings, slides, a jungle gym, see-saws, a merry-go-round, and perhaps even a complex "kid's castle" with turrets, bridges, crawl spaces, and rope ladders. However primitive or elaborate the setting you choose, now imagine young children and their caregivers there. Where are the children and caregivers situated in the scene? What are the children doing? What are the caregivers doing? How are they communicating with each other? Once you have done this imagining, please continue reading.

Our guess is that you envisioned most of the children as engaging in some sort of play. They were probably laughing, running, climbing, and participating in games. Some of the children may have been cautiously exploring the opportunities for play and assessing the possible dangers, while others were probably thrusting themselves wholeheartedly into the experience. At times, some of the caregivers may have been participating in the activities, but we suspect that you imagined them as typically sitting on a bench or standing off to the side of the action—observing, conversing with other adults, and occasionally offering some words of encouragement, warning, or praise.

If the children were playing happily in your imaginary playground, they may have joyfully cried out to the caregivers, "Look at me! Watch what I can do!" If any children became concerned or distressed, then they probably ran to a caretaker for comfort and reassurance. Once their needs were addressed, the children likely returned to their play.

In contrast to "playground," the word "supervision" probably stirs up very different memories and emotions for you. This time, we invite you to close your eyes and imagine a supervision scene. The scene may be an office in an agency, university training clinic, school, or private practice. Picture the supervisor and at least one supervisee. Are they sitting or standing? How close are they to each other? Envision their postures, gestures, and facial expressions. What are they doing and saying? Once you have taken a couple of minutes to picture the details of your imagined scene, please continue reading.

Our bet is that your imagined supervision scene was in marked contrast to your playground scene. Sadly, you may have found yourself envisioning a staid, uncomfortable, even distressing, scene in which a supervisor may be criticizing, embarrassing, or belittling a supervisee. Instead, we hope that you pictured a supervisor who was supportive, encouraging, and mentoring a supervisee committed to becoming more competent and self-aware as a clinician. Whatever you imagined, the words "creative" and "playful" are probably not the descriptors that you would apply to the typical supervision process. The purpose of this chapter is to invite you to re-visit your ideas about the clinical supervision process by engaging in exercises throughout this chapter that exemplify creative and playful supervision techniques. In spite of the many obvious differences between a playground and supervision, our goal is for you to explore the potential benefits of integrating creative and playful activities into supervision.

SUPERVISION AND PLAY THERAPY

The role of the supervisor is a delightful, stimulating opportunity to work with emerging therapists who see the world with fresh eyes. Many of you have or will walk that road on your professional journey and find that supervision is a wonderful opportunity to return to that sense of discovery and to keep renewing yourself. Supervision is also complex and demanding for several reasons. First, you are responsible for your supervisees' actions in therapy. If a supervisee is performing inappropriately, you may be ethically and legally accountable for that behavior (Falvey, 2002). Second, you are expected to familiarize yourself with the details of every case your trainees are handling. Third, you must provide constructive and comprehensive feedback, fully appreciating the individual needs, idiosyncrasies, and strengths of each supervisee. Fourth, throughout your interactions with supervisees, you must demonstrate a commendable level of professional expertise, therapeutic competence, and commitment to ethics. Finally, you are expected to facilitate the personal growth and professional development of your supervisees (Bernard & Goodyear, 2004). Successful supervision involves administering, evaluating, teaching, assessing, mentoring, and facilitating.

While we have incorporated technology such as video recordings, e-mails, and bug-in-the ear devices in our training and supervisory process, most supervisors of play therapists rely predominately on verbal communication when conceptualizing cases, giving feedback, and discussing treatment plans (Neill, 2005). With trainees of play therapy, the typical emphasis has been on understanding concepts, demonstrating therapeutic skills, and complying with external standards of professional conduct. For example, Ray (2004) has developed a supervision checklist of specific criteria for successfully performing play therapy.

Ironically, supervision, for the most part, has neglected the powerful tools of the play therapy process—creativity and play—in facilitating personal growth and professional development. Recently, Gil and Rubin (2005), along with other play therapists (Stewart et al., 2005, 2006), have promoted the use of play and creative activities to enhance the supervision experience. In this chapter, we offer imaginative exercises in which supervisees can express, discover, integrate, and reflect in modalities other than verbal communication. By inviting exploration, encouraging expression, and engaging in playful encounters, supervisors can help trainees discover and appreciate the power of play and the depth of nonverbal expression. Instead of attending only to external standards of information acquisition, skill levels, and professional conduct, creative and playful techniques of supervision can facilitate the emergence of innate talent that lies latent within trainees. Experiential activities can energize and inspire supervisees to immerse themselves in the art of play therapy. Creative and playful supervision can help supervisees acquire their own therapeutic identity, develop their own internal supervisor, achieve a sense of professional autonomy, and become empowered as therapists.

Of course, supervisors must prepare play therapists by training them to perform appropriately and effectively. However, we have no desire to create our therapists in a cookie-cutter fashion. Creative and playful supervision pulls for more collaboration in the supervisory relationship, encourages supervisees to become curious about their own potentials, illuminates the possibilities for continued professional development, and emphasizes the importance of discovery in the supervision experience. The ideal supervisory relationship is collegial, rather than a rigid hierarchy (Cresci, 1995). Play-based supervision, characterized by collaboration, encouragement, illumination, and discovery, encourages supervisees to develop an *inner* vision—a grounding intuition that helps them stay in contact with their clients and a guiding vision of their own potential as an emerging professional (Presbury, Echterling, & McKee, 1999).

Basic Principles

Before focusing on specific activities, we want to mention some basic principles of successful supervision. First, developing a relationship with a supervisee parallels the process of establishing a counseling relationship (Haynes, Corey, & Moulton, 2003). Therefore, you must always supervise with LUV. The acronym LUV stands for Listen, Understand, and Validate, the foundation of any successful helping relationship, whether it is therapy, supervision, or any other form of intervention (Echterling, Presbury, & McKee, 2005). When you offer LUV, you are actively *listening* to your supervisee's verbal and nonverbal messages, communicating your empathic *understanding* of the play therapy trainee's thoughts and feelings, and *validating* unconditionally the person's innate worth. If a supervisee doesn't feel heard, understood, and accepted, then your creative exercises, however elegant, can appear to be only scheming manipulations or, at best, meaningless gimmicks. As a play therapy supervisor, you are not the expert with all the answers, the sage who dispenses glib advice to neophytes. Instead, by offering your supportive presence, you offer a safe space, a psychological refuge during this challenging stage of your supervisee's professional development. Fundamentally, your relationship, embodied in your LUVing encounter with a trainee, is the most powerful clinical supervision tool of all.

Another basic principle is to recognize and truly value the power of creative play to enrich lives, promote relationships, foster growth, and facilitate development across the entire life-span. In play-based activities, your supervisees experience a sense of empowerment, recognize their untapped capabilities, and connect to sources of sustenance and nurturance; they build the scaffolding for a successful career in play therapy. However, we urge you to embrace, honor, and celebrate play not only with your therapy clients and supervisees, but also with colleagues, collaborators, consultees, students, family, and the entire community. Research offers powerful and convincing evidence that play has a pervasive and positive impact on neurological functioning (Schore, 2000; Play science—The patterns of play, n.d.).

A third essential principle is to focus on the strengths of your supervisees by highlighting their successful interventions and presuming their potential as therapists. Of course, new therapists often feel overwhelmed and inadequate. However, they also possess undiscovered strengths, overlooked talents, and unnoticed resources. As a supervisor, your task is to facilitate the emergence of their innate gifts that lie latent within them. By adopting this approach, you help supervisees acquire their own therapeutic identities, develop their internal supervisors, and learn to trust in their resources in the moment.

Supervision and Symbols—An Object Lesson

Reflect for a few moments about your experiences in supervision, both as a supervisor and as a supervisee. Identify characteristics of the supervision process that you value and choose one that you believe is particularly significant. Next, select an object that represents that quality. Now, generate questions and comments about supervision and the supervisory relationship by noting other characteristics of the object. If you initially selected the figure of an owl because it represents the value of wisdom in supervision, you may now wonder about other characteristics of an owl and how they might influence supervision. For example, you might note the vigilance of the owl and how or if that quality is desirable in supervision.

Similarly, in individual or group supervision, you can ask supervisees to select an object and describe the way in which it illustrates the quality that they value. Additional characteristics of the object are noted, and questions and comments about other attributes of the supervision process can be explored. The objects may be selected from a collection of miniatures or just from what the person has with them at the moment. Objects may be drawn, painted, sculpted, or can be provided by the supervisor or supervisees. Of course, if the supervisor is supplying the objects, is important to have artifacts representing a wide variety of cultures.

In figure 17.1, the first photograph shows three items: a gift, a running shoe, and a heart. The gift and running shoe were sculpted by chapter author Anne Stewart when conducting the object lesson in supervision sessions. The heart was on a shelf in the supervisor's office and was used by supervisees to represent aspects they valued in supervision. The second

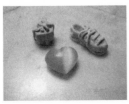 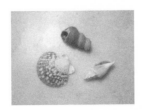 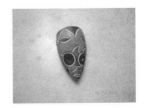

Figure 17.1. Object Lessons. Examples of Items Used in the Exercise.

photograph shows the use of a class of objects, in this case shells, which can be used to identify characteristics and also convey the community created by the supervision group. Other groups of items that are the same but different, such as rocks, leaves, cups, chairs, or keys, can be very useful for this activity. The last photograph shows an African artifact, highlighting the importance of having diverse cultural relics represented for supervisees.

The use of symbolic material to convey emotional experiences is a hallmark of play therapy. In the object lesson exercise, the use of an object permits you and your supervisees to engage in a similar creative process. The use of symbols may help you notice varied, even competing, interpretations about supervision experiences and perhaps realize some similarities across the negative and positive experiences. In all the exercises in this chapter, we encourage you, as the supervisor, to participate and share while making sure to maintain the focus on the supervisee's experience. You can modify these exercises for individual or group supervision.

Qualities of Successful Caregiving and Effective Supervision

We decided to use a familiar relationship to continue our exploration of playful supervision, a relationship that is well known and well researched by mental health professionals, namely, the caregiver-child relationship. Attachment theory and research offers compelling and rich explanations about the importance of this relationship, which enhances security and exploration in childhood and throughout life (Ainsworth, et al., 1978; Main, Kaplan, & Cassidy, 1985). An attachment theory and research-driven intervention called the Circle of Security educates caregivers to be appropriately responsive to their child's cues for safety and exploration; to increase their ability to reflect on their own and their child's thoughts, feelings, and behaviors; and to consider how their experiences affect their current caregiving (Marvin, Cooper, Hoffman, & Powell, 2002). These same patterns of interaction and reflection are useful to adapt to the supervisor-supervisee relationship. In the language of attachment and the Circle of Security, the supervisor should be bigger, stronger, wiser, and kind; whenever possible, follow the supervisee's need; whenever necessary, take charge.

Complementing an attachment perspective are other dimensions of the supervisory relationship that parallel the fundamental characteristics of successful caregiver-child relationships. These include using a developmental perspective, conveying positive and clear expectations for performance and behavior, providing frequent and constructive feedback, recognizing the power differential and, most importantly, acknowledging the reciprocal and dynamic *relationship* as the focus.

Developmental Perspective

Just as parents change how they interact and instruct their children at different ages, so play therapist supervisors adjust their ways of interacting as supervisees develop. Parents walking in the park with their 15-month-old are hurrying close behind, ready to catch the toddler. As the child gets older, parents may walk alongside, holding hands with their child, with the child intermittently racing off and returning. When the child is a teenager, parent and child are not likely to be walking together at all, but the parent is still watchful and very much needed.

Models of supervision consistently recognize the importance of the supervisor using a developmental perspective (Bernard & Goodyear, 2004). The supervisor is expected to assess the supervisee's level of knowledge and skills and provide information and challenges that are consistent with the supervisee's developmental capabilities, recognizing that supervisees require different supervisory environments across time. Supervision theorists have advocated various stages to describe the process of growth and the specific tasks and needs associated with the stages. The play-based exercises we present can be used across developmental levels from the novice to the master-level therapist. This is so because a therapist's awareness of self and others is a constant process of discovery and growth.

Positive and Clear Expectations

Caregivers instruct children in ethical issues and help socialize them. Play therapist supervisors not only aid their supervisees in skill development but are preparing them to be members of a professional community with its own standards of ethical conduct and practice. Strength-based supervisors, like affirmative caregivers, communicate positive and clear expectations for their supervisee's performance. This does not mean micro-managing the supervisee's behavior. Rather, the supervisor and supervisee jointly determine goals for the supervision process. The supervisor shares didactic and case information in a way that builds on what the supervisee is doing well and recognizes the knowledge they bring to the discussion. The supervisor is also prepared to modify supervision as the supervisee gains experience (Stolenberg, McNeill, & Crethar, 1994). The supervisor organizes the information to support the supervisee's attainment of interpersonal assessment techniques and intervention skills, as well as knowledge of conceptualization schemes, ethical considerations, and treatment goals.

Frequent, Timely, and Constructive Feedback

Caregivers spend a great deal of time offering feedback to their children. A primary activity of the supervisory relationship is the provision of frequent, timely, and constructive feedback. Supervisees often anticipate receiving feedback with a great deal of anxiety. The supervisor can help assuage this anxiety by establishing an atmosphere that values "learning in public" and by planning with the supervisee how, when, and what type of feedback will be provided. A supervision contract that specifies supervision goals as well as the mechanisms for feedback is very useful.

Power Differential

Healthy caregiver-child relationships have an appropriate power differential that corresponds to their roles and age-appropriate abilities in the family constellation. Unlike caregiver-child relationships, supervision relationships are adult-to-adult interactions, but the adults differ in terms of their status and knowledge, denoting power differences with which the participants must contend. Todd and Storm (1997) offer a thought-provoking discussion on the types of power relevant to supervision, such as position power and knowledge power, and question whether there is not an inbuilt contradiction in the idea of collaborative supervision. They challenge the supervisor to ask critical questions about power to ensure it is not used in an exploitive manner. They encourage supervisors to question whose knowledge is being privileged and how and where the knowledge power was generated. Being transparent about the impact of power can help you and the supervisee navigate your relationship with openness and be better equipped to explore the influence of gender, age, ethnicity, ability, sexual orientation, and culture in both the supervision and therapy relationships.

Of course, there are limits and cautions to consider in using a parent-child metaphor to describe aspects of the supervisory relationship. Parents are focused on the personal growth of their child, and supervisors attend to their supervisee's personal growth in the service of professional development, namely, creating a more skilled play therapist.

EXEMPLARY EXERCISES

Supervisors of play therapists come from a variety of mental health disciplines, each with an array of well-developed models to guide the supervision process. These are important discipline-specific models to employ in your role as a gatekeeper for the profession. In addition, we are offering a model from our shared field to categorize innovative exercises for supervision of play therapists. We selected Theraplay, a directive play therapy approach that uses the dimensions of structure, challenge, engagement, and nurturance to conduct the intervention (Jernberg & Booth, 1999). We selected Theraplay because its sessions include both the child and the caregiver (paralleling the supervisee and supervisor), are personal, fun, and focus on the relationship. We believe the four Theraplay dimensions—structure, challenge, engagement, and nurturance—can serve as a useful framework for organizing supervision activities.

Structure

Play gives children a chance to practice what they are learning.

—Fred Rogers, American television personality, 1928–2003

Structure refers to the caregiver's role of being "in charge" of critical aspects of the relationship and activities with the child. In Theraplay, the caregiver is expected to establish boundaries for the child's physical and psychological safety and to help the child understand the world. The caregiver is aware of the developmental status of the child and the corresponding developmental tasks and needs. The caregiver organizes the child's surroundings and experiences in ways that maximize learning and growth.

Applied to the supervision process, you are also "in charge" of establishing appropriate boundaries and creating opportunities for a psychologically safe relationship. Like the caregiver, you are expected to be consistent and responsive to your supervisee's needs, in the context of the trainee's professional development. In a manner congruent with your own theoretical orientation, you actively help define and clarify the supervisee's clinical experience. The following activities can assist you in exploring elements of structure in the supervisory relationship. The first exercise is a variation of an object lesson activity that provides a structured way to identify positive and negative attributions about the supervision process by drawing together.

Drawing Together

Invite students to think about all their supervision experiences. They may include times when they were the supervisor or the supervisee, as well as supervision in clinical or nonclinical roles. Ask them to identify one of their worst and one of their best supervision experiences. Instruct them to fold a sheet of paper in half. On one half they are to draw symbols that characterize their most negative supervision experience, create a title for the drawing, and date it. They are to repeat the process for their most positive supervision experience. Then, each person relates the meaning of the symbols in their drawings and tells how they believe the experiences are relevant for them in their current set of roles, demands, and relationships. This exercise is particularly useful in determining important interpersonal themes relevant to supervision, such as respect, autonomy, and dependence.

Rituals and Routines

Quality supervisory relationships, whether they are dyads or small groups, are learning communities. As with other communities, you can use routines and rituals to connect supervisees, affirm a collective identity, and celebrate the journey on which you have all embarked. As the supervisor, you can explore instructional approaches with supervisees that offer structure, meaning, and connectivity to their experience. Collaborating with your supervisees to create a supervision session agenda can help them know you intend to address their concerns and needs. The agenda should be followed consistently, but not rigidly. The consistent use of an agenda is intended to permit supervisees sufficient predictability to reduce their anxiety, and allow them to take risks and explore. Over time many groups begin to modify the agenda and make it uniquely their own. A sample session agenda, using the "What? So what? Now what?" framework, is shown below.

- Greeting ritual
- *What?* Report a lesson learned or treatment success story.
- *So what?* Share video clip(s), present specific request for feedback, discuss video clip(s), and share feedback.
- *Now what?* What do you need from the group to be ready for the week?
- Ending ritual

One supervision group identified an interest in solution-focused child interventions. After learning the scaling technique of asking a client to rate an experience from 1 (most negative) to 10 (most positive), the group modified the greeting in the supervision session to include a 1 (doing poorly) to 10 (doing great) scaling of how they were feeling as they entered the supervision session. Each supervisee held up fingers to communicate their self-rating and gave a brief explanation. They repeated the finger rating at the ending of the session and even used it in the hallway with one another. Another group reported their "lesson learned" content and then decided to share a new counseling technique that was related to the lesson. This expanded their technique repertoire greatly and was particularly meaningful because the techniques were linked to a relevant clinical context. You can help your supervision sessions to be predictable, as well as creative and fun, by designing routines or rituals that emerge from and reflect the strengths and talents of the supervisees. As in families, the use of rituals and routines offers supervisees a sense of connectedness and normalcy.

Haiku and Cinquains

Supervisees sometimes feel overwhelmed as they struggle to organize and make meaning out of their counseling and supervision experiences. Haiku and cinquains are particularly helpful as they provide a proscribed and compact format for supervisees to sort out their experiences. These poetic forms also help the supervisees use symbolism to relate and integrate their cognitive and affective understanding.

Haiku is a type of poetry from the Japanese culture that typically uses simple words to make observations about everyday things. The most common form is three lines, with five syllables in the first line, seven syllables in the second line, and five syllables in the third line. Haiku do not rhyme and are intended to paint a mental picture for the reader. A sample haiku, authored by Sharon Stewart, follows:

> Picking a symbol
> Holding it in heart and mind
> Unfolding its meaning

A cinquain is a five-line poem that also has a proscribed format that can assist the supervisee to order and express their experiences. It is created with the following design:

Line 1	One word	Subject or noun
Line 2	Two words	Adjectives that describe the subject or noun
Line 3	Three words	Verbs that relate to the subject or noun
Line 4	Four words	Feelings or a complete sentence that relate to the subject or noun
Line 5	One word	Synonym of the subject or noun

The following was playfully composed as an example by the chapter authors in a spontaneous duet:

> Play
> Exuberant, expansive
> Freeing, joining, transforming
> Olly outs in free!
> Homebase

Quotes

Quotes offer concise, and often pointed, observations about life and change—and therefore, can be very helpful starting places for supervisees to begin to reflect on their own beliefs and values. Ask your supervisees to find a quote to share that reflects their opinion or a question they have about a topic relevant to the therapeutic process. Topics such as children, play, families, parenting, change, uncertainty, and health are particularly helpful to explore. You can also provide quotes from different cultures and time periods or quotes that reflect extreme positions, permitting supervisees a way to identify and confront unexamined and uncomfortable assumptions that influence their viewpoint. The discussion board had the following directions.

Change   Read the list of quotes below about change. What quotations most closely fit your own notions about change? What is appealing to you about this way of conceptualizing change? In what ways has your family/ your supervision influenced your view of change? Think about a particular child client. What do you think he or she believes about change? In what ways are you interested in changing your ideas about change as you imagine yourself as a play therapist?

QUOTES TO CONSIDER

"They always say time changes things, but you actually have to change them yourself."—Andy Warhol

"Change, when it comes, cracks everything open."—Dorothy Allison

"Things do not change; we change."—Henry David Thoreau

"Nothing endures but change."—Heraclitus

"There is nothing like returning to a place that remains unchanged to find the ways in which you yourself have altered."—Nelson Mandela

The activity is well suited for electronic postings and threaded discussions. For example, we created a discussion board for supervisees to view a number of quotes about a series of play therapy–related topics and instructed them to select a quote, post their responses, and react and comment to other supervisees' observations. A variation of the activity can be done together in a supervision session and is called Inkshedding.

Inkshedding

Inkshedding provides supervisees an opportunity to organize their thoughts and emotional reactions to clinical events (in supervision or play therapy) or to complex constructs and principles. You could also do an Inkshedding activity after viewing a video segment. Following the stimulus, you invite supervisees to take one or two minutes to reflect on the material—it might be a quote, a clinical encounter, a supervision discussion, or a video. Next, ask them to write a five- to eight-sentence reaction that could include comments and questions. As each supervisee completes his or her reaction you pick it up and give it to another supervisee. The recipient reads the original comment and adds a reaction. Continue this circulation until every person's first response has been reacted to at least two times and then return the page to the original person.

According to developmental models, novice supervisees value directive, didactic, skills-based supervision with a high degree of structure (Falender and Shafranske, 2004). In addition to wanting and needing skills for their toolbox, beginning clinicians are likely to manage anxiety about performing well by looking to supervisors to "take charge." Therefore, playfully attending to this developmental need within the supervision session and supervisory relationship can reduce anxiety and help build a strong working alliance. Structured activities remind supervisors, particularly when supervising beginning clinicians, to offer suggestions regarding clinical techniques and client conceptualizations, not in an authoritative manner, but in a didactic, consultative style.

Challenge

> In play a child always behaves beyond his average age, above his daily behavior. In play it is as though he were a head taller than himself.

> —Lev Vygotsky, Russian psychologist, 1896–1934

Caregivers and supervisors encourage the growth and development of their respective charges. Caregivers notice naturally occurring ordeals and sometimes introduce taxing but developmentally appropriate tasks that require the child to stretch—to develop a new skill, to use an acquired skill in an unfamiliar context, to learn new information, or to combine information in a novel way. Likewise, the supervisor notices conditions that arouse tension and uncertainty for the supervisee. The supervisor may also create circumstances that produce anxiety, while simultaneously providing constructive feedback and emotional support for the supervisee. The intent of challenging tasks is to help children or supervisees successfully navigate the difficulty in the midst of a caring relationship, and in so doing, build or restore their confidence.

It's in the Bag

J. Edson McKee, one of our colleagues, created this activity that offers a fine metaphor for therapy and supervision. The exercise requires an ambiguous three-dimensional figure about the size of a breadbox and hidden in a bag. To create the object, gather together wood scraps of various shapes, round pegs of varying lengths and widths, dowels, pieces of plastic, segments of foam rubber, and other small objects of undefined shape. Next, assemble these objects willy-nilly fashion, using duct tape, glue, or string. The resulting object should be an abstract figure that defies easy description and geometric classification. Finally, hide the object in a bag with a drawstring.

When you bring the bag, with the contents hidden inside, to your supervision session, ask for a volunteer whose task it is to describe the object to the others. That person cannot peek into the bag, but can reach inside to feel the item while offering instructions on how to draw it. The other supervisees must draw a picture of what is in the bag, based on the description that the volunteer gives. The drawers may ask questions of the volunteer, but they cannot show their renditions to anyone else.

Once the others have completed their drawings, the describer also sketches a depiction of the object. Then, all the supervisees can compare their illustrations with the others. Invite the participants to reflect on the experience of performing this task. What were the more successful questions? What descriptions were particularly helpful for picturing what's in the bag? How is this activity like therapy? How is it like our supervision?

When you conclude the discussion, close the drawstring and put away the bag. Your behavior will dismay the participants. Someone always asks, "Aren't you going to let us see what's in the bag?" And, of course, the best part of the activity is coping with the realization that they don't get to see what's in the bag, because no one ever does.

Original Work

In the Original Work activity the supervisees are asked to use sculpting material to make a symbol of a characteristic they value, and that they believe they bring to the supervision relationship. Without comment, they are to hand their completed creation to the person on their left. Each recipient is to look over the symbol and wonder what characteristic the creator had in mind. Without changing the original, they are to use the materials to add something and pass it on to the next person. The object can be passed one to three times and then is returned to the person who first made it. It is suggested that you take about two minutes with each creation before passing it on.

It is critical that people do not talk during this time and that additions are completed without altering the original form. When the object is returned, each person reveals the characteristic that is symbolized and shares reactions to the process. You may pose the following questions:

- What do you enjoy about the additions from others? Which additions are more appealing? Which are less appealing to you?
- What was easy or challenging about adding to the work of others?

- What meaning do the changes have for you?
- What reaction is your original work having to the additions?
- What situations in supervision can you recall or imagine in which it will be great to have these additions?

Original Work is a provocative exercise to explore how a supervision community accepts and integrates feedback.

Mask

A common game that supervisors and supervisees play is, "What you don't know won't hurt me" (Kadushin, 1968). In this game, or way of relating, both persons are interested in presenting only a favorable picture. The result can be a superficial, overly social relationship. The Mask activity provides an opportunity to identify and share the ways we prefer to be known, as well as the personal strengths, insecurities, and questions we hold private. Supervisors and supervisees cut out a mask and glue it to a tongue depressor. Using pictures and words from magazines and art materials, such as markers, pipe cleaners, feathers, glitter, buttons, and sequins, you decorate both sides of the mask. On the side of the mask that others view, you create a picture of how you present and on the side you see when holding up the mask, you create a picture of the professional self that you see. Invite the group to put up their masks and look at each other, first with the side showing how you prefer to present and then with the "masked" side showing. Discuss your reactions to showing and viewing each side, and explore how the presentation impacts supervision and counseling relationships. You may want to display the masks and refer to them in the course of the supervision process, noting the accomplishments and growth of the supervisee, particularly in areas that they believed were not well developed or perceived as weaknesses.

Getting to Know You

The Getting to Know You activity can be done at any time in the supervision relationship. You can begin by describing how we all tend to introduce ourselves in rather scripted ways, usually stating our name, occupation, and professional affiliation. While our introductions change somewhat across differing contexts, they offer narrow ways of engaging in dialogue. In contrast, Getting to Know You provides a novel way to share who you are and to get to know others. The exercise can help us remember that we all hold many roles and have many stories, in addition to the one we are presenting to each other at the moment. The activity can be done in pairs or with each person presenting to all. Supervisees are asked to complete the following sentence stems symbolically or literally.

My river is . . .
My mountain is . . .
My family legacy is . . .
A characteristic of the supervision relationship I value is . . .
My name is . . .

The group is encouraged to comment on similarities and differences after the introductions are offered. This can be a beneficial activity to use when supervisees are having difficulty recognizing strengths and seeing the complexity and healthy striving in their own or other supervisees' struggles. The issue of having an overly narrow and problem-focused perspective may parallel supervisees' conceptualization of their client. Getting to Know You can assist supervisees in constructing a more complex picture of their client's world.

Cultural Collage

A critical component of supervision and therapeutic interventions is the ability to be culturally sensitive and responsive. This activity provides an opportunity for supervisees to identify important influences and traditions in their own development and in their client's life. The supervisee constructs a personal cultural collage using images and words from magazines. It is useful to have a dialogue with your supervisees about culture: What do they believe culture is, what is their culture heritage and identity, and how do they see culture manifested in their family celebrations and traditions, food, music, or religious practices? Engage in a discussion about the images and words and about the emotions that accompanied the construction of the collage. You might ask supervisees to tell what images or words they are most surprised they placed in their collage, who they believe would enjoy seeing and hearing about the collage, what images and words are most significant for you to understand as their supervisor, what else is important to know about themselves and their culture that I might not know by viewing their collage, and what are they most proud of in their cultural collage.

Supervisors can use these challenge activities to encourage risk-taking and increase motivation in the developmental process. Stoltenberg, McNeill, and Delworth (1998) describe a model for professional growth that addresses supervisee motivation across all levels of development. They articulate the supervisee's journey from a state of high motivation and anxiety, to a period of extreme fluctuations in motivation and confidence, to occasional doubts about effectiveness that do not immobilize. The challenge activities provide supervisors and supervisees opportunities to identify and confront areas for growth and to construct confidence.

Engagement

> Play is our brain's favorite way of learning.

> —Diane Ackerman, contemporary American author, 1948–

Theraplay interventions are designed to actively draw the child into playful interactions. The exchanges help the child learn to communicate, to be close, and to enjoy interpersonal contact. The role of the caregiver is to enthusiastically invite the child into the interaction and maintain his or her interest and arousal. Supervisory interventions that are focused on engagement provide opportunities for supervisees to explore personal information in novel ways and practice communicating. Emphasizing engagement in activities provides a venue for the supervisor to convey his or her commitment to and belief in a supervisee's abilities by designing opportunities to draw the supervisee into playful exercises. As you can see, the dimensions of structure, challenge, engagement, and nurturance are intertwined, and all are important ingredients in building a secure and supportive supervisory relationship.

Supervisionland

In this activity you and your supervisees select or draw pictures of animals to create a supervision "scene," named Supervisionland. Ask supervisees to reflect on their supervision experiences, look over a collection of animal pictures, and choose ones that display qualities believed to be crucial for high-quality supervisory experiences. (You can use clip art, greeting cards, or draw the animals for the scene. Certainly encourage supervisees to add any to an existing collection.) Figure 17.2 shows some animal drawings and a scene backdrop used in our Supervisionland activity.

All participants are invited to create the scene by placing their animals in Supervisionland. The Supervisionland scene can just be an area on the floor or desktop, a piece of poster board, a picture or photo of a jungle, forest, or seascape—or some combination of all these environments—drawn by the supervisees. Supervisees share their ideas about important qualities for supervision through the pictures they selected. The supervisor encourages supervisees to explore their fears, anxieties, and hopes for growth by noting the animal characteristics. Supervisees are also encouraged to view the selections in the context of all the animals in Supervisionland. For example,

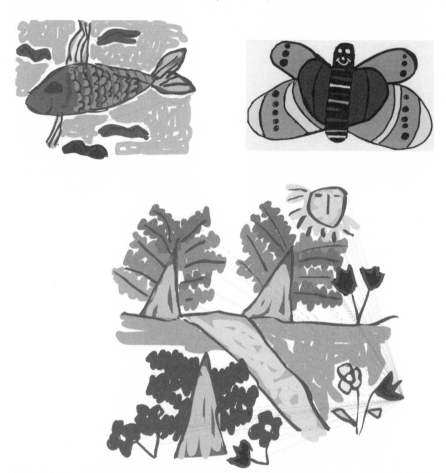

Figure 17.2. Supervisionland. Examples of Items Used in the Exercise. Select or Draw Pictures of Animals to Create a Supervision "Scene."

one supervisee picked an image of a bird, stating his fear of "being left out on a limb." The supervisor acknowledged that concern and, interestingly, described how he had selected the same picture to convey his hope of providing a safe place, a nest from which the supervisee could venture out. Figure 17.3 shows the bird drawing selected by both the supervisor and supervisee.

This activity is helpful to use early in supervision to assess supervisees' expectations and concerns. At the end of the supervision period supervisees are asked to contribute an image to add to the Supervisionland collection, thus leaving their own legacy in the supervision scene.

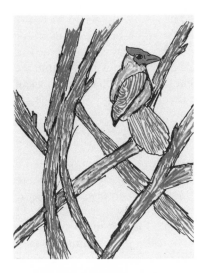

Figure 17.3. Supervisionland. Bird Drawing Selected by Supervisee and Supervisor.

Play Therapy Charades

Play therapy (PT) charades use the traditional game of charades, in which a person acts out a clue for a word or phrase, but uses the field of play therapy for generating the items. The supervision group is divided into two teams, and a time/scorekeeper is designated. The whole group must review and agree upon hand signals and gestures to be used in the game—this may actually be an interesting phase to process, as many family-of-origin rules often appear and can be sources of controversy! For example, how do you show plural, letter of the alphabet, or past tense? Decide on the number of rounds to play, and give out ten to twenty slips of paper. Independently, the teams generate and write down words and phrases on the pieces of paper. The phrases may be quotes ("Birds fly, fish swim, and children play."—G. Landreth), titles of play therapy books, leaders in the field, names of theories or concepts, techniques, or toys. To help make sure the items are solvable you may want to suggest that the teams only include items that almost all the people on your team are familiar with and that phrases be no longer than six to eight words. After that, your collective imagination is the only limit!

A player from Team One draws a slip from Team Two and reviews it for a short time (again, supervisees may have strong opinions about how this is done). The timekeeper tells the player to start. Team One then has three minutes to guess the correct answer. If they figure it out, the timekeeper records how long it took. If they do not figure it out in three minutes, the timekeeper announces that the time is up and records a time of three minutes. Team Two then takes their turn, and play proceeds the same way. PT charades usually continue until every player has had a chance to "act out" a phrase. The score for each team is the total time that the team needed for all of the rounds and the team with the lowest score wins the game. You may want to modify this to a cooperative game format by having the group, whether in teams or not, strive to beat their previous record or just eliminate the time and score keeping from the game.

Tag Team Role Playing

Supervisees are invited to identify an instance in a play therapy session where they felt stuck or ineffective. You and/or other members of the supervision group are assigned roles to play out. The supervisee with the question may rotate between playing the role of the play therapist, child or parent, observer, or supervisor. In Tag Team Role Playing the persons acting out the role play may ask for assistance by calling for a time out (signaling like a coach). At a time out, the person may just ask for an immediate suggestion about what to do next or may ask to sit out and have another group member step in, i.e., tag team for them as the role play continues. The tag team members do not critique or question but just step in assuming the role at that moment. The game can also be played to permit observers to call a "time in" in order to join in the role play. (When we play this version, the person being asked to leave the role play has the right to decline to step out.) Supervisees may also find it very helpful to role-play the situations they believe they successfully navigated in order to consolidate their gains. In another variation, supervisees may role-play the situations they are most afraid will occur. For some supervisees this will be the "aggressive" child, for others, the "withdrawn" child, and for others, the "clingy" child. Role playing permits the supervisee to practice play therapy skills in a safe and caring relationship—an excellent condition for learning.

Puppets

Puppets are used in play therapy supervision to help supervisees develop playfulness, creativity, and spontaneity. Puppets can be used at any time to interact with supervisees to add excitement and surprise to the dialogue. Supervisees may use the puppets to role-play themselves and their client in scenes from the play therapy room or from the child's school or home life. Supervisees can further explore their beliefs about the child's family by naming other supervisees to role-play family members. Supervisees, acting in the family roles, select puppets and create a story with a beginning, middle, and end. The actors are to decide on a title and a moral for the story. Supervisees are told that the story must be original and should be rehearsed. The supervisor and supervisees not in the play act as the audience. After the story is performed, you and other audience members, also using puppets, interact with the puppets in the play in character. Staying within the metaphor of the play, you question the characters and provide opportunities for them to talk with each other. For example, "How does the bunny feel about being left in the cave?" "What character seems to have the most power?" "Which other character wants power, too?" "Tell me what will happen next."

Sand Tray Supervision

In this activity you invite the supervisee to construct a sand tray of the child and family. Tell the supervisee to pick a miniature that best reflects their thoughts and feelings about the child and other family members, and arrange them in the sand tray. Ask them to give a title to the tray. Next you ask the supervisee to pick a miniature that best shows their thoughts and feelings about themselves in relationship to the child and family, and again title the scene. After each construction it is helpful to begin with a simple comment, such as, "Tell me about this child and family" or "Now tell me about how you see you, in relation to the child and family." You may also inquire about how the supervisee came to compose the titles for the sand tray and, lastly, invite the supervisee to select a miniature to represent you and place it in the tray and generate a title. Posing circular questions that presume that "everything is somehow connected to everything else" (Tomm, 1988, p. 6) can help different perspectives and connections open up. You might pose questions like, "Who in this scene is most worried?" "What does that person do when he is worried, or not worried?" "Who will be likely to notice that worry and find a way to help?" or "Who, do you guess, actually wants to have the most hope for the child, but is afraid to show it?"

Staying in the metaphor of the sand tray to ask questions and pose comments can yield intriguing and illuminating observations about the beliefs the supervisee holds about the child and family. (It is preferable to have a sand tray and a collection of miniatures to do this supervision activity, although you can replace or augment miniatures with magazine or greeting card images, found objects, personal sculptures, or drawings.) Variations of this activity abound. Of course, the directions can be modified to fit the developmental level of the supervisee and the issue they would like to explore. They can also be changed to select miniatures to represent the relationship between people in the family, or to depict the child and family at particular time periods or during specific events, or in the future, when the current issues have been resolved. Consider adapting other techniques from family therapy, such as family sculpting, for engaging supervision.

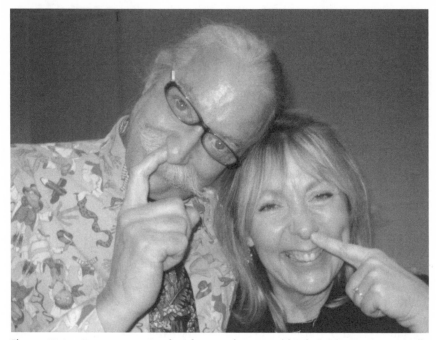

Figure 17.4.   Engagement. Patch Adams and Anne with Their Fingers Strategically Placed.

Engagement offers the supervisor a chance to get to know and to delight in the supervisee. The work we do is gratifying and demanding, and it can take its toll on our emotional resources. Engagement activities can replenish the supervisee and supervisor and give you permission to be silly and serious, skilled and not knowing, apart and connected, all at the same time. Above is a photograph of chapter author Anne Stewart with Patch Adams in a pose that communicates how simple it can be to engage with each other. Just because we do serious work does not mean we have to take ourselves seriously.

Nurturance

Play fosters belonging and encourages cooperation.

—Stuart Brown, MD, contemporary
American psychiatrist

Caregivers provide comfort for their children. They help soothe and calm their children's worries and are emotionally available, attuned, and responsive to the child's needs. A child that learns a caring adult will be available to respond to their needs will develop the ability to self-soothe and become increasingly self-sufficient. While reaching out with nurturing activities may not be a supervisor's immediate inclination, this type of activity can be very helpful in building a connection with supervisees who are reacting to supervision with hostility or off-putting behaviors, as well as supervisees who present as pseudo mature. The supervisor must consistently respond to the supervisee's insecurities, doubts, and fears, and not be deterred by possible miscommunications about their needs. Over time this support, in the form of nurturance and confrontation, will help the supervisee to quiet uncertainties and increase their self-awareness and autonomy.

Helping Hands

You can easily adapt this intervention for use with individuals or groups. Briefly talk about how all of us need and offer helping hands to one another. Give each person a pencil and paper, and invite the supervisees to draw the outline of one of their hands. On each finger, they then can make a drawing or write the name of who or what has helped them in their professional growth thus far. They can also make another Helping Hand to describe five ways that they have been a resource to others. You do not need paper and markers to do this activity. Supervisees can just show their hands and describe the help they have received and given.

Helping Hands invites supervisees to explore how they have been making a positive difference for others, as they grow and change themselves. It encourages them to bring into their consciousness that they are playing an active role in contributing to the development of others.

Circles of Support

This exercise is quite powerful. It is best done with a group of six or more. First, divide the group evenly and instruct half them to form an inner circle facing each other and to close their eyes. Direct the remaining supervisees to form an outer circle, positioning themselves right behind someone in the inner circle. Tell those in the outer circle to think back to when they were an infant and identify a positive phrase they wished would have been said to them when they were babies.

Next, the people in the outer circle lean forward and whisper that phrase in the ear of the supervisees in front of them. The inner circle stays in place, while the people on the outer circle step to their right behind the next person in the inner circle and whisper the message again. This continues until the outer circle participants have moved back to their original spots.

The outer and inner circles reverse places and the new inner circle members close their eyes while the outer circle members start whispering positive messages to those in front of them. The circle exercise is repeated so everyone has an opportunity to hear positive messages and to deliver them to others.

Hold a discussion following this activity for participants to talk about their early recollections, how they felt about themselves in the past and present, and how these messages are relevant to the current supervision process. This exercise was introduced to us by our friend and colleague Evangeline Munns, author of *Theraplay: Innovations in Attachment-enhancing Play Therapy*.

Pocket Pal

In this activity supervisees make their own transitional object. Participants are instructed to think of a person who has been a source of support for them, at any time in their lives. They then think of a message, stated or unstated, that the person has conveyed, such as, "You are a treasure," "Your smile brightens the world," or "You can do anything!" Supervisees then write the message on a Popsicle stick or meditate and imagine the message onto the wood. Supervisees decorate the stick to create a "pocket pal." The supervisees may or may not share the actual message, but the supervisor further explores by asking them to imagine when they might benefit from hearing the message, where they could strategically place their pocket pal to be reminded of the message, and what helps them believe the message. This activity can also be done as a message on a stone.

That's What I Like about Me!

That's What I Like about Me! gives supervisees practice in generating positive self-statements and building self-esteem. Participants pair off and take turns asking and responding to the question, "What do you like about yourself?" In this structured activity, the conversation is limited to identifying and witnessing self-affirmations. For a period of two minutes, one person asks the question, "What do you like about yourself?" The responder names a characteristic or quality she enjoys. The person asking the question responds with, "What else do you like about yourself?" No other inquiry is permitted during the two minutes. It is surprisingly difficult for people to name many things they value about themselves. It also can be particularly difficult for the person asking the question to refrain from engaging in a conversation or offering praise such as "Yes, I like that about you, too." Following the two minutes each of questions and answers about what the supervisees like about themselves, the pairs and group have a conversation about the content they identified and about how comfortable or uncomfortable it felt in each role. The group examines how the reactions they experienced are relevant to the supervision process.

It is important for all therapists to continue to examine their own personal issues and find ways to be nurtured by others and ourselves as we are trying to help others. These playful exercises afford us, as supervisees and supervisors, imaginative ways of looking at ourselves that can bring us personal discoveries and also connect us to others and build our learning, and playing, communities.

CONCLUSION

As you come to the close of this chapter, and this book, we invite you to recall one of those moments in your life when you have been completely caught up in the creative process or wholeheartedly engaged in play. At that instant, you were engrossed in the experience, absorbed in the here-and-now, and entirely immersed in the flow. You are never alone when you are fully present because it is precisely at those moments that your nurturing caregivers—their voices, values, strengths, and ways of being—emerge. All creativity and play, even in solitude, is communal.

Now, remember one of those times when you felt that you were at the peak of your therapeutic powers. At that moment, you were empathically resonating with your client, dancing gracefully the transcending dance of change, and embodying the collective wisdom of your internalized supervisors. Sensing their presence, standing on the foundation they offered, and harkening back to the chorus of their voices, you are never performing solo when you are truly therapeutic.

As a supervisor, you are called to be a dedicated mentor, skilled instructor, and talented model. Adding the role of creative playmate brings richness, depth, and discovery to your supervision. Through play, your supervisees learn by heart how to be truly therapeutic and, although they develop their own inner vision under your supervision, they will never play alone as therapists.

REFERENCES

Ainsworth, M. D. S., Blehar, M. C., Waters, E., & Wall, S. (1978). *Patterns of attachment: Psychological study of the strange situation.* Hillsdale, NJ: Erlbaum.

Bernard, J. M., & Goodyear, R. K. (2004). *Fundamentals of clinical supervision* (3rd ed.). Boston: Allyn & Bacon.

Cresci, M. M. (1995). How does supervision work? Facilitating the supervisee's learning. *Psychoanalysis and Psychotherapy*, *13*, 50–58.

Echterling, L. G., Presbury, J., & McKee, J. E. (2005). *Crisis intervention: Promoting resilience and resolution in troubled times.* Upper Saddle River, NJ: Merrill/Prentice Hall.

Falender, C., & Shafranske, E. (2004). *Clinical supervision: A competency-based approach.* Washington, DC: American Psychological Association.

Falvey, J. E. (2002). *Managing clinical supervision: Ethical practice and legal risk management.* Pacific Grove, CA: Brooks/Cole.

Gil, E., & Rubin, L. (2005). Countertransference play: Informing and enhancing therapist self-awareness through play. *International Journal of Play Therapy*, *14*, 87–102.

Haynes, R., Corey, G., & Moulton, P. (2003). *Clinical supervision in the helping professions: A practical guide.* Belmont, CA: Thomson Brooks/Cole.

Holloway, E. L. (1995). *Clinical supervision: A systems approach.* Thousand Oaks, CA: Sage.

Jernberg, A., & Booth, P. (1999). *Theraplay: Helping parents and children build better relationships through attachment-based play.* San Francisco: Jossey-Bass.

Kadushin, A. (1968). Games people play in supervision. *Social Work*, *13*, 23–32.

Main, M., Kaplan, N., & Cassidy, J. (1985). Security in infancy, childhood, and adulthood: A move to the level of representation. In I. Bretherton & E. Waters (Eds.), Growing points of attachment theory and research. *Monographs of the Society for Research in Child Development*, *50*(1–2), 66–104.

Marvin, R., Cooper, G., Hoffman, K., & Powell, B. (2002). The Circle of Security project: Attachment-based intervention with caregiver-pre-school child dyads. *Attachment and Human Development*, *4*(1), 107–24.

Neill, T. K. (Ed.) (2005). *Helping others help children: Clinical supervision of child psychotherapy.* Washington, DC: American Psychological Association.

Play science—The patterns of play. (n.d.). Retrieved June 1, 2007, from nifplay .org/states_play.html.

Presbury, J., Echterling, L. G., & McKee, J. E. (1999). Supervision for innervision: Solution-focused strategies. *Counselor Education and Supervision*, *39*, 146–55.

Ray, D. C. (2004). Supervision of basic and advanced skills in play therapy. *Journal of Professional Counseling: Practice, Theory, & Research*, *32*, 28–41.

Schore, A. N. (2000). The self-organization of the right brain and the neurobiology of emotional development. In M. D. Lewis & I. Granic (Eds.), *Emotion, development, and self-organization* (155–85). New York: Cambridge University Press.

Stewart, A. L, Benedict, H., Bratton, S., Drewes, A., et al. (2005). Excellence in training: Sharing exemplary practices in the education and supervision of play therapists (workshop at the Association for Play Therapy Conference, Nashville, Tennessee, October 10–15).

Stewart, A. L, Benedict, H., Bratton, S., Drewes, A., et al. (2006). Excellence in training: Sharing exemplary practices in the education and supervision of play therapists (workshop at the Association for Play Therapy Conference, Toronto, Canada, October 9–14).

Stolenberg, C., McNeill, B., & Crethar, H. (1994). Changes in supervision as counselors and therapists gain experience: A review. *Professional Psychology: Research and Practice, 25*(4), 416–49.

Stolenberg, C., McNeill, B., & Delworth, U. (1998). *IDM: An integrated developmental model for supervising counselors and therapists.* San Francisco: Jossey-Bass.

Todd, T., & Storm, C. (1997). *The complete systemic supervisor.* Boston: Allyn & Bacon.

Tomm, K. (1988). Interventive interviewing: Part III. Intending to ask lineal, circular, strategic, or reflexive questions? *Family Process, 27*, 1–15.

Index

abuse: juvenile/substance, 99; sexual, 120
abused, children therapists, 252
acceptance, 102, 106
Ackerman, Diane, 297
active listening, 72, 97, 170–71
active utilization quadrant, 45–46
activity: bridging, 50–51; engagement, 302; simulation, 101; to touch deeper/unconscious feelings, 278. *See also* exercises; supervisory activity; techniques
Adams, Patch, *302*
ADHD. *See* attention deficit hyperactivity disorder
Adlerian: personality priorities, 170; play therapy, 40, 44; technique, 241
adolescents, with borderline, 251
adult-centric, counseling, 69
adult-centricism, avoiding, 76
Advanced Seminar in Art Therapy, 199
African-American culture, 203
aggressive children, 129–42; case study on, 132–33; countertransference issues and, 142;

empathy/attachment and, 130; etiology of, 129, 142; gender differences in, 130; limit setting for, in playroom, 141; studies of, 131; understanding, 129; viewed as "bad kids," 142
alcoholism, 99
Allen, J., 140
Allen, Robert, 277
Allison, Dorothy, 292
American Counseling Association convention, 15
anger, 106
APT. *See* Association for Play Therapy
art: countertransference, 121–22, 255–56; registered, therapist, 256; therapy, 97, 101, 254; therapy program at George Washington University, 256. *See also* expressive arts
Art for All the Children: Approaches to Art Therapy for Children with Disabilities (Anderson), 101
articles, play therapy supervision, 211
Asian culture, 203–4

309

About the Editors

Athena A. Drewes, PsyD, MA, RPT-S, is a noted author and co-editor of *School-based Play Therapy* (2001, Wiley & Sons) and *Cultural Issues in Play Therapy* (2005, Guilford Press). She has almost 30 years of clinical experience in working with children and adolescents across all types of treatment settings. She is director of Clinical Training and APA Internship at the Astor Home for Children. Dr. Drewes has supervised colleagues and doctoral psychology interns for over 12 years in play therapy, encouraging and assisting many in becoming registered play therapists and registered play therapist-supervisors. She served six years as director of the Association for Play Therapy, is a registered play therapist and play therapist-supervisor, and is adjunct professor of Play Therapy at the graduate level at Marist College (Poughkeepsie, New York) and Sage College (Albany, New York). She is founder and director of the Play Therapy Institute, LLC; and founder and past president of the New York Association for Play Therapy.

Dr. Drewes has written numerous articles and book chapters on play therapy, is on the editorial boards of the *International Journal of Play Therapy* and *Teaching and Education of Professional Psychologists*, and is a national and international presenter and trainer on play therapy.

Jodi Ann Mullen, PhD, LMHC, NCC, RPT-S, is faculty member at the State University of New York at Oswego in the Counseling & Psychological Services Department, where she is the coordinator of the Graduate

Certificate Program in Play Therapy. Dr. Mullen is a registered play therapist and play therapist-supervisor. She is the author of several manuscripts on play therapy and supervision. Her book (co-authored with Dr. Jody Fiorini) *Counseling Children and Adolescents through Grief and Loss* (Research Press, 2006) is the recipient of "Book of the Year" honors by the *American Journal of Nursing*. Dr. Mullen is a board member of the New York Association for Play Therapy and on the editorial board for the *International Journal of Play Therapy*.